Bioscience Ethics

Bioscience ethics facilitates free and accurate information transfer from applied science to applied bioethics. Its major elements are: increased understanding of biological systems, responsible use of technology, and curtailment of ethnocentric debates more in tune with new scientific insights. Coined by Irina Pollard in 1994, bioscience ethics has become an internationally recognized discipline, interfacing science and bioethics within professional perspectives such as medical, legal, bioengineering and economics. The fundamental feature of this book is its breadth, which is important because bioscience ethics interweaves many diverse subjects in the process of gathering specialist scientific knowledge for bioethical review. It contains chapters which embrace topics affecting human reproduction, end-of-life care and euthanasia, others which challenge human-dominated ecosystems, and review population growth, economic activity and warfare. A background section describes the evolution of ethical consciousness, explores the future and proposes that the reworking of ethical boundaries can enhance mature decision-making in harmony with changing technology.

IRINA POLLARD is an Associate Professor in the Department of Biological Sciences at Macquarie University in Sydney. In the 1990s, she initiated and developed new ways of communicating science described as bioscience ethics. Her research activities have generated a deep concern for social justice and, as a result, she is active in community education and serves on local and international Institutional Ethics Committees. Through UN-affiliated organizations, she is occupied with international bioscience-bioethics education projects via active membership of UNESCO's School of Ethics and, more recently, as the Chair of the Australian Unit of the International Network of the UNESCO Chair in Bioethics. In 2007 she was elected to the Board of Directors of the International Association of Bioethics. She also founded the Bioscience-Bioethics Friendship Co-operative (BBFC) web portal at http://www.bioscience-bioethics.org/ which provides free admittance to educational material in the areas of stress physiology, reproduction, toxicology/teratology and environmental ethics, and access to other useful links for those interested in bioscience and bioethics.

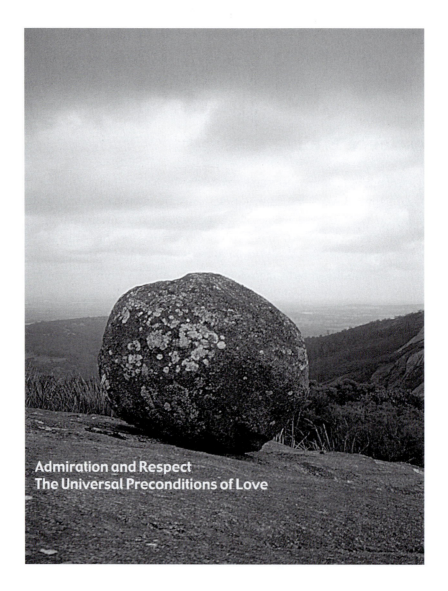

Admiration and Respect
The Universal Preconditions of Love

Bioscience
Ethics

IRINA POLLARD

Macquarie University, New South Wales,
Australia

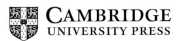

7/09

CAMBRIDGE UNIVERSITY PRESS
Cambridge, New York, Melbourne, Madrid, Cape Town, Singapore, São Paulo, Delhi

Cambridge University Press
The Edinburgh Building, Cambridge CB2 8RU, UK

Published in the United States of America by Cambridge University Press, New York

www.cambridge.org
Information on this title: www.cambridge.org/9780521768283

First published 2009

Printed in the United Kingdom at the University Press, Cambridge

A catalogue record for this publication is available from the British Library

Library of Congress Cataloguing in Publication data
Pollard, Irina.
Bioscience ethics / Irina Pollard.
p.   cm.
Includes bibliographical references and index.
ISBN 978-0-521-76828-3 (hardback)
1. Medical ethics. 2. Bioethics. I. Title.
R724.P64 2009
174′.957–dc22   2009007322

ISBN 978-0-521-76828-3 hardback
ISBN 978-0-521-74527-7 paperback

Contents

Preface

The ethical dimension of science is significant because all of us will need to participate, as citizens, in making informed choices about its uses and abuses. Biological education, while consistent with new knowledge, ought also to be relevant to real-life experiences within sociocultural and ethical contexts. The indiscriminate use, abuse and misunderstanding of science's valuable technological developments are, beyond doubt, a matter of ethical concern and collective responsibility. To adequately respond to the challenges that our technological-based predicaments have created, a deeper understanding of biological systems is essential. To this end, the new transdisciplinary field dubbed 'bioscience ethics' provides unique opportunities for advancing biological understanding within the scaffolding of ethics. Without free and accurate access to scientific, medical and technological expertise – factors which drive present-day social change – the search for a bioethics in tune with modern reality is severely disadvantaged. Bioscience ethics provides a source of information that bridges the gap between applied science and applied ethics. The concept does not displace bioethics; rather it aims to assist its growth. As the interface between scientific endeavour and its application into acceptable forms of bioethical consensus, bioscience ethics demands increased understanding of biological systems, the responsible use of technology and curtailment of ethnocentric debate in tune with scientific insight. The fundamental feature of this book is its breadth – by integrating ethics with the life sciences and by emphasizing that the human condition is the product of past and present circumstance, it highlights the ethics that emerging scientific insights may involve. Publications such as my introductory text, *Life, Love and Children: A Practical Introduction to Bioscience Ethics and Bioethics* (developed for open-access educational purposes), have generated growing interest in bioscience ethics by students and academics as well as the general public. This book responds to the growing interest by adaptively integrating traditional reductionist insights within broader cross-disciplinary levels of bioethical significance. My hope is that, with deepened biological understanding, new standards of social conduct, more in cooperation and harmony with the environment and ourselves, will evolve.

IRINA POLLARD

Acknowledgements

Any enterprise of breadth rests heavily on the scholarship of others. Therefore, I would like to thank all authors from the extensive published literature whose material I have freely used but, owing to space constraints, only a selection is provided in the Further reading. Predominantly I owe a debt to my partner Roger Hiller who critically read all my drafts, insisted on clarity of expression, and who generously gave expert guidance throughout the book's development. It's been instructive to see how Roger's well-judged assessments resulted in important content/textual modifications which so effectively highlighted the intended essence of my writing. I'm also considerably indebted to my son Morgan Pollard for engaging me in probing discussions, especially in the environmental sections. I also extend my thanks to numerous friends and colleagues who helped me focus my thoughts throughout the laborious writing process, and to the students who gave enthusiastically of themselves during their reading of the subject as taught at Macquarie University. I especially owe a debt to bioscience ethics students and staff who strongly supported my fledgling subject, initially taught as an introductory vacation unit, and insisted that bioscience ethics needs to be expanded and recognized in any science curriculum. I also want to acknowledge friends, of like mind, who in the course of various collaborative educational projects within UNESCO's School of Ethics and elsewhere, provided valuable opportunities to stretch my interests in bioscience ethics. In this regard I particularly want to thank Darryl Macer for being an excellent friend and invaluable colleague. To all, I extend a warm thank you.

The original scientific illustrations are an integral part of the book's text and for these I owe a special thanks to the scientific illustrator and artist Barbara Duckworth who, without fail, was able to create meaningful illustrations from my roughest sketches. I'm also very grateful to Ray Duell for skillfully generating eloquent electronic diagrams based on my amateur drafts and for his ongoing assistance in computing matters essential in the preparation of this volume. Ray's IT expertise is astounding, as can be demonstrated by inspecting our web-based education portal, freely accessible at http://www. bioscience-bioethics.org/.

Finally, I want to acknowledge my two editors at Cambridge University Press – Alan Crowden and Dominic Lewis – for enthusiastically embracing bioscience ethics and assisting in its promotion. Thanks are also due to all at Cambridge University Press who helped to bring this book to fruition. For me the journey has been both challenging and enlightening.

1

Human origins, natural selection and the evolution of ethics

Bioethics can serve no useful ends if it is to be merely a watered-down version of contemporary biology ... Bioethics must be based on modern concepts of biology and not on unsupported introspection.[1]

Technologies, all byproducts of science, have redefined how we live, work, fight, relax and communicate with one another. They have not only given us knowledge and provided a previously unimaginable technologically based standard of living, but also unprecedented coercive powers. Humans can now choose to command forces in the service of differing social, economic and political goals, and also, predictably, any potential consequences of their choices. Paradoxically, it's not the science but the use or abuse of science's gifts that challenge and demand mature intellectual appraisal. By commanding technological powers way in excess of our Stone Age brain's emotional capabilities to responsibly contain that power, we find ourselves at odds with our evolutionary heritage. We seem uncertain in which direction to head and how to achieve the behavioural goals that provide the adaptability requisite for survival and future wellbeing.

Our predicament may reflect that we are, in essence, essentially the same animal that evolved approximately 30 000–35 000 years ago. Within a comparatively short evolutionary period, we have successfully adjusted from a nomadic lifestyle living in small, closely genetically related groups, to living within settled villages and have weathered, more or less, the stresses of nationally based industrial societies. Now we need to negotiate a complicated,

---

[1] Potter, V. R. (1971). *Bioethics: Bridge to the Future*. Englewood Cliffs, New Jersey: Prentice-Hall, p. 4.

interconnected, information-based global society. In addition, there are definite environmental warnings that our very destiny may be on the line – the choice between responsible survival and biological extinction is ours to make. We can no longer refute that the way we are multiplying, consuming natural resources, using energy, condoning institutionalized violence and producing waste has fundamentally changed the balance of our global environment. Significantly, the 'naked ape' is now forced to calculate the likely odds of the species' survival within differing future scenarios. Fortunately, well-developed human instincts are already embodied in our genes as we place special value on social attributes such as caring and sharing. These important qualities gave our ancestors strong survival values as we evolved socially. Beyond the powers of the rational mind, our remarkable brains house faculties that embrace love, compassion, solidarity and a sense of fair play. Caring survival skills can be easily observed even in the desperately deprived, such as among destitute homeless kids who routinely share their meagre food and drink – as well as their drugs of comfort. However, it is hard to fundamentally appreciate how dramatically different our socioecological environment is today compared to that in which we adaptively evolved.

This book is about caring and sharing knowledge; it is about people, kids, scientific achievements and monumental scientific failures. Its purpose is to provide a practical interface spanning knowledge gained from modern scientific endeavours and existing bioethical discourse. Before ethical and moral philosophy can be of leading assistance, a good working knowledge of biological systems is essential. My hope is that, by vitalizing interests which facilitate the acquirement of wisdom based on biological understanding, new social values, based on such discernment, can be developed.

Modern science, ethics and evolving bioscience ethics

Science is descriptive, dealing with facts and requiring verification, whereas ethics (formally a part of philosophy) is prescriptive, dealing with what ought to be and depending upon justification. It follows, therefore, that science is ethically neutral while its application is not; that is, the ethics in science do not reside in the science itself but in its conduct and application. When science was in its infancy there was little contradiction between the science and the ethics; that is, 'science ethics' differed little from any other kind of ethics. Modern science, however, is a disseminated resource that is changing the way we live and so can no longer be claimed to be in effect neutral. Although it is now established that scientists can no longer claim that science is neutral but must consider the ethical and social aspects of their work, there still remains the need to bridge essential differences between science and its technology on the one hand, and its social consequences on the other. The bridging process is the province of bioethics. Bioethics refers literally to 'life ethics' and grew out of a vast scholarly literature which had accumulated over centuries in the philosophical and theological traditions. The ever-present risk is that in the process of bioethical/philosophical discourse, crucial scientific knowledge may be inadvertently left out, misunderstood, distorted or subsequently lost because, clearly, speed of change is not of the essence when formulating and justifying human values. To illustrate – compare the discussion of a specific ethical issue such as stem cell research in, for example, a medical journal, a theology journal and a philosophy journal, and note the strikingly different processes of ethical argument. These differences present real barriers to the individual who is concerned with influencing practical decisions, to decide how bioethics should be applied, or even whether it should be applied at all. These differences also present real problems in national politics where questions of how much consensus must exist on an ethical principle before its enforcement becomes a responsibility of the state. How large must a minority be before tax funds collected from all ought to be denied to uses that the minority finds ethically reprehensible? Logic dictates that it stands to reason that scientific evidence should be taken into account when making socially important decisions, but is it? Could it be that to protect the corruption of scientific understanding is the reason why the discipline of bioethics has fragmented into several areas of concentration, such as gender-specific ethics, medical ethics, environmental ethics, forensic ethics, to name but a few? A related difficulty has been that some scholars draw distinctions between ethics and morals as concepts, while others use the terms interchangeably. From the historical perspective, morality is a body of specific rules or guides to human behaviour, whereas ethics is the intellectual justification and organization of those rules – some of which are in agreement with modern scientific insights, while others are not.

All scientific knowledge and applied technology requires ethical consideration to ensure that it is used appropriately and responsibly. However, the question of whether we have adequately identified our bioethical responsibilities relative to our scientific understanding is dependent on whether we have access to current scientific research. At the 1997 American Association for the Advancement of Science held in Seattle, my colleague Steven Gilbert and I launched 'bioscience ethics' – a term I had previously coined and used informally. Bioscience ethics has taken off since and has developed into the accepted interface bridging applied science and applied bioethics. Bioscience ethics assists by promoting biological understanding useful in the development of ethically responsible decision-making in tune with present-day reality; or, if preferred, by combining the 'normative' with the 'informative' in the scientific context. Bioscience ethics[2] facilitates this bridging process by dismantling present-day restrictive subject boundaries that curtail full and clear information transfer across relevant disciplines. The major elements of bioscience ethics are increased understanding of biological systems, responsible use of technology, and reassessment of ethnocentric debate more consistent with new ecological and sociomedical insights. Bioscience ethics does not replace bioethics in any shape or form; rather it facilitates informed decision-making in matters of science and its applications.

In its most basic respect, bioscience ethics aims to democratize esoteric science by making it comprehensible to the scientifically untrained but socially concerned individual. Rightly, it is up to society to decide whether a technological application is ethically acceptable; however, appealing to scholarly philosophical and/or theological discourse, distanced from the scientific workbench, is not always the most efficient way to bargain with the realities created by modern scientific innovations. Likewise, the solution to modern ethical problems cannot always be found within an abstract system of principles to be chosen, or rejected, or even imposed from above. In the final analysis, the sum of us must decide which bioethical principles, values and beliefs are most appropriately applied to a particular biological problem. To this end, accurate, updated biological understanding must be provided if responsible ethical positions are to be reached, especially when judgements are to be made about scientific matters. To this end, the minds of scientists trained to utilize their analytical, logical skills to investigate natural phenomena can usefully be of practical service. More importantly, scientists socialized to see and interpret the world around them in ways that their training demands have an ethical obligation to contribute to the social discourse from which bioethical values are derived. Although scientists at work ask fundamental, ethically neutral questions devoid of value judgements, it cannot be assumed that science lacks emotion. Evidently, science's application must be judged and evaluated before deriving new values from scientific insights; therefore, scientists (being human) experience exhilaration at a discovery, grief at an inappropriate application, and otherwise engage their minds in matters of passion and ethics. In truth, scientists are prone to be over-burdened with a personal and collective responsibility because many of the present-day problems were created by the misapplication of the science to which they are so dedicated. Ironically,

---

[2] Bioscience-bioethics education portal at www.bioscience-bioethics.org/.

many of the solutions to our technologically based predicaments again lie in the scientists' practical skills and biological understanding.

The business of human survival has always been, and still is, one of mature ethical debate within science-based endeavours involving decisions of life and death. Thus, the business of bioethics is well placed to decide whether any specific scientific innovation has anything to say about ethical imperatives and, in true democratic spirit, provide methodical justification in tune with the demands of present-day survival. In this context, a new bold bioethics argues that scientific evidence is to be taken into account when making socially important decisions. Self-evidently, bioscience ethics and bioethics (colloquially dubbed bioscience-bioethics) may seriously challenge traditional (human-centred) ethical and moral theory, but that can only be of advantage because challenge generates energy which, in turn, fuels cultural evolution in diverse and unexpected directions. It would, therefore, be inappropriate for this book to espouse theological or doctrinal assumptions, and it does not, although there may be a confluence of ideas in many instances. Paradoxically, bioscience ethics builds on biological imperatives but is driven by social, psychological, secular and theological predicaments. The book's chapters link a series of interrelated topics concerned with procreation, health and the environment – issues particularly suitable when emphasizing science's power over our individual lives. For example, chapters sorted under the overall heading 'human-dominated ecosystems' rework environmental priorities by adjusting ethical boundaries distanced from their ethnocentric roots. The chapters concerned with procreative biology highlight the personal and the transgenerational issues.

As long as our culture continues to reflect advances in science and technology, there is an obligation to make science accessible to everyone. Many of us have no clear sense of the wholeness of scientific practice, despite the fact that we are living through an explosion of science education made suitable for those with little or no background in the sciences. I would like to begin by briefly examining our origins and what is known about the evolution of human ethical consciousness. A better understanding of our past improves understanding of our present selves and highlights major areas for thought.

The hunter–gatherer *Homo sapiens*

The human brain's evolution can be divided into three distinct ancestral stages (the 'triune' brain – a term popularized by Paul MacLean, 1990), in which each evolutionary stage solved different physical survival functions and behavioural environmental problems. These are the primitive (or reptilian) brain, the early mammalian (or limbic) brain and the new mammalian brain (or neocortex). The primitive brain (also called the basal ganglia) is largely controlled by the unconscious autonomic nervous system, and embodies a significant core of automatic survival functions, including sentiments of which we are not necessarily aware. Basic functions relating to instinctive behaviour patterns of self-preservation include the desire for pleasure, choosing a mate, breeding, fighting, fleeing, territorialism, social hierarchy ('pecking order'), selection of leaders, status maintenance, tendency to follow precedent, resistance to change, awe for authority, compulsiveness, ritualism, prejudice and deception. It may seem puzzling, but behaviours such as dominance displays, flocking, schooling, herding and associated instinctive behaviours are socially effective lifestyle functions that reduce violent inter-actions between members of a species and are life-enhancing behaviours under most circumstances. We carry our primitive reptilian brain, consisting in the main of the brainstem, basal ganglia, reticular activating system and the midbrain, around with us largely unchanged.

The early mammalian or limbic brain that arose in the transition from reptiles to mammals about 150 million years ago embodies the first layer of the cortex responsible for our social and family behaviours as mammals. It underlies the subjective experience of emotional feelings that guide functions bordering on defence, food and sex, as well as activities related to the expression of the semi-conscious emotions and feelings linked to attachment and care of offspring – obligatory functions for the preservation of the species. Accordingly, the limbic brain's primal activities (such as the 'fight or flight' fear response) relate to the production of powerful emotions that incite further the objectives derived from the primitive portions of the brain. Limbic-gener-ated emotions and their corresponding reactions are, typically, immediately independent of thought reactions to perceptions as relayed by the senses. This may explain why certain judgements, such as political or religious dogmas or any other strongly felt inspirations, may be so overwhelming that they remain in the face of logic and contradiction.

The latest evolutionary development is the new mammalian brain or neo-cortex, which evolved over the last 60 million years and is most notable in primates, particularly humans. Its extensive neocortical development encom-passes conscious mental activity, and this made reasoning, abstract intelli-gence, mathematical thinking and decoding of sensory information possible, as well as many other new talents such as music, language, meditation, dreaming and expanded memory. Substantial brain reorganization occurred during the evolution of the neocortex, where flexing and packing against the cranium made possible the development of new pathways connecting midbrain regions to the neocortex and providing many new evolutionary opportunities. That music, for example, is the product of natural selection is not debated despite the existence of conflicting ideas as to its precise purpose. Popular hypotheses include that music promotes social cohesion in group activities such as war or religion, and that its evolution is driven by the pacifying effect it has on infants. Effectively, then, portions of the triune brain handle functions and behaviours that are common to the animal ancestors that share it, but these functions have also evolved together to produce collective agreement in thought and emotion to insure good quality survival of the species (see section on Neuroethics below, p. 16).

Despite our appreciation of our brain's deep evolutionary history, we are still unsure as to when in prehistory our ancestors negotiated the divide from ape to human. Until recently, most researchers believed that the transition took place when humankind systematically started to make stone tools for immediate and future use. Such behaviour implies a capacity for human-like conceptual and abstract thought, contrasting with the thinking processes of the other primates which seem to be mainly perceptual (i.e. limited to the experience of the immediate senses). The first tools were simple, sharp stone flakes and shaped cobbles, known as Oldowan technology, and appeared around 2.5 million years ago in East Africa. The age of these flakes closely matched those of the then earliest known fossils of the genus *Homo*, to which modern humans belong. Recent fossil discoveries in Kenya have, however, pushed back the record of upright-walking hominids to about 4.2 to 3.9 million years ago. Another difficulty in using stone tools as a mark of humanness is that pygmy chimpanzees, or bonobos, also make and use similar tools. Nevertheless, the emergence of the first good evidence for a species closely resembling us seems to be at least 2 million years old.

Genetic anthropologists have identified a trend of accelerating change in the evolutionary lineage leading to modern humans from ape-like ancestors – a trend that is ongoing. Following the emergence of the first ancestors of the *Homo* species, the ape-sized brain began to experience a 40–50% enlargement, which was repeated three times. It may have been that mutational benefits acquired through the evolution of binocular vision, necessary for the hunting lifestyle, subsequently led to the selection of a larger brain whose excess potential was advantageously redirected towards abstract thought, mathematical ability and so on. This interesting hypothesis, of course, is debatable; however, scientists have recently discovered a region of overlapping genes that evolved extremely quickly in our ancestors and that may explain why human brains are dramatically larger than those of other mammalian lineages. The genes in question are active in cells that appear early in embryonic development and assist in forming the cerebral cortex and its connections to other parts of the developing brain. Whatever the aetiology, radical brain expansion did open up new evolutionary potentials in intellect and culture. It has been suggested that the era of tool making also saw the emergence of the elements of social organization seen in modern hunter–gatherer societies, including division of labour, sharing food resources and sophisticated language. In this scenario, the Oldowan tools (approximately 1.4 million years old) were made by a protohuman hunter–gatherer society whereas the species *Homo sapiens* used to define humans with fully enlarged brains and sophisticated culture appeared in the fossil record some 60 000 years ago. Fully modern humans are typified by forms prevalent since the last interglacial period about 35 000 years ago.

Modern humans are the only surviving species of a more diverse family of hominids and are now most closely related to the living African apes as determined by the common ancestor from which humans and chimpanzees evolved. At the outset, two species descended from a common ancestor start out with identical DNA but, as the generations go by, random changes accumulate and the longer the two species have been separated, the greater the difference in their DNA. Differences in DNA are expressed as a percentage rate and are referred to as the 'molecular clock'. Comparing human and chimpanzee DNA gene sequences reveals that the DNA of humans and chimpanzees corresponds more closely (1.6% difference or 98.4% similarity in DNA sequences) than would be expected, given the considerable morphological differences between the two species. Then again, this small 2% difference still leaves the equivalent of 14 million nucleotide differences, distinguishing the 20–25 000 protein-coding genes of humans from those of chimpanzees. As any geneticist knows well, a small number of nucleotides can make a very big difference. For example, one wrong base pair can give you sickle-cell disease; one malfunctioning gene can make all the difference (Chapter 10). It is apparent that subtle reshuffling of DNA was sufficient to have given us, over an estimated 5 million years – or ~250 000 generations – a species capacity that has never existed before, and that has transformed the world.

We also know, from DNA studies measuring the frequency of certain genetic markers in populations, that *Homo sapiens* has great variation in local form (demonstrating polymorphism of many genetic characters) but remarkably low overall genetic difference, even between geographically distant human populations. This means that within its single gene pool there could be more variability within one population than between individuals from different populations or races. Such genetic data lend support to the notion that all modern human populations are descended from a recent single ancestral population (the 'out of Africa' and 'mitochondrial Eve' models), and confirms the scientific reality that we are all members of the same race of people. Mitochondrial DNA clones itself rather than recombining, so is passed to the next generation only by the mother. Since mitochondrial DNA also evolves 10 times faster than nuclear DNA, it conveniently provides an independent molecular clock to reveal an individual's maternal ancestry.

Our close extinct relative, *Homo neanderthalensis* (Neanderthal man), who flourished in Europe and western Asia between about 200 000 and 30 000 years ago, possessed many similarities to humans and had a brain volume greater than that of modern humans. The archaeological evidence also points to a uniquely advanced Neanderthal culture, including sophisticated burial practices. Certain genetic evidence indicates that the population that left Africa some 100 000 years ago interacted with another early human group that had been in Europe for much longer. DNA sequencing of fossil remains may in future reveal whether or not modern humans harbour an archaic Neanderthal imprint.

We still don't really understand some vital periods in our own past. Why did human creativity shown in art, music, sophisticated tools and spirituality suddenly flourish 35 000 years ago when our brains had evolved to the modern size some 65 000 years earlier? Human anatomy and physiology has changed little in the past 35 000 years, yet human culture has changed dramatically. Cultural change represents a recent kind of evolution to support the transmission of learned knowledge across generations in the least possible time. Whatever one generation learns can now be passed onto the next by guidance, instruction, education, ritual, tradition and even indoctrination; all of which ensure continuity in culture. Richard Dawkins, in *The Selfish Gene* (1989), suggested that we are no longer only shaped by our selfish genes but also by ideas which he called 'memes'. The concept of the meme, analogous to the gene, is now known as 'dual inheritance theory' or 'gene-culture co-evolution theory'. In the case of culture, the inheritance mechanism is social learning where members of a particular community learn ways to think and behave from influential members of their community acting as role models. Different thinking processes have different consequences for the patterning of cultural change through time. Peter Singer, in *The Expanding Circle* (1981), suggested how culture may have genetically selected for compassion as tribal society expanded beyond its original bounds of the family. On the other hand, cultural preferences, such as attitudes and styles, are not specifically encoded in the genes, so these attitudes and fashions can readily be reversed. It seems that social flexibility may well have become our greatest asset in the struggle for survival.

While bipedal walking, cooperation in family and tribal units, long educa-tion, self-consciousness and sophisticated language were evolutionary pre-requisites, the essential characteristic of *Homo sapiens'* intelligence was, and still is, creativity. Many believe that our species' creativity, more than any other element, gave rise to artistic expression and ethical rules. That is, in biological terms, human uniqueness resides primarily in our brains with one of its products being culture. Our brain size has more than doubled in the past 2 million years to a volume of some 1500 cubic centimetres. This steady growth in brain size and complexity made possible a steady growth in intel-ligence, and an increasing mastery of the world. But size isn't everything. What also matters is how the brain is structured, with the human brain's uniqueness lying in its flexibility. Flexibility and intelligence is demonstrated by the ability to face problems in an unprogrammed and creative manner. But the full, transgenerational benefits of a good solution to a particular dilemma can only be reaped by communicating and sharing the knowledge with the rest of the tribe.

It is believed that the key change depended on some fine-tuning of the larynx, making sophisticated languages possible. Before this vital structural change evolved, human groups spoke a protolanguage that linked items in the environment to words which could be linked to one another in simple series. But the simple chain of words could not allow the expression of complex ideas such as cause-and-effect relationships. Such ideas became possible only when a grammar emerged to organize words into sentences. Grammar offered huge benefits, such as a comprehensive modelling of the world and abstract thinking that was not tied to immediate action. As a consequence, planning became possible once humans could contemplate the choice of options most likely to be successful. We became empowered to anticipate a wide range of behaviours in different environmental situations relating to the need for aggressive self-preservation, or peaceful cooperative living. It is believed that the analytical, conscious mind was born out of intellectual flexibility together with an innate lifelong love for learning, exploring and playing. So the early hallmark of human evolution was that this exceptional species had the capacity to reason, to reflect on its actions and to discourse with each other. During the brain's subsequent evolution, consciousness opened up other unique possibil-ities of conscience, perchance favourable to the expansion of ethics.

Among human evolutionary theorists it is popularly believed that human development was advanced not just by the enlargement of the neocortex but, in particular, that part known as the frontal lobes. The frontal lobe is the largest of the four lobes constituting each of the two cerebral hemispheres. It is responsible for voluntary control over most skeletal muscles and significantly influences personality. It is also associated with higher mental activities, such as planning, judgement and conceptualization. When comparing the skulls of *H. sapiens* and *H. neanderthalensis*, one notices a striking difference. Typical of Neanderthal people was the low and narrow forehead, indicating a small frontal lobe, and highly developed parietal, temporal and occipital lobes, with the total brain size exceeding that of modern humans by an average of 100 g. Intelligence is a cooperative function of the cerebral cortex and does not depend critically on sophisticated frontal lobe circuitry. The frontal lobe's contribution is creative and voluntary initiative, resulting in our advanced ability to respond to challenging situations with novel solutions. So the human evolution of rationale will also provide us with the basis of freedom which could then be used in symbolic activity (art, for instance), or to initiate planning, make purposeful use of the imagination and solve problems by reasoning. The net result was not only unparalleled biological advancement as a species, but also incomparable technological power. It may be speculated that the problems that such awesome technological power may have provoked a counterbalancing survival strategy based on reasoning, ethical reflection and the development of moral rules (see section below on Neuroethics, p. 16). In the past century, we have experienced giant advances in technological inventiveness and ruthless use of technological power. It can only be hoped that in the twenty-first century, a critical mass of humans will demand humane reconciliation by creatively engaging in social change, furthering our evolution toward a mature species. It is possible that the material wealth now enjoyed by a significant proportion of people, particularly in industrialized nations, will provide the leisure necessary for intellectual and spiritual advancement; freedom from want may provide a breathing space for our further evolution.

Ethics – our evolutionary heritage

Ethical codes have arisen through the interplay of biology and culture. The human brain – the cortex in particular – is more than an instrument responding to the environment. There are parts of the cortex's frontal lobe that interpret what is received, incorporating it into the development of judgement, volition and consciousness of self and others. From these abstract qualities arose the ability to choose between alternative behaviours which accelerated the development of a collective awareness, or ethics. Collective awareness reinforced by freedom of behavioural choice may well have promoted an ethical order of fitness-enhancing behavioural preference to be used to best advantage in personal and social relationships.

Ethical choice depends on the capacity to foresee the results of actions and an acceptance of individual responsibility; that is, ethics is a guide to the most adaptive method of exercising our freedom of choice. In this view, freedom and responsibility are aspects of the same phenomenon and are characteristic of the human condition. As individuals, we each have a very low fitness unless we associate with our fellows for our personal gain, so we live in social groups and we cooperate because it is the most beneficial strategy. At the same time, these social groups must, for their survival, restrain from shameless self-centred acts and refrain from deceitful manoeuvres. However, Nature has again guided the evolutionary course of the human brain to advantage. The amygdala (located in the front portion of the temporal lobe of the cerebral cortex) originally played a central role in the acquisition and processing of fear but is now also crucial for processing emotions indispensable in social communication. It is here that judgement on the emotional significance of all incoming information is made and emotional memories are stored, conveniently close to the elaborate connections of the enlarged prefrontal cortex. The biological consequence of amplifying the amygdala's function may have been that the primal fear of attack was moderated by feelings of shame and guilt. Shame and guilt about hurting others is an innate biological trait and an essential part of the human ethical repertoire.

Other important functions of the human brain, which facilitate novel social interactions, can be readily identified. In the course of human evolution, sex, for example, has developed from a purely procreative activity into a variety of recreational activities central to the function of society. The advantages of retaining sexual receptivity at times when conception is not possible are obvious. Such a strategy is an evolutionary device to maximize parental care of the young by maintaining long-term relationships associated with comfort and sexual pleasure for the highly sexed human. Even early human societies understood this and developed many ways of preventing unwanted conceptions (Chapter 9). Other examples of human culture having their origins in biology can be seen in the ways that biological 'taboos' against incest are culturally reinforced or why exogamy (marriage outside the close kin group) is often encouraged as a means of solidifying political, social and economic relationships. Thus, we are enhancing our fitness in two ways. Culturally, we use marriage bonds to establish beneficial social arrangements and biologically to avoid inbreeding, with its fitness-reducing consequences.

Since ethics developed alongside the enlargement of the original family group, it seems as if the expansion from a closed kinship morality (purely altruistic) to an inclusive ethics was crucial in advancing human evolution. The balance of evidence suggests that human evolution was advanced in situations where the recipients of favourable natural selection were groups of people duty-bound to one another by leadership, dialect, geography, rituals and cultural traditions. Cultural group selection can reward altruism and other forms of virtue by strengthening the group, even at the expense of the individuals. In biological terms, the appearance of unselfish traits in individuals boosted the group's survival. The natural world is full of elaborate forms of cooperation which extend far beyond the boundaries of mere relatedness. Modern computer simulations suggest that extensive cooperation is an evolutionary stable strategy as it produces a benign environment in which everybody thrives. Nature is not predominantly 'red in tooth and claw' because savagery is not a beneficial strategy and is not the usual direction of evolutionary change (Chapter 12). In human evolution, group selection may have been accelerated with the raising of domestic animals which, by providing food and other products, supported a larger population in the Mesolithic Age, beginning about 15 000 years ago. Larger groups still were favoured with the advent of agricultural practices in the Neolithic Age, beginning around 10 000 BCE,[3] further increasing food production necessary for an expanding human population. Group selection would also have incorporated group selfishness – could it be that racism is a contemporary remnant of such group egocentrism?

It may also be that our extraordinary intelligence is the product of natural selection exerted by coordinated and cooperative social groups fiercely competing against each other. Over our evolutionary history, Machiavellian intelligence must have favoured those cooperators who tactically outmanoeuvred competitive social groups. Put bluntly, conspecific conflict, as opposed to environmental selection, may well have been the major player in advancing and shaping human intelligence. In the modern context, however, institutionalized warfare is no longer a fitness-enhancing behaviour; instead it is a losing strategy (Chapter 14). In the modern context, we need to manoeuvre innate cooperative behaviour towards peaceful coexistence skillfully.

We now know that race is a convenient social construct rather than a biological reality. Describing ourselves as Caucasian, Asian, African – or whatever – is simplistic and seriously corrodes understanding and appreciation of our genetic diversity and commonality. At the most basic level, skin colour has been used as a surrogate for 'race'. Although each of us carries a set of genes that affects the colour of our skin, this is only an infinitesimal fraction of our genome. Modern genetics has enabled scientists to study human variation using thousands, rather than a few colour-encoding genetic polymorphisms,

---

[3] BCE – Before the Common Era – is used throughout the text but the reader is welcome to substitute the equivalency BC.

and so contribute to a serious discussion of population histories, ethnic categorization and race. Allele frequencies in populations can be compared to assess the extent to which populations differ from one another, and it is now clear that humans vary only slightly at the total DNA level both within and between differing populations. All studies based on different types of genetic variation are in accord and support an evolutionary scenario in which anatomically modern humans evolved first in Africa, accumulating genetic diversity. A small subset of this African population then left the continent, and founded anatomically modern human populations in the rest of the world.

Our evolutionary heritage is the continuum of intellect and consciousness, where the earliest intellectual deliberations grew out of extracting theoretical values from practical life. The record of human activity gives us the impression that ethical practices were first applied in science and medicine. The healer of disease and injury, even in the earliest societies, was an individual who possessed exceptional talents and ethical qualifications. We see health concerns hinted at when the oldest known human statuettes, dating from the first age in which works of art appeared, represented women. These magnificent Palaeolithic figurines are known as fertility figures or 'Venuses' and had the attributes of their sex considerably emphasized or enlarged. Scholars have interpreted this type of art as symbolizing a belief in transference of a power recognized in nature to an image considered to have an equivalent potency. An important concern for early *Homo sapiens* must have been fertility, which enabled both them and animals (which were valued for their flesh, skins, bones, horns, etc.) to reproduce. It is reasonable to postulate, therefore, that for the hunter–gatherer a deepening understanding of the wisdom and beauty of Nature may have played the central role in the evolution of ethical thought. It may be useful to remind ourselves that 'aesthetics' has its root in the Greek word '*aisthetes*' meaning 'one who perceives', illustrating the wisdom of integrating science, ethics and art with Nature. Holistic ethics (also sometimes called ecocentric ethics where the entire ecosphere is considered) was practised in ancient traditions and has survived in several forms as, for example, the Dreamtime of the Australian Aboriginal peoples (see Chapter 15 on Gaia's evolving physiology for a modern holistic interpretation of Earth).

Recorded history gives us more insight into our very recent evolution. Much is made of the Sumerians of Mesopotamia (the ancient country between the Tigris and Euphrates rivers, now Iraq) who, in about 3000 BCE, left behind a vast legacy of 'firsts' inscribed on clay tablets in cuneiform script. Theirs was the first recorded example of a palace-driven urban society cooperative with government. The Sumerian legacy also included an early record of ethical thought. The ethical concept had to do with restoring justice and freedom to the citizens of

Lagash, a Sumerian city-state. But human civilization had been developing for several millennia before the written record began, so that the evolution of premonitions of human ethical thought on topics such as truth, justice, freedom, mercy and compassion began long before their written record.

Relationships between Nature, science, medicine and ethics continued to occupy our ancestors for another 2000 years or so until the sixth century BCE, when another cultural leap for humankind took place. Pythagoras and the Ionian philosophers in Greece, Confucius and Lao-Tsu in China, Buddha in India and Zoroaster in Persia were all reworking the status quo and formulating new principles of liberation and conduct. The Greeks, for example, began to turn away from mythological explanations of the world around them and to seek instead physical causes. The realization that environmental phenomena are affected not by the Gods, but by processes inherent in natural law, was significant, because it re-shaped people's culture, predisposing them to the subsequent development of experimental science. At the heart of Pythagorean thought, for example, was that numbers could serve as ethical archetypes and the description of reality in terms of mathematical relationships could provide insight into human behaviour, reflecting properties inherent in Nature herself. To the Greek legacy must be added the later contributions from the Islamic, Jewish and Christian traditions. Accumulated intellectual insights paved the way for the development of science-based medicine in surprisingly modern terms and boosted ethical thinking, as demonstrated by giants such as Hippocrates (c. 460–377 BCE) – nicknamed the 'Father of Medicine' – and Aristotle (384–322 BCE). The Hippocratic Oath, the ethical standard for physicians, remained virtually unchanged until the last half of the twentieth century. Aristotle distinguished in his *Treatise on Ethics* between the statement of truth and the execution of an action; that is, it is not enough to want to do good, but necessary to do good.

It is important to remember that the Hippocratic tradition is a western-based discussion separate from equally powerful eastern-based traditions, especially those of ancient China and India. The practice of medicine in the time of the Buddha, for example, took place against the backdrop of traditional Indian physiology and medicine, which had its own code of ethics. Many of the most famous doctors were wandering Buddhist monks who practised their calling in surprisingly modern terms, with their medical responsibilities extending even to the facilitation of a happy death. A comparison of the major religions and philosophies of the world shows that, despite their largely independent origins, the essence of their ethical codes is remarkably similar. This suggests that the philosophers, prophets and law-givers responsible for these ethical codes understood which norms are consistent with long-term biological survival. Once these norms are adopted they become part of the cultural tradition and are culturally inherited, and sometimes modified, from generation to generation.

Two factors prepared medieval Europe for the new science of the seventeenth century. These were the translation of Greek and Arabic scientific texts of the twelfth and thirteenth centuries into Latin, and the development of universities in the west, which used these translations as the basis of a science curriculum. The English scientist Roger Bacon (1214–94) is accredited with being the founder of experimental science. He insisted that humans can understand natural laws in terms of 'cause and effect' relationships. From his time onwards, the scientific method meant that reasoning (hypothesis) had to be confirmed by demonstration (experiments).

Neuroethics – unravelling the neural basis of moral judgement

The neurobiological foundations of emotion are attracting mounting interest within the neurosciences owing to advances in functional neuroimaging technology. Modern brain imaging began in the 1970s with computed axial tomography scans and many advances have since been made. In the earlier days of neuroimaging, studies focused on structure–function relationships, such as the primary sensory and motor regions of the brain. Today neurological studies probe at our deepest thoughts, define our complex cognitive behaviours and judge our rational decision-making and consciousness. Neuroimaging reveals the structure of the living brain through technologies such as computer-assisted tomography (CAT) scans or magnetic resonance imaging (MRI). Brain function is revealed through positron emission tomography (PET) scans, single photon emission tomography (SPECT) scans or functional magnetic resonance imaging (fMRI).

With fMRI it is possible to identify patterns of neural activity associated with storing and retrieving sequences of complex events, attitudes and emotions. Emotion plays a pivotal role in ethical experience by assigning value to events, objects and actions. Ethical choice depends on our capacity to foresee the results of actions and includes the acceptance of individual responsibility. Some of the most fundamental questions about our unique evolutionary origins and social relations are centred on issues of altruism and unselfishness. Most academics agree that ethical codes have arisen through the interplay of biology and culture. The human brain – the cortex in particular – is more than an instrument for shaping the environment. In addition to receiving and linking the heard, seen, smelled and felt sensations, there are parts of the cortex's frontal lobe that interpret what is received, incorporating it into the development of judgement, volition and consciousness of self and others. From these abstract qualities, it is believed, evolved altruism or seemingly unselfish behavioural characteristics; that is, the willingness to choose cooperative over alternative behavioural options. As described above, this opened opportunities for the development of a collective awareness, or ethics, which, subsequently, gave way to an ethical order of fitness-enhancing behavioural preference to be used to best advantage in personal and social relationships.

Converging lines of evidence from evolutionary biology, neuroscience and experimental psychology have demonstrated that ethics is indeed hardwired into our brains – effectively blending modern empirical testing with ancient wisdom. As a consequence, a fresh concordance between secular-based science and spiritual practice has provided new possibilities for the advancement of mental and social wellbeing. Most remarkably, from a partnership between neuroscience and bioethics, a distinctly new field of 'neuroethics' was born, bringing to the forefront new thinking on ethical, social and legal matters. With the aid of fMRI, scientists have established that when subjects are viewing scenes suggestive of ethical emotions, a common network of brain areas that includes the prefrontal cortex and temporal regions, the thalamus, hippocampus, amygdala and hypothalamus is strongly activated. Significantly, brain activation is consistently more powerful when responding to stimuli that evoke ethical or moral emotions compared with the processing of neutral or unpleasant stimuli. Equally significant is that brain imaging studies also indicate that our brains have evolved to make altruistic (unselfish) behaviour psychologically rewarding, and to make us perceive selfish behaviour as anti-social and undesirable. Engaging in altruistic behaviour – or merely the thought of doing good – invokes the thrill of a cascade of 'feel good' neuro-hormones such as dopamine (the messenger of the brain's reward system), β-endorphin (our natural opiates) and oxytocin (the 'cuddles' or social bonding, fantasy and imagery hormone). These studies strongly suggest that altruism is an evolutionarily conserved genetic programme, rewarding adaptive societal behaviour.

It must also be pointed out, however, that technology is developing at an ever-increasing rate and, in tandem, forcing ethics to adapt swiftly in order to keep up with this expansion. In the next few decades, we will have unpre-cedented opportunities to improve health and wellbeing, but also have increasing power to annihilate ourselves and our fellow passengers on Earth. Experts have estimated the risk that humankind will be wiped out by some technological disaster – nanotechnology, biological warfare, nuclear – to be 20–50% in the next century. However, this is already possible with existing technology so we have to become more resourceful by applying our collective energies from the combined pool of intelligence and sense of adaptive responsibility. As our neocortex has rapidly evolved so have our powers of reasoning – we have built tools and weapons, we have explored space, mapped the human genome and split the atom. Unfortunately, however, while intellectual brain power has advanced, the brain's older limbic structures (driving emotions, fears and destructive impulses) have basically remained unchanged. This discrepancy has warped adaptive communication between the old and the new.

In the above context, it is not dignified to accept the gifts provided by our intellectual intelligence and neglect to recognize matching emotional responsibilities. It is only fair, if *Homo sapiens* is profiting from an improved intellectual intelligence quotient (IQ), that this gift is counterbalanced by an improved instinctive awareness conveniently referred to as emotional intelligence or emotional intelligence quotient (EQ). In the twenty-first century, it is below human dignity to devalue great scientific advances irresponsibly, such as, for example, using familiarity with the nuclear chain reaction to build a bomb. An in-tune EQ describes the aptitude and skill to perceive and assess the emotions of self, others and groups. A well-developed EQ signals, neurologically, that the brain's homeostatic system has adopted an advanced steady state – one more responsive to the physical and social environments and, therefore, more adaptive in terms of ethical control over changing circumstances.

Evolving bioscience-bioethics

The history of bioethics over the latter part of the nineteenth century has been the development of a secular ethic. Bioethics advanced through differing secular cultures united by peaceable reflection and discussion, but without possessing a common ethical viewpoint. It was the oncologist Van Rensellaer Potter who, in 1971, first coined the word 'bioethics' in his book *Bioethics: Bridge to the Future*. Since the term 'bioethics' means 'the study of life ethics', there can be no one doctrine that is bioethics. Importantly, 'world ethics' must be seen against the diversities of cultural views and prevailing conditions. The modern bioethical movement started with the civil rights movement and racial concerns but quickly spread to serving the, now technologically based, medical profession. Since World War II, phenomenal advances have occurred in all fields of human endeavour, but most evidently in medical knowledge and scientific skills.

Science, through medicine, has provided precise quantifiable benefits for humanity. Since the mid-nineteenth century, developed countries have experienced one of the most dramatic changes in the history of the species – a near doubling of life expectancy at birth from around 40 years to nearly 80 years. The rate of improvement in life expectancy is even higher in developing countries, with an increase from around 40 years in 1950 to 63 years in 1990. Whether we are becoming healthier as we live longer is, of course, open to debate. It is well documented that, as life expectancy increases and fertility declines, the impact of chronic degenerative diseases rapidly increases; thus, directly juxtaposing quality against quantity of life trade-offs. Nevertheless, the power of medicine to prevent Nature from taking her course has massively extended life, and with that power has come a considerable extension of ethical choice. Once it became possible to keep patients alive by artificial respiration and to improve resuscitation techniques, doctors were faced with new dilemmas. The emergence in the mid-1960s and the early 1970s of a number of technological advances in organ transplantation, long-term haemodialysis and ventilators sharpened these ethical dilemmas. The twenty-first century has already been identified as the 'biotechnology century', in which the major advances of science include genomics (the science concerned with the mapping, sequencing and analysis of the complete set of genes from an organism) and the mapping of the complete human genome. This latest gene technology revolution is accelerating social change and bioethical controversy. There is much debate about ownership and exploitation of genetic materials, patent laws and the experimental limitations that should be imposed by domestic/international law. Modern biotechnology has the potential to solve many of the world's problems involving food supply, health and the environment (Chapter 10). However, as with all powerful new technologies there are risks, both real and perceived, along with the benefits.

Can traditional bioethics satisfactorily encompass the explosion of biological and medical technologies? The most widely accepted theory of biomedical ethics, and the one most seen in textbooks, is by Beauchamp and Childress (1994). They defend the four-principles approach to bioethics: beneficence, non-malfexperience, autonomy and justice. Within medical ethics, autonomy is often discussed in relation to human rights, and incorporates the concepts of confidentiality and informed consent. The two sides of ethical behaviour, to do good and not to do harm, are encoded in beneficence (doing what is best) and non-malficence (causing no harm). In 1998, Darryl Macer reworked and simplified these bioethical principles by condensing the discipline to its essentials of 'bioethics is love of life'. Macer's proposition is that all inner motivation and strength for ethical behaviour comes from love – or the biological imperative for humane survival. By balancing the four principles, self-love (autonomy), love of others (justice), loving life (non-maleficence) and loving good (beneficence), one has the vehicle to express personal values according to the desire to love, and, dare I suggest, realize the dictates of healthy neuronal activity. However, when we ask two people to do this complicated balancing act, the outcomes invariably differ. But the differences are healthy for bioethics because, just as diversity of species provides biological stability, diversity of ideas provides cultural security. To secure a sustainable future, we need to promote bioethical maturity. A modern society is bioethically mature when it has learned to balance responsibly the benefits and risks of new technology and reject inappropriate applications.

An alternative, more encompassing, theory of bioethics incorporating the group point of view, is the ethics of care. Caring means an emotional commitment to, and willingness to act on behalf of, persons with whom one has a significant relationship. This ethic was recently revised in feminist writing, where it was argued that women predominantly display an ethic of care, in contrast to men who predominantly exhibit an ethic of rights. Now that we must think in terms of the global community, the principles of an ethic of care form an integral part of the book's text and are supported by bioscience-bioethical principles. Translating care into action requires a new educational framework, one which creates an acceptance of the ethical obligation that each one of us is to a considerable degree custodian of subsequent generations. Self-responsibility, on the other hand, means more reliance on autonomy by owning information so we can make our own informed decisions about our health and other important matters. Chapter 7 is devoted to this theme and documents recent medical evidence that control of our destiny drives physical, psychological and social wellbeing. This newly documented data has generated vigorous ethical debate regarding the practical implications of approaching health care removed from the holistic context of life.

In the course of the twentieth century, people all over the world have become acutely conscious of their rights as well as their persistent violation. Violation is inevitable if we are not mindful of individual and collective responsibility, without which neither rights nor other values can be effectively safeguarded. Safeguarding of rights involves bioethics, but this by itself is insufficient because rights comprise claims but do not imply the responsibility for satisfying these claims. For responsible individualism to work, reform must come from a critical mass of grass roots support. But how can grass roots support factor in an in-depth understanding of complicated biological information so that ethically responsible positions can be developed? Without free and accurate access to scientific, medical and technological expertise, enduring reform is not achievable. If we wish to revise closely held traditional values in the search for a bioethics in tune with present-day reality, then we have to accept that science and technology is the factor which drives present-day social change. And this is where bioscience ethics completes the picture.

Like the children's game of 'cat's cradle', bioscience ethics has fixed elements (increased understanding of biological systems, responsible use of technology and reassessment of ethnocentric debate), but since it is shaped by scientific developments, its inner configuration is infinitely accommodating. In science, new data can modify – or even overturn – established theory, law or dogma. This is how scientific research provides a self-corrective mechanism free from out-of-date constraints. Bioscience-bioethics balances this recognition in the development of social and behavioural tools in harmony with the principles of the bioethically mature society. Ultimately, bioscience-bioethics involves not only familiarity with Nature's principles but also respect for rights and responsibilities, which include abstract qualities such as truth, gratitude, guilt, love, communication, consensus and compromise – effective mechanisms for dealing with ethical pluralism. New applications generated by innovative science and technology profoundly affect established mores that, in turn, power new ideas as to how best manage changing conditions. Fundamental to this process, if the bioethical discussion is to be relevant to our knowledge-based lives, is the search for high biological understanding. Commitment to transform society will not come through superficial short-term fixes but through long-term commitment to education and humanitarian-scientific reform. By integrating ethics into the life sciences, bioscience ethics highlights issues that relate directly to our lives and bring to the bioethical discussion an awareness of the biological dimension on which tradition and technological application function. In the final analysis, therefore, bioscience-bioethics promotes cultural resilience, social flexibility and sustainable survival skills.

Traditional education in the sciences is mostly confined to facts, concepts and mechanisms. Reference to ethical judgement remains with the individual teacher – some include issues of concern, others do not; thus, in biology for example, bioethics is taught in a 'hit and miss' fashion since the discipline does not demand bioethical debate. On the other hand, traditional education in disciplines such as economics, engineering, law, the arts, for example, do not demand knowledge of, or debate of, matters of scientific concern. Yet changes in society brought about by science and technology have affected human relationships and practices in fundamental and often irreversible ways. Because of our power over Nature, there is an increasing need to re-evaluate the positive and negative effects of science and technology in the modern context. There is also an equal need to raise students' awareness – no matter what the subject – about bioethical predicaments resulting from new scientific insights and technological applications. Fortunately, modern university students no longer accept the 'empty vessel to be filled with factual information' view and are demanding that the processes of knowledge acquisition be tempered with understanding, wisdom, participation and ethical responsibility. Optimism was also expressed because of a perceived acceleration in the diversity of human enlightenment and increasing global collaboration in facing our environmental predicaments.

Citizens rely on governments to protect their safety and promote their health, but governments can do this only if sufficient knowledge can be accumulated to guide policy. For example, there is a positive ethical duty to use medical records for the benefit of the whole population in answering important epidemiological questions, or to protect the health of others. One non-negotiable requirement of bioscience-bioethics is that of veracity, which can well be illustrated by the 'mad cow disease' example. Scientists have argued that, although there was no proof of a link between CJD (Creutzfeldt–Jakob disease) and BSE (bovine spongiform encephalopathy), it could not be eliminated. Politicians conveniently took no evidence for a link to mean that there was no risk, even when unusual cases of CJD began to be described in young people late in 1995. In the decade since the BSE epidemic began in British cattle, governments have tried to push scientific advice aside when it did not suit them. At the heart of the BSE example lies a failure to be open with the public. For government ministers to act as though they believe that the public should be 'reassured' rather than informed about uncertainties is insulting and also potentially disastrous. People have a right to the facts, and should develop a critical understanding of the world in which they live. Scientific knowledge grows in a climate of balanced acceptance of uncertainties, the need to preserve what has been proven and tested, and the courage, when the environment changes, to adjust to new realities. After all, there is the risk that, if we as a people maintain obsolete values and beliefs, we also maintain outdated goals and behaviours. I am hopeful, therefore, that this book will bring new points of view and generate enthusiastic discourse about how to promote adaptive biocultural diversity in the ethical debate.

Principles of bioscience ethics for discussion

- To incorporate current scientific insights of practical significance within a cultural context is an aim of bioethics. Bioscience ethics is the interface ensuring that such scientific information is not omitted or corrupted in this process. In your opinion, is a good working knowledge of biological systems essential before the philosophy of bioethics can adequately be addressed? Justify your point of view.

- Many among us perpetuate the perception that life in the 'natural state' is solitary, brutish, unclean, short and mean, implying that there are few natural rules of justice to soften or restrain 'nature red in tooth and claw'. Is this view justified or does it signal a destructive evolutionary strategy adopted by *Homo sapiens* – the most gifted of creatures?
- By acquiring the power to reason, humans exchanged personal freedom for personal security – do you agree or disagree?

2

Sex determination, brain sex and sexual behaviour

'I should see the garden far better,' said Alice to herself, 'if I could get to the top of that hill: and here's a path that leads straight to it – at least, no, it doesn't do that' (after going a few yards along the path, and turning several sharp corners), 'but I suppose it will at last. But how curiously it twists! It's more like a corkscrew than a path!'[1]

Alice's confusion brings to mind Nature's dance of unexpected twists and turns which may, or may not, provide favourable conditions for achieving reproductive success. The twists and turns are not automatically in synchrony with species' requirements to persist through time. All life forms compete to maximize their reproductive success by counterbalancing conflicting interests and calculating cost and benefit analyses. Humans, and their Quaternary companions in evolution, exist today only because they are the descendants of those that successfully reproduced in past environments. Future generations, if they are to survive, will need to do the same and adapt to rapidly changing environmental conditions – not an easy ask.

The foundation of normal adult reproduction is set during fetal life. Sex, as all other functions, is the product of dancing genetic and epigenetic variables so complex that under normal conditions developmental instructions seem to appear from one adaptable informational unit. While genetics focuses on how organisms retain traits by inheriting genes from their parents, epigenetics refers to additional methods of biological inheritance that do not directly relate to the inheritance of collections of genes. More specifically, it refers to reversible, heritable changes in gene expression that regulate physiological

---

[1] Carroll, L. (1872). *Through the Looking-Glass*, Chapter 2. London: Macmillan.

and/or behavioural characteristics without a change in DNA sequence. Characteristically, modulated gene expression represents a response to environmental dynamics. Behaviour is the result of genetic-environmental interactions over time, and the most common behaviours in any particular environment are more successful, in evolutionary terms, compared to available alternatives. However, there are aspects of early development which, if uncorrected, may have long-term effects upon the individual. Behavioural, dietary and other adverse epigenetic effects during critical periods in development may permanently impose a vulnerability to physical and psychological illnesses in the offspring (Chapter 3). When epigenetic influences adversely affect the sexual differentiation of the fetal germ cells, then a changed genetic programme may be expressed in the offspring of a subsequent generation. Conversely, reproduction under good conditions creates a positive force in shaping human identity.

Sex determination

During embryonic and fetal development, males and females take distinctly different paths in forming their typical (and sometimes not so typical) sexual characteristics. In mammals it is the presence, or absence, of fetal testes which determines the sex of the conceptus. The subsequent differentiation of the accessory sex structures follows the primary differentiation of the gonad, whose endocrine secretions in turn influence their development. Thus each step in the process of sexual differentiation is dependent on the preceding one, and under normal circumstances chromosomal sex agrees with the phenotypic sex – or the observable characteristics of the individual. Normal sexual development is an orderly sequential process divisible into developmental stages known as chromosomal sex, gonadal sex and phenotypic sex.

Chromosomal sex

Chromosomal sex is established at fertilization when the sperm provides either an X chromosome, resulting in a 46XX embryo, or a Y chromosome, resulting in a 46XY embryo. The Y chromosome is essential for the development of males; for example, the karyotype of XXY (Klinefelter syndrome) is male and XO (Turner syndrome) is where a female is born with only one X chromosome instead of the usual two. In humans (as in all mammals), no matter how many X chromosomes are present, a testis will develop as long as the sex-determining region of the Y chromosome is also present. Klinefelter's syndrome individuals are male in general appearance with underdeveloped testes and enlarged breasts owing to developmental impairment by products of the extra X chromosome. Turner's syndrome individuals are underdeveloped females, possessing infantile sex organs and are frequently sterile. This is because in both men and women, infertility can arise from an incorrect number of X chromosomes.

As a rule, genes and chromosomes come in pairs – sex chromosomes are an exception to this rule. Females have two X chromosomes and a set of autosomes (AA) or non-sex chromosomes. Males have only one X chromosome, a male-specific Y chromosome and a set of autosomes. Therefore, one X chromosome in each cell must be randomly inactivated early in female embryonic development – a process known as X-dosage compensation, which works to equalize the expression of X chromosomes in both sexes.

The human Y chromosome is one of the smallest human chromosomes and is divided into two portions, a long and a short arm. The short arm contains a sex-determining region, termed *SRY* in humans and *Sry* in mice, that encodes a testis-determining gene. *SRY* diverts the bipotential embryonic gonad from the default ovarian pathway to that of testis differentiation and masculinization. Decisive evidence of the role of *Sry* came from transgenic mice possessing the normal female XX chromosomes plus *Sry*. These developed into males with normal testes and subsequent normal male copulatory behaviour; however, spermatogenesis was absent. Other gene families on the Y chromosome affect normal spermatogenesis and certain aspects of sexually dimorphic traits, such as increased growth rate of male embryos. The process of normal male phenotypic differentiation is a complicated one as it depends on the presence of *SRY* together with the participation of many X-linked and autosomal genes common to both male and female embryos.

Genes controlling ovarian differentiation are located on both X chromosomes (because normal differentiation of the primordial gonad into an ovary occurs only in the presence of two intact X chromosomes) and an unspecified number of autosomal gene families.

Gonadal sex

Until a human embryo is about 5 weeks old it lacks any kind of sex organs, and 12 weeks later male sexual development is completed. At approximately 5 weeks of gestation, when the embryo is about 8 mm long, a ridge of cells, the gonadal ridge or genital crest, destined to develop into the future testis or ovary, grows out of each mesonephros, the temporary excretory organ of the embryo. The gonadal ridge cells will differentiate into the somatic (body) cells of the future gonad: in the male, these are the Sertoli and interstitial Leydig cells and in the female these are the granulosa and theca cells. The primordial germ cells, destined to differentiate into oocytes and spermatozoa, arise from an entirely different location outside the embryo proper, the allantois or dorsal endoderm of the yolk sac. The primordial germ cell migration, guided by chemotactic signals, coincides with the formation of the gonadal ridges which they invade. Once inside the gonadal ridges, the germ cells multiply by mitotic divisions. The undifferentiated gonads now have all the cellular components necessary to develop into either testes or ovaries.

Around 6–7 weeks of gestation, human fetal gonads show the first microscopic signs of tissue differentiation, but only in gonads destined to develop into testes. Differentiation of the ovaries occurs a few weeks later than the differentiation of testes. It can, therefore, be assumed that the SRY gene is expressing at, or prior to, the time of differentiation of the male-supportive Sertoli cell lineage, but from the time of conception there are clear differences between potential ovaries and potential testes. For example, the XX and XY gonads differ in their rate of development even before the Sertoli cells start to differentiate. This growth discrepancy commences soon after fertilization as early cleavage is faster in male conceptuses, and male newborns are normally heavier and bigger than their sisters. It has been suggested that the crucial function of the sex-determining region of the Y chromosome is to accelerate the development of the male fetus in order to set the conditions in which the Sertoli cells can develop. It is essential for the testes to differentiate early in development because, unless the germ cells are enclosed inside the seminiferous cords, they either degenerate or enter the first stages of meiosis. If meiosis is initiated, then differentiation of egg cells occurs in a genetically male fetus and an ovary will develop. Factors retarding fetal growth incorporate the inherent risk of a desynchronization of sequences critical to male sexual differentiation. While a female fetus can afford to develop at leisure, becoming a male is a race against time, highlighting perhaps the first competitive event in a male's life.

Phenotypic sex

Phenotypic sex denotes the development of the reproductive tract through which, in the adult, the germ cells will eventually travel. Each embryo originally develops two sets of potential reproductive tracts, the mesonephric or Wolffian duct, and the paramesonephric or Müllerian duct. The Wolffian duct has the potential to develop into the male reproductive tract, including vas deferens, epididymis, seminal vesicle and ejaculatory ducts, while the Müllerian duct can give rise to the female reproductive structures, including the oviducts (Fallopian tubes), uterus and upper part of the vagina. In any embryo, depending on the genetic sex, one set of ducts develops while the other regresses.

The somatic cells of the fetal testes produce two classes of hormones. The first is Müllerian inhibiting hormone (MIH), a glycoprotein of Sertoli cell origin which demolishes the Müllerian (or potential female reproductive) tract, and conditions the seminiferous epithelium. The second is testosterone, a steroid of Leydig cell origin which stabilizes the Wolffian (or potential male reproductive) tract, and directs the development of the external genitalia. MIH is not solely responsible for Müllerian duct regression, as steroid hormones also influence the process. When remnants of Müllerian duct persist, there is usually also cryptorchidism, a failure of the testes to descend. Another physiologically important function of MIH is connected with the further morphological differentiation of Sertoli cells and the formation of junctional complexes that allow the development of anatomical and functional subdivisions of the adult seminiferous epithelium. With completion of the seminiferous cords, a second stage of development in the fetal testes commences. Starting at approximately 8 weeks of gestation, the steroid-secreting interstitial or Leydig cells differentiate between the sex cords. They secrete testosterone, which causes the Wolffian duct to develop into the male reproductive tract.

Until the eighth week, the external genitalia are identical in both sexes and have the capacity to develop, from rudiments common to male and female embryos, in either direction. Under the influence of testosterone these rudiments are converted into male genitalia; in the absence of testosterone the female genitalia are formed. Figure 2.1 depicts successive stages in the development of undifferentiated human external genitalia through the crucial 12–14-week point at which male and female fetuses can be distinguished by ultrasound inspection of the external genitalia.

In the male, testosterone is responsible for Wolffian duct virilization, while a metabolite of testosterone, 5α-dihydrotestosterone (DHT), stimulates the development of the male external genitalia as well as the bulbourethral and prostate glands. In the absence of testosterone and DHT, the female reproductive tract and external genitalia develop. At this time the endocrine differentiation of the fetal ovary, as evidenced by the beginning of estradiol synthesis, also occurs. Estradiol is not essential for female phenotypic development but is involved in the differentiation of the primordial follicles.

Prior to the synthesis of any hormone by a tissue, enzyme differentiation is necessary. For instance, as illustrated in Figure 2.1, the urogenital sinus and genital tubercle can, on acquiring 5α-reductase, convert circulating testosterone to DHT. Similarly, in the fetal testis the progressive increase in 3ß-hydroxysteroid dehydrogenase activity is reflected in increased testosterone synthesis from its precursors pregnenolone and androstenedione. In the fetal ovary, estradiol production reflects increased aromatase activity. It follows,

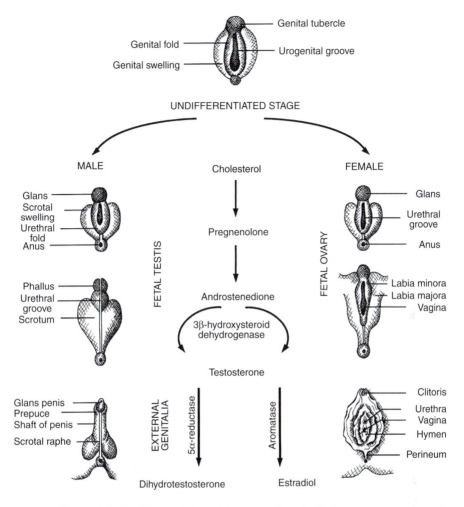

Figure 2.1 The differentiation of the external genitalia from common primordia consisting of undifferentiated labioscrotal folds that are located on either side of the urogenital groove. In the female these folds remain separate and become the labia minora and majora. In the male they fuse to form the corpus spongiosum and the scrotum. Typically, by 12–14 weeks, male and female fetuses can be distinguished by inspection of the external genitalia. (Reproduced from Pollard, I. (1994). *A Guide to Reproduction: Social Issues and Human Concerns*. Cambridge: Cambridge University Press, Fig. 2.1, p. 28, with permission.)

then, that changes in the rates of only a few enzymatic reactions at a critical time in development may have profound consequences for sexual differentiation. Initially, the Leydig cells synthesize testosterone as an autonomous function of the steroidogenic cells, but later in differentiation, when functional receptors for luteinizing hormone (LH) and follicle stimulating hormone

(FSH) are present, testosterone and estrogen synthesis is regulated quantitatively by these gonadotrophins; either gonadotrophin releasing hormone (GnRH) from the fetal pituitary and/or chorionic gonadotrophin (hCG) from the placenta. It is during the development of the fetal hypothalamic–pituitary–gonadal axis that male and female fetuses are vulnerable to epigenetic influences. These influences have the power to modify fetal GnRH secretion and permanently modify the endocrine feedback axes controlling fertility in the adult.

Errors of sexual differentiation

Errors of sexual differentiation were among the first human birth defects to be recognized. Since antiquity, individuals with genital anomalies have been deified or ridiculed. Anomalies which result in abnormal sexual dimorphism may be caused by intrinsic defects in gene expression and/or epigenetic modification of normal gene expression. Intersexuality describes the phenomenon of being born with an ambiguous reproductive system. True hermaphroditism is an intersex condition in which both an ovary and a testis are present in the same individual, or one or both gonads contain histological features of both (ovotestis). The diagnosis of true hermaphroditism can be made when histological examination confirms an ovotestis by demonstrating distinct tubules in the testicular component and follicles in the ovarian component of the gonad. In the majority of ovotestes, the ovarian and testicular tissues are arranged end-to-end, with a histologically distinct line of demarcation between the two types of gonadal tissue. True hermaphroditism is an error in development that may have resulted from an embryo whose cells were a mosaic of 46XX and 46XY cells, or where a component of the *SRY* sex-determining region had been translocated to the X or other autosomal chromosome site. The relative amount of *SRY* transposed would determine the amount of testicular development in an individual whose karyotype is female (46XX).

Pseudohermaphroditism, on the other hand, is a condition where the individual's gonads agree with the chromosomal sex (normal karyotype 46XY or 46XX) but have the external characteristics of the opposite sex. For example, male pseudohermaphrodites have normal testes but incomplete masculinization of the Wolffian duct system and external genitalia. Female pseudohermaphroditism occurs when normal ovaries are present but the body is partially masculinized.

As we have seen, gonadotrophin-dependent testosterone synthesis further regulates the growth and differentiation of the external genitalia and descent of the testes. Hypospadias is the medical term that describes the continuum from small anomalies in penis morphology of no functional concern, to severe cases of ambiguous genitalia. Ambiguous genitalia in a newborn pose immediate problems of gender assignment, rearing and prolonged health concerns since certain forms of hermaphroditism are accompanied by a high incidence of gonadal malignancy. A particular hereditary form of hypospadias arises where testosterone synthesis is normal but 5α-reductase is deficient owing to a genetic error. This form has been extensively researched from case studies of individuals living in the Dominican Republic where the incidence of male pseudohermaphroditism is unusually high. Although this form of pseudohermaphroditism is not a life-threatening anomaly, it is socially and clinically significant when moderate to severe. The severe cases are always raised as girls because at birth each child has a labial-like scrotum, a blind vaginal pouch and a clitoris-like phallus. The testes and derivatives of the Wolffian duct system, such as the epididymis and the vas deferens, are normally differentiated. At puberty, however, there is an absence of breast development and in a proportion of the boys the voice breaks, muscle mass increases, the phallus enlarges to become a penis and spermatogenesis is initiated. The postpubertal psychosexual orientation is often masculine although early female childhood conditioning can cause some conflicts. Late virilization in these boys may be caused by the combination of higher levels of plasma testosterone at puberty than during embryogenesis and by the presence of some residual 5α-reductase activity. DHT is an androgen that is ten times more potent than testosterone and, consequently, local 5α-reduction in target tissue possessing 5α-reductase can greatly amplify the androgenic signal.

Pseudohermaphroditism and related anomalies may also be caused by random exposure to unsuspected developmental disturbance. Exposure to certain chemicals at critical times in development may significantly elevate the risk of structural, biochemical and immunological anomalies in both sexes. Of particular concern are chemicals which possess androgenic or estrogenic properties that may be introduced therapeutically, or inadvertently derived from the environment. The 'Dice syndrome' (the roll of the dice) describes the random exposure of any individual to unsuspected disturbing influences of environmental origin. A special form of Dice syndrome is iatrogenic disease, meaning originating from the physician and, by extension, any intervention unintentionally deviating a developmental process. A classical example is that of the synthetic non-steroidal estrogen, diethylstilbestrol (DES) promoted for the treatment of women at risk of miscarriage, intrauterine fetal death, toxaemia and preterm birth. In 1971, a statistical association was found between maternal ingestion of DES and the occurrence in the daughters of a rare form of clear cell adenocarcinoma of the vagina and cervix. Subsequently, a link between prenatal DES exposure and a variety of other abnormalities in the reproductive tract of both the male and female offspring was established. Between the late 1940s and its prohibition in the early 1970s, an estimated 6 million individuals (the majority in the USA) were affected by prenatal exposure to DES.

Compounds possessing estrogenic activity may also disturb differentiation of the central nervous system (CNS) which may, subsequently, affect psychological and behavioural development with long-term consequences (see next section). Although many behavioural studies are inconclusive, an overall picture has emerged indicating that prenatal exposure to specific synthetic compounds, particularly DES, may feminize male-orientated behaviour (manifested as, for example, decreased interest in contact sport and decreased scores in visuospatial tasks) and defeminizes certain aspects of female CNS functions (manifested as, for example, decreased verbal skills). These conclusions must, however, be regarded within specific social rather than physiological contexts since they were based on selected average behaviour patterns of an Anglo-Saxon population living in middle-class America. Psychological conditions such as depression and anxiety disorders, however, are significantly more frequent in DES-exposed persons when compared to non-exposed controls. On the other hand, compounds that possess androgenic activities may also pose a risk if taken before or during pregnancy. Prominent among these are progestogens – synthetic steroidal compounds included in some birth control prescriptions and certain naturally occurring plant steroids.

Phytoestrogens are naturally occurring plant substances that have weak hormonal activity and are normally harmless constituents of our diet. However, when used in phytotherapy (medical treatment using plants), increased understanding about their biological functions is required. Ginseng (*Panax ginseng*), for example, is a popular ingredient in many herbal prescriptions because its efficacy has been passed down over thousands of years since its discovery in China's mountain provinces of Manchuria. Originally it was consumed for its restorative qualities and promoted as an anti-stress, anti-ageing drug; now it is a popular energizer for many undergoing physical or mental exertion who use ginseng as an alternative to 'pep' pills or caffeine. Its principal active constituents are steroids, termed panaxocides, that stimulate the secretion of adrenal hormones, in particular cortisol and sex steroids, which explain its energy-boosting character (Fig. 2.2). It is believed that these hormonally active compounds assist the body's adaptive response by increasing resistance to stress. Regardless of efficacy, it is unwise to contemplate self-therapy with biologically active substances without also considering their

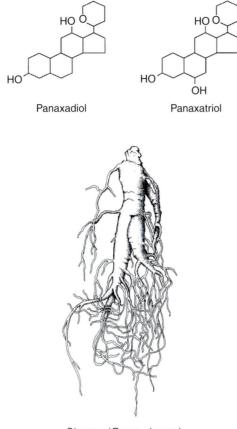

Ginseng (*Panax ginseng*)

Figure 2.2 The chemical structure of panaxadiol and panaxatriol glycosides found in *Panax ginseng* and the ginseng root. (Reproduced from Pollard, I. (1994). *A Guide to Reproduction: Social Issues and Human Concerns*. Cambridge: Cambridge University Press, Fig. 16.3, p. 317, with permission.)

potential effects on fetal growth and development. Many herbal products, including ginseng, have the ability to stimulate the hypothalamic–pituitary–adrenal axis, posing serious concerns about their safety during pregnancy and lactation. A good recipe is to be knowledgeable about bioactive substances and use in moderation.

Brain sex determination

The brain is also a sexually differentiated organ. In the female, the cyclical pattern of secretion of the pituitary gonadotrophins LH and FSH control the normal ovulatory or menstrual cycle. In the male, on the other hand, maintenance of spermatogenesis is not cyclical and depends upon a steady secretion of pituitary gonadotrophins that drive testosterone synthesis. The hypothalamus of both sexes evolves toward the female cyclic secretion of gonadotrophins unless the endocrine hypothalamus is exposed to androgens during prenatal development which results, after maturation, in an irreversible differentiation of the nervous system with a tonic, constant secretion of LH and FSH. In this the hypothalamus mirrors the differentiation of the gonads and, importantly, the organizational effect of the adult brain takes place by specific hormonal exposure early in life. In the newborn female rat a single injection of testosterone results in the absence of cyclical gonadotrophin release and anovulation in adult life owing to the establishment of a tonic (male) secretion pattern. In humans, brain exposure to testosterone has to occur at critical periods between 16 and 28 weeks' gestation for the various organizational effects to become irreversible. There are possibly several critical periods covering different organizational effects, both anatomical and physiological. Good evidence also exists that, for human brain organization toward maleness to occur, circulating fetal testosterone is converted within the brain by the enzyme aromatase to estradiol; thus, in effect it is the estrogen estradiol that masculinizes the brain in male fetuses. However, dihydrotestosterone (DHT) may also have a role in the organization of masculine behaviour in primates.

Although the brains of males and females are sexually differentiated in the fetus, appropriate physiological, psychological and behavioural traits are not maximally expressed until specific brain areas are activated by the hormonal milieu found at puberty and during adulthood. This is because development of the CNS is dependent upon an orderly sequence of hormonal influences; an early organizational stage integral to the development of the nervous system coinciding with sex determination, and a later activational stage which is controlled by gonadal steroids at puberty. For example, while the brain's control over aggression is masculinized by testosterone early in development, the adult expression of this function also requires high levels of testosterone. Interestingly, the activational effect of testosterone does not work through conversion to estrogen but acts directly or via conversion to DHT. It must be highlighted, however, that a purely neuronal basis of human sexuality is distorted, as sexual diversity is part of the natural order. During establishment of the brain's intricate circuitry, there are numerous ways that epigenetic variables may influence developmental programming, enhancing – or weakening – the connections linking social environment with structural, functional and behavioural development.

The socialization of human sexuality

Sexual behaviour is dependent for its expression on genetic coding but is vulnerable to modifying epigenetic influences during critical periods in differentiation. In the area of sexual behaviour, the individual must be studied in the context of evolutionary history, individual genotype and environmental development. This is because natural selection has incorporated a flexible strategy of sexual behaviour which relies on cerebral control rather than strictly hormonal command. Inherent behavioural flexibility is adaptive and may explain why, despite consistent effort, scientific attempts to explain diverse sexual behaviours biologically have met with little success. The extent to which our behaviour follows the dictates of our genes, or is the expression of conscious resourcefulness of our thinking brains, is not known, but is the subject of much interest and controversy.

On the whole, significant human survival strengths can best be understood by referring to mechanisms which have maintained social and physiological flexibility across generations. The opportunistic switch from brute hormonal to cerebral control provided the ability to accommodate change and, eventually, the capacity for judgement, spontaneity and free will. Perhaps the most striking characteristic of this newly acquired flexibility in *Homo sapiens*' evolution has been the socialization of sexuality. Because we are a socialized species, the assumption that the purpose of human sexuality is purely reproductive is false. Human sexuality serves other essential purposes, such as communication, bonding, touching, self-esteem and social organization. Copulation has a greater social significance than just transmission of genotype, as even a cursory study of the history of contraception reveals. For thousands of years humans have tried to prevent pregnancy. Pregnancy prevention, as practised in early societies, included prepubertal coitus, prolonged lactation, delayed marriage, celibacy, withdrawal, the use of abortifacients, vaginal pastes, menses-inducing tampons and various substitutes for heterosexual intercourse. Socialized sexuality in this context reminds us of our varied cultural heritages. Writings over the last few hundred years have forcefully demonstrated evolving socially acceptable views of what was deemed to be 'masculine' or 'feminine', and these represented a continuum from homosexuality to heterosexuality or, in biological terms, a normal continuum of alternative phenotypes. From the human standpoint: sex chromosomes determine sex; gender identity (also called 'innate gender') acknowledges awareness, or belief, in one's maleness or femaleness; gender/sex role is the public manifestation of gender identity, including appearance, behaviour and sexual orientation but excludes desire which may be multiform and not always reproductive.

Sexual orientation

Biological explanations of sexual orientation have broadly focused on genes, hormonal events in utero, and maternal immune responses that are thought to inscribe sexual orientation on to the neural circuitry in the brain. However, no consistent hormonal, immunological or genetic differences have been found between gay, straight, bisexual or asexual preference. All the proposed models are open to criticism because of their implied reliance on developmental abnormalities within the select cohorts of subjects examined, rather than in the healthy population at large. Consequently, many scholars are challenging the view that a single theoretical model is capable of explaining a phenomenon as complex as human sexual orientation or trans-sexualism (see next section). This view rejects normal sexual orientation as being a simple bimodal male–female distribution. Instead, a basic behavioural scaling reflecting flexible genetic predisposition in combination with epigenetic inputs allows for the expression of a range of sexualities. This range is in better accord with actual genotypic and accompanying neuroendocrine variation. According to this hypothesis, the continuum spanning possible human sexuality has its aetiology defined in terms of male- or female-mediated forms of selective marking that enable certain target gene(s) to switch through the incomplete to the fully penetrant state. Such a mechanism can result in an epigenetically driven continuum of orientations ranging from asexual, through graded bisexual, to homosexual.

By distancing ourselves from preoccupation with the gay and lesbian communities (with its implied reference to developmental abnormalities), we can focus on adaptive mechanisms underpinning alternative forms of sexual expressions. Because individuals exist in an environmental continuum, adaptive preconceptional and prenatal programmes have biological significance as they ensure a generational preparedness for the prevailing conditions. Lifestyle factors existing before conception and during fetal life are likely to continue throughout pregnancy and beyond; thus, preparedness may facilitate the offspring's adaptation by anticipating postnatal life from prenatal conditions.

A transgenerational legacy of adaptation is maintained because the steady-state control values of many mammalian physiological/metabolic feedback systems are not rigidly programmed genetically but are set, in part, on the basis of the prevailing environmental conditions during critical periods in development. A good example is the hypothalamic fine-tuning which regulates thyroid function. This setting is established by the maternal hormonal environment during a critical period around the time of birth and persists for life. Under normal conditions, a developmental flexibility serves to fine-balance the offspring's systems with the adapted hormone levels of the mother. Equally, processes that fine-tune brain sex determination may also shape the establishment of alternative sexualities under the influence of stress. In the male, stress-induced alteration of adrenal function may suppress testosterone synthesis during critical periods of gonadal differentiation and this, in turn, may affect the brain differentiation crucial to adult male heterosexual behaviour. Early studies of stress during pregnancy and resulting human sexual orientation relate, directly or indirectly, to war influences. An unusually high proportion of males born in Germany during and immediately after World War II were homosexual. Other retrospective studies record that 9–12 months prior to conception, mothers of gay men experienced levels of stress scores two and a half times as high as those of mothers of heterosexual sons, and nearly two-thirds of the mothers of gay men recalled stressful episodes during pregnancy compared with one-third of mothers of bisexual men and less than 1% of mothers of heterosexual men. It may be assumed that the extreme distress of war would affect not only pregnant women, or women about to conceive, but men as well.

The phenomenon of genomic or parental imprinting suggests that the soma, or body, influences developing germ cells during gametogenesis by selectively marking or imprinting them. At fertilization, this imprinting influences the direction of the conceptus's growth and development. Genomic imprinting demonstrates that DNA is not passed on through the generations intact and that environmental influences can also produce inheritable changes in the way DNA works.

Fraternal birth order can also affect sexual orientation, since men with many older brothers are more likely to be gay while the number of step-brothers and adopted brothers has no effect. The 'maternal immune hypothesis' posits that a maternal immune reaction is provoked by male fetuses and becomes stronger after each pregnancy with a male fetus. The relevant fetal antigen might be one of the male-specific, Y-linked, major histocompatibility antigens, often referred to collectively as H-Y antigen. The hypothesis is that mothers of sons produce anti-H-Y antibodies during pregnancy that interfere with the masculinizing effects on future sons.

Variable endocrine environments during critical periods in development may likewise increase the incidence of homosexuality in women. A good example, already described in the section on errors of sexual differentiation (p. 30), relates to the adult daughters of DES-treated mothers who exhibit markedly increased incidences of bisexual and homosexual behaviour. As described earlier, for masculinization of the fetal brain to occur, testosterone is first converted to estrogen, so it is possible that the synthetic estrogen DES may have prenatally androgenized brain differentiation in women who then have a higher incidence of homosexual feelings. Since the 1940s, soon after the sex steroids had first been synthesized, there were many attempts to prove a definitive neurohormonal theory of sexual orientation which could be associated with 'natural masculinity' and 'natural femininity'. However, there is no statistically valid study based on random sampling of the entire male or female population that links sex steroid levels with homosexuality. An excess preoccupation with the science of homosexuality may underlie an intention to control and/or eliminate it in future, an attitude that could gain traction if a gay gene, or genes, were to be discovered.

Transgender and gender recognition

> I was born fourteen years ago, when I was fifty-two years old. Not born again; not reborn...just born. A long gestation period, and a difficult one, full of pain and joy, achievement and failure. I jumped because I was pushed but if I hadn't been pushed I think I would eventually have jumped anyway. No wonder I adopted the butterfly as my symbol. I emerged from the confining chrysalis of masculinity to be the female person I had always known myself to be, despite years of avoidance, denial and sublimation.[2]

A transsexual is a person whose gender identity is at conflict with his or her genetic sex and physical appearance. In the majority of cases, physical appearance of the genitals is a reliable indicator of sexual identity. In a minority, incongruity between anatomical sex and experienced gender identity is so pronounced and persistent that transsexuals may seek treatment to, as far as medically possible, physically change their bodies and live as members of the other sex. However, a growing recognition that sex and innate gender need not be related has led to an increasing number of transgendered who transition but refuse surgical intervention. Thus, the concept of what it is to be a man or woman is gradually being modified from the physical to the mental.

Past and ongoing studies on chromosomes, hormones and brain structure/function relationships have not provided reliable and replicable insights into how a person's gender identity is moulded. As already noted, human sexual differentiation is a multistep, sequentially interrelated process in which genetic information is translated into the phenotype of a person who subsequently

---

[2] Cummings, Katherine. (2001). My story: the life and loves of an XY woman. *Polare* **41**, 27.

establishes a male or female identity and awareness of sexual orientation. Research in this field is hampered by the prior assumptions of many scientists and clinicians who classify transsexualism as an abnormality in need of revolution. With the aid of new technologies, however, neuroscientists are beginning to replace 'pathology' with direct observations of brain sex plasticity. Cerebral lateralization studies have revealed that alleged masculine patterns of brain functions (meaning that the brain usually uses predominantly one hemisphere to accomplish a cognitive task) can be found in anatomical females; similarly, alleged feminine patterns of brain functions (meaning that the brain will have proportionally greater contributions from both hemispheres to accomplish a cognitive task) can be found in anatomical males. These cerebral lateralization studies reinforce the natural continuum of physiologically overlapping phenotypes and must replace the popular but overly simple dimorphism. Other methodological difficulties stem from the implicit but biologically incorrect concept that gender identity and homosexuality are interconnected. As a result, the word 'transsexual' has lost popularity in favour of the preferred term 'transgendered'. A transsexual can in fact be homosexual, bisexual, heterosexual or asexual. Since the terms transsexual and transgendered are currently in common use, they will be used here interchangeably.

Although it is still widely held that the two genders are natural and immutable, transsexualism has a long history and exists in all societies and ethnic categories. Moreover, in societies that can tolerate lack of correspondence between gender and genitals, there is no documented transsexual discrimination. Cross-cultural perspectives on gender demonstrate the many ways that biological brain gender can be used as a blueprint for maintaining community wellbeing. A well-documented example comes from the 'two-spirit people' (once referred to by the discredited generic term 'berdache') identifiable among many North American and Canadian First Nation Indigenous groups. Two-spirit refers to third gender people and implies a masculine spirit and a feminine spirit living in the same body. Such people are respected for being both male and female, which makes them more complete and, thus, better balanced when performing specific social functions in their communities. For example, in some groups, male-bodied two-spirits were active as healers and conveyers of oral traditions, made pottery, wove, and fulfilled other special functions in connection with festivities and dance. Conversely, female-bodied two-spirits typically took on roles such as chief, councillor, trader, hunter, raider and peace messenger. The above thinking is also reflected in the ancient Greek tradition. Plato, when discussing the power of love, maintained that originally the sexes were not two but three in number; there was man, woman, and the union of the two, from which the name 'androgynous' survives but nothing else.[3]

In the South Pacific islands of Samoa, as many as one family in five may have a son who is a *fa'afafine* – literally meaning a male who is like a female. *Fa'afafines* are boys who are typically nominated by their families as 'excess' males and grow up from an early age as girls. *Fa'afafines* are usually well educated and are among society's most respected members as they devote themselves to education, health, social welfare and the preservation of traditional Samoan culture. There is also a long history of transgender acceptance in Asia where, for example, cultures in the Indian subcontinent include individuals assigned male at birth but who later live as a third gender referred to in Hindi as 'hijra'.

Western and some other dominant extant cultures require a medical diagnosis of transgenderism, which may be settled only after years of continuous gender identity confusion and 'remedial' assistance. However, autobiographies and personal accounts repeatedly describe feelings from early childhood of being locked inside a body in which they do not belong. The awareness of being different as a child, which may be accompanied by bullying and teasing at school, highlights a genuine problem that is deserving of understanding and appropriate sociomedical management. Instead, social banishment even well into adulthood is the experience of many, an experience made worse by certain social elements that maintain that a life of overt transsexualism is synonymous with immorality.

In practical terms, there are two basic approaches to identifying a person's sex for community and legal purposes. First is the uncomplicated straightforward approach that exclaims 'it's a boy!' or 'it's girl!', as indicated at birth by the infant's genitalia. The second is a more complex biological approach. Transgender research (as for sexual orientation) has broadly focused on genes and hormonal events in utero that may point to causal, or multi-causal, factors facilitating, or inhibiting, the development of the neural circuitry on which gender identity is inscribed. The psychoneuroendocrine theory holds that brain exposure to an abnormal concentration of sex hormones during fetal and early postnatal life is a major determinant of gender identity and, subsequent, transgenderism. Alternatively, there are known gene variants which affect sexual differentiation of the brain. Repeat polymorphic variants of such genes increase the susceptibility for male-to-female transsexualism.[4] In particular,

---

[3] *Collected Works of Plato*, 4th edn. (1953) (Translated by Benjamin Jowett.) Oxford: Oxford University Press.

[4] Repeat polymorphisms refer to variations in the length of certain DNA segments where a few letters of the genetic code 'stutters' or repeats in the same order several times.

one repeat variant found on the estrogen receptor, or $ER\beta$, gene, which acts as a gateway controlling the flow of estrogen, was significantly associated with the frequency of male-to-female transsexualism. The more frequent the repeats or stutters of the $ER\beta$ gene, the greater the incidence of transsexualism. However, long allele repeat variants are also relatively common in the general population, so many variants cannot be a primary cause of transsexualism, but certain combinations may well be a contributing cause.

On the basis of epidemiological evidence, sex and gender identity are not an option of personal choice; rather they are derived from interacting genetic and epigenetic elements. Gender roles, on the other hand, can be changed and under reassignment (with or without surgery) it becomes possible to bring innate gender and gender role into congruence. Male-to-female (M–F) transsexuals are individuals classified as males at birth who went from a male designation to a female designation and vice versa for female-to-male (F–M) transsexuals. It is estimated that transgender prevalence is of the order of 1 in 500 but may even be more frequent. Transgenderism is typically self-diagnosed at a very young age and lasts a lifetime and, hence, at any given time is much larger than the number of officially diagnosed cases. Given this relatively high incidence, medical and public health communities as well as governmental institutions must seriously consider practical ways of improving social welfare and legal rights issues as they concern the transgendered. To date, legal rights issues of transgendered have largely concentrated on changing birth certificates and other personal documents, the right to marry, entitlements to government benefits, and protection under anti-discrimination legislation.

For transsexuals, transitioning from the gender of birth is a stressful physical and social process, and some medical professionals express considerable doubt about the desirability of facilitating gender transition, especially with gender assignment surgery. On the other hand, a unisex appearance/lifestyle is problematic in a gendered world where sex or gender has to be declared for sociological and legal purposes. Most is known about M–F transsexuals. This may be because of a greater willingness to share experiences, or because male-to-female transsexuals are more conspicuous socially, or because, historically, transwomen had been socialized to be more assertive and demanded greater access to gender clinics catering to their specific needs.

Before gender clinics recommend gender assignment surgery, several conditions have to be satisfied. One clear pattern of similarity among the M–F transgendered is that an estimated 93% began cross-dressing in their mother's or sister's clothes when first experiencing anxiety over their sexual ambivalence. Such a universal behaviour appears to be an early realization that their contrived appearance as boys is deceptive and in need of eradication. As adults, transitioning typically commences with living as women and developing their bodies to resemble those of biological females. Before gaining access to assignment surgery, both transwomen and transmen have to demonstrate certainty of gender identity, taking appropriate steroidal sex hormones, maintaining regular contact with their physician, and living publicly according to their gender identity.

In the past two decades, surgical techniques have improved radically, but gender realignment is still heavy surgery involving reshaping the whole body and constructing genitals to appear normal and, as far as possible, function normally. Transwoman surgery involves removal of the testes, male accessory glands and almost the entire penis. The inverted penile skin, with preserved blood and nerve supplies, is used to line the neovagina after a cavity is created in the pelvis. This procedure (known as vaginoplasty) forms a fully sensate vagina and clitoris. The labia majora are made out of the scrotal skin, while the labia minora are constructed by pleating the junction of the penile and scrotal skin. The operation also repositions the urethra so that water passes directly into the bowl during urination from a sitting position.

Transman surgery involves bilateral mastectomy, or removal of the breasts, shaping of a masculine chest, and removal of all the internal female sex organs. Genital reconstructive procedures (phalloplasty) involve the use of either clitoris (often enlarged by testosterone treatment and freed by metoidioplasty) or tissue grafts from the arm, thigh or belly and an erectile prosthesis. In a metoidioplasty the enlarged clitoris is released from its position and moved forward to more closely approximate the position of a normal penis. The urethra needs to be re-routed through the phallus to allow urination through the reconstructed penis and the labia majora are united to form a scrotum into which prosthetic testicles are inserted.

It is evident that sex and gender determination can be viewed in a number of ways, whether as biology, lifestyle, accomplishment and/or ways of being. Recognition of the above view exchanges the either/or gender dichotomy hypothesis for the notion of a natural continuum. Acceptance of diversity may herald a new, less dogmatic era, acknowledging that gender is only one part of sexuality, inseparable from feelings of identity and desire. In closing, it seems appropriate to quote again from one of Australia's most politically active transgendered intellectuals, 'People love people and gender is incidental',[5] suggesting that sex can be an expression of love unrelated to reproduction and, conversely, that love can exist without sex (and often does).

[5] Cummings, Katherine. (1992). *Katherine's Diary: The Story of a Transsexual*. Melbourne, Australia: William Heinemann, p. 213.

Principles of bioscience ethics for discussion

- Ethics probe: many consider that research into the origins of sexuality is an unwanted distraction from the real issues of concern, such as anti-gay and transgendered violence and discrimination. Can scientific knowledge magnify problems or difficulties instead of achieving a desired goal?
- To what extent is it regressive to follow existing mores, rather than facilitating social change toward a more tolerant and open society which would ultimately benefit all? Discuss ethical approaches that should successfully challenge societal prejudices and discrimination against singles, gays and others living outside the social norm.
- As our knowledge of brain development increases, we are able to alter its function, and it becomes important to integrate neuroscience and neuroethics into the foundations of learning. Point to a diversity of neuroethics which may provide an adaptive entry into the realm of communication and culture.

3

Inappropriate lifestyle and congenital disability in children: basic principles of growth, toxicology, teratogenesis and mutagenesis

> I am very much for human rights but I think for the dignity of the human being, it is necessary not only to emphasize the rights, but also the responsibilities.[1]

The emergence of intelligence and discernment in our thinking brain provided a degree of autonomy in forward planning, tool-making, imitation and teaching. Acquisition of sophisticated language made it possible to understand mental states in others, which helped in the creation of a unique hominid social, political, economic, ethical and spiritual order. This chapter describes normal development and how epigenetic influences (that is, all the environmental variables which modulate gene activity) might derail it. Harmful epigenetic influences can trigger intrinsic gene defects (mutations) or adversely modify normal gene expression, resulting in impaired growth and development. Good health, far from being a natural state or universal right, is a matter of achievement, a consequence of privilege or good luck even. It is for this reason that health is defined in the Constitution of the World Health Organization (WHO) as being a state of 'complete physical, mental and social wellbeing, not merely the absence of disease or infirmity'. This definition succinctly emphasizes the positive aspects of a fully realized genetic potential. Good health can, therefore, be seen as the result of a positive environment supported by socioeconomic advantage. This and the subsequent two chapters are concerned

---

[1] Theologian Dr Hans Kung on *A New Ethic of Human Responsibility*. ABC Radio National – The Religion Report Transcript 9 December 1998, page 1 (www.abc.net.au/rn/talks).

with ways that everyone can improve – maximize – their own and their children's genetic potential. Very few of us come close to fully expressing our genetic potential, but with increased biological understanding we can move closer to enjoying our innate distinctive capabilities.

Parenting is one of the most difficult and responsible tasks that we are ever likely to undertake, yet society takes it for granted that parents intrinsically know what to do. Analysis of relationships between parents and their children has been sadly under-represented in the traditional philosophical repertoire of ethical concerns. The cynic would argue that there is a perfectly simple explanation as to why children's needs and wellbeing are frequently bypassed; children have no vote, no political power and no financial independence. Because good health is made more accessible by science and positive social change, we are now facing significant new educational challenges and bio-ethical responsibilities. Good parenting is a practical subject for which mothers and fathers are accountable. Simone de Beauvoir's 'ovarian' work effectively unmasked the mystique surrounding women's 'natural' place in society when she analysed social problems arising out of gender inflexibility, particularly in the home. Now it is up to the committed sum of us who (regardless of sex or gender) must demand the preservation of children's wellbeing so that they, in turn, uphold their parental responsibilities across the generations.

Responsible parental behaviour should follow from the recognition of the obligatory dependency of children on their adult contacts, and from an identification of the dangers that parents themselves sometimes present to their children. These dangers may originate from a parent being uninformed about basic biological principles, and it is in this context that bioscience ethics can be of assistance. Therefore, this chapter describes briefly the basic principles of toxicology, mutagenesis, teratogenesis and delayed development; essential knowledge before reviewing the ethics of parenting.

Patterns of human growth

The foundation for normal adult reproduction is set during fetal life. Sex, as are all other functions, is the product of genetics and environment working as one complex informational unit where their separate contributions cannot be isolated under normal conditions. Prenatal and postnatal development takes place in an environmental context; that is, the continuum of the individual's changing surroundings and life experiences. Epigenetic influences become more evident the older an individual becomes. Age, education, experience, conditioning and disease all shape appearance, thought, emotion and behaviour.

Development starts in the ovaries and testes of the parents where the cells destined to become gametes are first differentiated as distinct germ-lines. These distinct lines combine at fertilization to forge the generational link between parent and offspring. Therefore, when reviewing our life history we need to consider more than the traditional highlights, such as age-related fertility decline and mortality. We need to take account of the entire succession of physical, physiological, behavioural, intellectual, emotional and spiritual change through which each individual passes from conception to death. Basic biological characteristics, such as epigenetically induced changes in the rate of prenatal or postnatal growth patterns and variations in the attainment of sexual maturity (puberty), need to be evaluated in addition to genetic endowment. The underlying mechanisms of how we change in shape, form and function from the helpless baby to the fully formed adult are some of the most fascinating aspects of our history. Although studies of the genetic mechanisms of growth are still in their infancy, sufficient is known about them to be able to use them as diagnostic tools in monitoring the health of individuals and populations. Understanding the correlation of cultural, behavioural, economic and environmental factors with health and wellbeing is one of biology's greatest challenges (Chapter 7).

Much of the success of the human species stems from the large body size, an exceptional brain and an extended period of childhood. This gives us the metabolic and ecological advantages of greater size relative to many other species. The ability to think our way through problems, and the time to develop behaviours through play and learning makes us successful, social, problem-solving adults. Another feature of human success is our adaptive flexibility (plasticity) of growth in response to environmental or ecological stress. In the face of adversity such as famine, for example, we are able to reduce or stop growth altogether and catch up, to varying degrees, during times of plenty. How this adaptive flexibility is regulated genetically and endocrinologically (hormonally) is not clear. Growth, at its simplest, is the increase in size of the body or its parts, while maturation refers to the timing and tempo of progress towards the mature biological state. Both growth and maturation vary with the specific system under consideration, whether endocrine, nervous, reproductive, skeletal, immunological or behavioural. In other words, the outcomes of growth and maturation are the development of functional competence – the result of complex interactions among genes, endocrine secretions, energy and nutrient supplies, and environmental variables. These interactions begin well before conception and continue prenatally and postnatally.

The embryonic/fetal periods and embryo staging

Prenatal life is the time from fertilization of the oocyte to the birth of the baby. The mean duration is 38 weeks or, more precisely, 264 days, with a range of 254–274 days. Growth and development during this time is accompanied by the sequential appearance of new tissues and their remodelling, involving degradation of existing structures and replacement with new formations. Individual embryos cannot be arranged in the order of their age because any given example may be more advanced in one respect while being delayed in another. So, for the purpose of obtaining a relative measure of the level of development, comparisons with a selected series of embryos, numbered in the order of their developmental stage, can be useful. The internationally accepted Carnegie system of staging, for example, concerns the embryonic period, with the scheme consisting of 23 developmental stages based on external and internal morphological appearances. Each stage depends mainly on specific features that appear or change rapidly, such as the number of paired somites, the differentiation of the nervous or vascular systems, the early appearance of the eye, or the form of the emerging limbs.

The transition from the embryonic to the fetal period typically occurs at 8 weeks post-fertilization, when the greatest length is approximately 30 millimetres. The technical criterion for the end of the embryonic period is, however, the initial formation of marrow in the humerus (the single long bone in the arm which extends from the shoulder to the elbow). By the end of the embryonic period, all organ rudiments should already have been laid down. This is also the time during which most congenital anomalies first become apparent. Once the basic structures are formed, it becomes increasingly difficult to alter them structurally. The subsequent fetogenic period is the period largely devoted to body growth, histocytological differentiation and functional maturation of organs and organ systems. Insults during this period predominantly cause growth retardation, developmental delay and functional deficits, particularly neurobehavioural as the brain matures relatively late in development.

A satisfactory staging system for the fetal period is not yet available, so the fetal period is conveniently considered in terms of trimesters of approximately 13 weeks each. Figure 3.1 is a schematic diagram of human development with specific critical periods marked. Critical periods in intrauterine development are those periods during the development of organs, or organ systems, when they are most sensitive to external influences. Exposing an organ to a toxic substance or other disturbing influence during its particularly vulnerable critical period results in maximum developmental damage. As concerns the

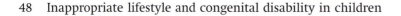

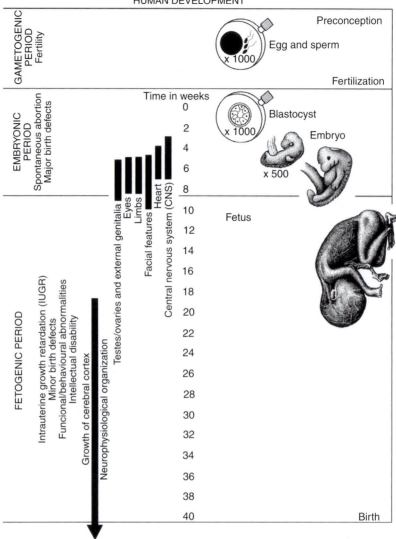

Figure 3.1 Schematic diagram of human development from preconception to birth. The processes involved in the normal development of human and other mammals can be characterized as follows.

Early development: fertilization requires about 24 hours to complete and involves a series of changes in sperm and egg physiology before finally the fusion of the male and female pronuclei forms the zygote or conceptus. In the early stages of development, cells destined to form the extraembryonic (placental) membranes and those of the embryo begin to differentiate.

Embryonic period: organogenesis is the most complex stage of development and is characterized by the formation of all organs and organ systems of the embryonic development of the central nervous system (CNS), it is important to emphasize that human brain development is exceptional and multiphasic, extending over the entire prenatal period and through the first 2–3 years of postnatal life. The first phase of brain growth is one of neuronal multiplication which is followed by the second and major growth phase of glial cell proliferation when axons grow, dendrites branch extensively, synapses form, neurotransmitter systems develop and myelination proceeds. Thus, in essence, neurons multiply in the first trimester of intrauterine life but the major growth phase is during the third trimester and continues after birth. Brain growth in weight is approximately a quarter complete by birth but attains about three-quarters of its adult weight by 2 years. There is, obviously, a finer-grained chronology within the above overview as, within a single brain region, subpopulations of neurons develop at different rates and at different times. Importantly, different parts of the CNS form at different stages of development and there are many critical periods where neurotoxins can exert their deleterious effects. The degree of damage and how this might influence selective attention and information-processing abilities across the developmental continuum is greatly influenced by factors such as the timing and pattern of fetal exposure, as well as individual differences in genetic susceptibility of the conceptus.

Ultrasound has been used for the assessment of intrauterine growth. Using modern transvaginal ultrasound scanners, the embryo can be identified reliably less than 4 weeks after conception and its length measured. The subsequent rapid and accelerating growth of the fetal crown–rump length can be measured by either transvaginal or transabdominal ultrasound scans up to about 10 weeks post-conception (or 12 weeks after the last menstrual period). At 12 weeks post-conception, a rapidly increasing number of fetal structures

Figure 3.1 (*cont.*)
body. Each organ or organ system has a particular time during pregnancy when it is being formed, the critical period being marked by vertical bars. During the critical period of intrauterine development, the embryo or fetus has the greatest sensitivity to environmental influences. Striking advances during the third week are the development of somites, the heart, the neural folds and the major divisions of the brain, the neural crest, and the beginnings of the internal ear and the eye.
Fetogenic period: important developments are general body growth, histological and functional development of organs, and the histological development of the central nervous system (CNS). Brain development, however, occurs during the entire period of fetal differentiation and through the first 2 years of postnatal life.

Drug abuse during gametogenic, embryonic and fetogenic periods may harm normal growth and development in the offspring and increase its chances of being born with birth defects, low birthweight and mental/behavioural deficits.

can be seen with clarity and can be measured. Normal growth charts exist for many of them. In addition to measuring these individual structures, the ratios between some, such as the head and abdomen circumference, or head circumference and femur length, can be computed and are of particular value in identifying growth-retarded fetuses. In growth retardation, soft tissue growth, such as that of the abdomen, tends to be affected early, while limb growth, and especially head growth, is preserved until later in the disorder. Ultrasound is the most effective tool for the assessment of intrauterine growth of the fetus but this technology cannot tell us anything about the genetic mechanisms which control fetal responsiveness to the external environment and which provide additional fine-tuning of its genetically programmed development.

The placenta as the maternal–fetal interface

Implantation is the process whereby the embryo penetrates the uterine endometrium (decidua), resulting in a functional juxtaposition of the embryonic and maternal blood systems. Following implantation, the process of placentation enables the fetus to survive within the uterus. At this time, the two most conspicuous extraembryonic tissues are the chorion and the amnion. The chorion consists of an outer layer of villi (made up of the syncytiotrophoblast and adjacent cytotrophoblast tissues) which integrate with the maternal decidua to create the placenta. The amniotic cavity safely houses the conceptus. The basic structures of the placenta are the chorionic villi which are its functional units. As seen in Figure 3.2, villi of the chorion penetrate deeply into the uterine tissue whilst enlarging and branching extensively. They become highly vascularized as fetal blood vessels become established within them. The villi, in turn, are bathed by maternal blood which flows continuously through the maternal (intervillous) space (sinus).

The properties of the placenta promote the efficient exchange of molecules between mother and fetus by establishing metabolic diffusion gradients and carrier-mediated transfers. The effectiveness with which gradients can function depends on the placental blood flow rates, placental metabolic activity and factors affecting them. Placental growth is dependent on the state of maternal nutrition during early placentation. This in turn affects growth of the embryo so that, in general, fetal weight in late gestation is directly related to placental weight. The fetus uses the uptake of nutrients (glucose, amino acids and lipids) via the umbilical circulation to fulfil two major requirements: for growth to build new tissues, and to provide substrates to fuel energy metabolism. The placenta also plays a crucial role in the synthesis and metabolism of hormones and peptide growth factors that direct appropriate signals to the

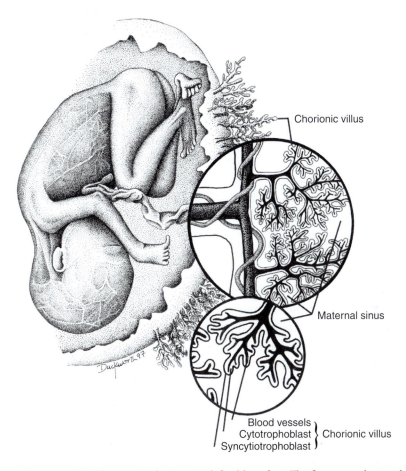

Chorionic villus

Maternal sinus

Blood vessels $\Big)$
Cytotrophoblast $\Big\}$ Chorionic villus
Syncytiotrophoblast $\Big)$

Figure 3.2 The placenta as the maternal–fetal interface. The fetus uses the uptake of nutrients via the chorionic villi to fulfil two major requirements: for growth to build new tissues, and to provide substrates to fuel energy metabolism. Circled enlargements show the umbilical vessels and branches of the extensive chorionic vascular bed of the fetal compartment within the maternal intervillous spaces.

placenta itself, and to maternal and fetal targets driving the succession of endocrine events and the timing of parturition. These metabolic processes are dependent on the interaction of genetic and epigenetic influences.

Abnormal prenatal growth patterns, fetal programming and long-term health consequences

Normal intrauterine growth is considered a good marker for fetal wellbeing; the same is true for postnatal growth. There are, however, aspects of early development which, if uncorrected perinatally, may have long-term effects upon the individual. Fetuses have mechanisms by which they adapt to deterioration in environmental conditions brought about by drug abuse, disease, nutritional deprivation and non-adaptive lifestyles. Adaptation is subject to genetic variability and if the limits of genetic adaptability are exceeded, fetal growth restriction and/or organ damage may result. Should epigenetic influences adversely affect the sexual differentiation of the fetal germ cells, then a changed genetic programme may be perpetuated in the offspring of a subsequent generation. Conversely, reproduction under good conditions creates a positive force in shaping human identity.

Intrauterine growth retardation (IUGR) is the most common term used to refer to the consequences of inadequate growth in the fetus. Another way is to describe the uterine growth-retarded infant as being small-for-gestational age, or small-for-dates. Small-for-gestational age means a birthweight below the tenth percentile of intrauterine growth curves – in general 2500 g or less – but it excludes infants with malformations, chromosomal aberrations or prenatal infections. Inadequate birthweight may also result from prematurity; that is, preterm delivery where the duration of pregnancy was less than 37 weeks rather than poor fetal weight gain for a given duration of pregnancy. Fetuses that are larger than the cut-off value may also be growth-retarded, but not identified. These would be fetuses whose intrauterine growth was genetically programmed to result in a larger than average size, but whose growth rate was slowed by intrauterine factors. In general, the lowest risk of neonatal death and the greatest likelihood of optimal physical and intellectual development is in children 3000 g or more at birth.

As explained above, the environment experienced from preconception to birth exerts a profound influence on physiological function and, as a consequence, also on the risk of disease in adult life. Since normal development can be disrupted by harmful epigenetic influences, those individuals who survive their prenatal challenges may be destined to struggle with long-term health consequences. For instance, strong epidemiological associations exist between impaired growth during fetal life and infancy, and an increased risk in adulthood of developing certain diseases of adaptation such as cardiovascular disease, hypertension, cancer, asthma, type 2 diabetes, schizophrenia and depression. A great deal has been learned since David Barker and colleagues (University of Southampton, UK) first proposed that suboptimal intrauterine growth may alter fetal development in ways that predisposes the offspring to a range of diseases in adulthood.

As nutrition directly or indirectly influences epigenetic processes that finetune growth, the nutrient supply to the fetus is a prime determinant in establishing the offspring's long-term health prospects. The phenomenon variously referred to as 'fetal programming', 'developmental programming of adult health and disease' or just 'programming' occurs when the normal pattern of fetal growth is disrupted in response to unfavourable intrauterine conditions. Essentially, programming takes place when normal placental signalling is disrupted. However, little is known about the mechanisms whereby variable stressful challenges programme the future trajectory of development. Hormones regulate fetal growth and tissue development, so changed endocrine indices are likely to have a central role in intrauterine programming. The strongest candidates involved in fetal programming are the glucocorticoids, or stress hormones, because they are growth inhibitors able to affect the development of any organ system, and their concentration in utero is elevated by all nutritional and other stressful challenges known to have programming effects. Glucocorticoids can act directly on genes and indirectly through changes in the bioavailability of other hormones (such as insulin, insulin-like growth factors and thyroxine), and have persistent differential effects on the hypothalamic–pituitary–adrenal (HPA) or stress axis (Chapter 7). The HPA axis is highly sensitive to programming during fetal development and thus, in turn, influences physiological function throughout the course of life. Importantly, there is good evidence that programming of HPA activity might underlie some of the long-term effects that are observed following harmful prenatal influences. It is believed that fetal programming is an adaptive evolutionary strategy in mammals that confers some survival advantage in utero, albeit at an increased risk of adult-onset degenerative diseases.

Endocrine changes might be both the cause and the consequence of intrauterine programming but how such programming is implemented remains unclear. As described in Chapter 2, epigenetic inheritance refers to heritable changes in gene regulation without a change in DNA sequence that may, under certain circumstances, endure across several generations. Epigenetic marking such as DNA and histone methylation are considered likely mechanisms to induce long-term programming effects. Methylation is a process whereby marks are set in chromatin to programme gene expression differentially, resulting in the activation, repression or silencing of the gene. Folate functions as a major methyl donor for nucleic acid synthesis; it is thus influential in methyl group availability for DNA synthesis and normal tissue growth, integrity and repair – including the proliferation of neuronal progenitor cells in the developing brain. Methylation, however, might not be the only method of chromatic remodelling, and ongoing studies may well discover a wider range of epigenetic programming mechanisms.

The risk of developing diseases of adaptation can be intensified further by environmental risk factors such as drug abuse, obesity, physical inactivity, prolonged anxiety and increasing age. The type of fetal growth impairment and consequent expression is dependent upon when the insult occurred and how long it lasted. For example, if a fetus was exposed to a severe insult during the first phase of cellular multiplication, this would result in an overall decreased number of cells. The effects of this reduced cell number are irreversible and result in symmetrical IUGR. Chromosomal abnormalities and severe viral infections early in pregnancy are examples of insults that may cause symmetrical IUGR. However, a fetus exposed to an insult late in pregnancy, during the stage of cell enlargement and differentiation, will usually have asymmetrical IUGR. This infant will suffer from a decreased size of cells but not (with the exception of the brain which has, as described above, several critical, or vulnerable, periods during pregnancy) a decreased number of cells. Asymmetrical IUGR usually spares the vital organs, for example brain and heart, necessary to survive intrauterine life, at the expense of organs, for example liver, lungs and kidneys, that are necessary for extrauterine life. Interestingly, brain growth appears to be affected last. This 'brain-sparing effect' appears to be characteristic of the human species and may be a genetically determined mechanism to preserve the intellectual function at the expense of other functions. The long-term prognosis for a fetus with asymmetrical IUGR is more favourable than the prognosis for the fetus who suffers from symmetrical IUGR. The infant with symmetrical IUGR is at greater risk of long-term neurodevelopmental and cognitive dysfunction owing to decreased total brain size.

Growth retardation in the fetus is known to be related to many factors associated with the maternal constitution and health, and with the quality of the maternal internal and external environments. Maternal nutritional deprivation or undernutrition adversely affects fetal growth, as do lifestyle factors such as drug abuse (Chapter 4). In many cases, postnatal exposure to the same harmful environmental factors which stressed the fetus in utero continue to jeopardize the wellbeing of the already vulnerable infant. On the positive side, however, early assessment of fetal growth retardation can reduce further harm by appropriate medical and nutritional intervention to the newborn. Early intervention is crucial since postnatal catch-up growth in certain categories of infants who have been retarded in utero is possible. That is, should nutrition and favourable environmental conditions coincide with the first months of life – a period of very high growth velocity – even the very low birthweight (less than 1500 g) infant may experience a growth rate similar to that of the full-term infant. It is believed that infants who experienced catch-up growth of height and head circumference have probably realized their full physical and intellectual potential, and their slower intrauterine growth need not be an enduring disadvantage. Because of the progressively decreasing growth in head circumference (equals brain size) after the first 6 months, the chances for catch-up growth after intrauterine or early postnatal growth retardation diminish with increasing age.

It is, therefore, important to re-emphasize that the heritability of complex systems, such as behavioural and personality characteristics, are all the result of genetic and environmental influences interacting as one informational system. By studying transgenic animals, scientists have been able to gain a clearer idea of the influence of specific genetic predispositions on behaviour. A genetic predisposition involves inherited physiological factors which influence behaviour. These include brain chemistry – the neurological structure with which we are born – where the combined action of several different genes, each with small but cumulative effects, produces a certain genetic predisposition. A genetic predisposition directs, but does not necessarily control, behaviour. Some genetic predispositions remain latent until a triggering event or set of circumstances occurs. For instance, a particular predisposition may be activated by distress, illness or lifestyle choices (such as smoking). Positive and negative experiences have the power to alter our brain's chemistry and function permanently in extreme cases. The reader is also referred to the discussion on psychosocial stress and its harmful effects on postnatal growth and development (Chapter 6, Stress and psychosocial short stature).

Toxicology: basic principles

Toxicology is the science of poisons. A poison, or toxicant, is a substance that is harmful to living organisms because of its detrimental effects on tissues, organs, or biological processes such as reproduction. Whether a substance is toxic depends upon various factors or conditions: for example, the route or site of toxic exposure, the amount (dose) of the substance incorporated, the duration (total time period) per exposure incident, and the frequency (rate) of exposure. Therefore, it is possible to classify toxic exposures on the basis of acute versus chronic and local versus systemic presentation. In human toxicology, the degree of harm done by a poison is not only dependent upon the route, dose and frequency of exposure but is also strongly dependent on the individual's genetic resilience, developmental stage and health status. For example, gametes (eggs and sperm), embryos and fetuses are more vulnerable to toxic insult when compared with children who are, in turn, generally more susceptible than are healthy adults.

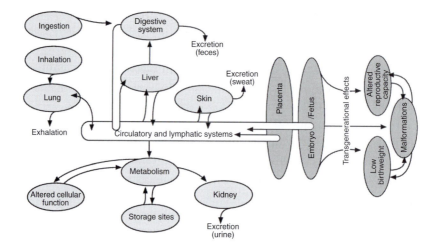

Figure 3.3 Pale ellipses are diagrammatic representations of the major sites of exposure, distribution, metabolism, storage points and elimination of toxic substances in the body. Dark ellipses represent fetal exposure to toxicants via the placental interface and possible long-term effects.

When discussing exposure sites for toxicants it is helpful first to consider the major routes by which life-sustaining substances enter, are distributed, metabolized and finally eliminated from the body. The pale ellipses in Figure 3.3 provide a diagrammatic overview of the major sites of exposure, distribution, metabolism, storage points and elimination of substances, including toxic ones, in the body. Toxic substances enter the body by the same routes as nutrients and oxygen; that is, via the lungs, the digestive system and the skin. The circulatory and lymphatic systems then carry these substances around the body and expose them to the body's cells. The liver is the body's main processing and detoxification site, whence nitrogenous and toxic wastes are delivered to the excretory system for elimination by the kidneys.

Cells in the body's tissues and organs use the nutrients to maintain the processes of life such as respiration, metabolism, growth and reproduction. The immune system is made up of specialized cells that travel in the circulatory and lymphatic systems. The lymphatic system is a transport system consisting of a network of vessels that extend throughout the body and collect lymph from the tissues to deliver it back to the blood circulatory system. The lymph is filtered as it circulates through major lymph glands situated in the neck, armpits and groin, trapping invading bacteria and other debris. The destruction of specific pathogens (bacteria, viruses) is an important function of the immune system. However, when considering pathogens, drugs and other toxicants, the major routes of intentional, or accidental, exposure listed above have to be adjusted to include additional routes of entry, such as vaginal, rectal, intravenous and intramuscular.

The route by which toxic substances are introduced into the body is strongly dependent upon their physical and chemical properties. The lungs are most likely to take in toxic gases or very fine, respirable solids or liquid particles like dust, radioactive particles and toxic aerosols. Solids usually enter the body orally, while absorption through the skin is most likely for liquids or semi-solids in solution like emulsions, sludges and creams. Because chemical interaction between different substances may affect their individual toxicity, the biological effects of two or more toxins – or drugs – administered together can be very different in kind and degree compared with either of the substances alone. When two substances have similar physiological functions, their effects may be simply additive, or they may be synergistic; that is, the total effect is greater (sometimes by many orders of magnitude) than the sum of the effects of each separately. Potentiation occurs when a substance enhances the action of another substance and antagonism when a substance decreases the effect of another substance; that is, has opposing biological effects. The term used to refer to a substance which is foreign to the living system is 'xenobiotic'.

By their very nature, drugs are xenobiotics which alter biological processes, so the potential for harm is almost always present. The major consideration when prescribing drugs in medicine is to establish a dose that has an adequate therapeutic effect without unacceptable side effects. However, the present discussion does not concern itself with predetermined supervised medication; rather it deals with voluntary, unsupervised behaviour causing preventable disability in children. Biological responses to harmful xenobiotic chemicals include mutations, cancer, birth defects and effects on the immune system. Immunosuppression can cause the immune system to lose its ability to control infectious agents and neoplastic cells to give rise to cancerous tissue. Often the effects of xenobiotic exposure are subclinical in nature, but have profound long-term effects on ageing and reproductive function. Some pollutants, even at low doses, may adversely affect human physical growth. Common harmful xenobiotic materials in the environment are heavy metals such as lead and mercury, pesticides, plasticizers and many other industrial chemicals, drugs and pharmaceutical products.[2] Should there be no lasting harmful effect from

---

[2] For a discussion of the reproductive effects of industrial chemicals and pesticides of the group of dioxin-like compounds, including the polychlorinated biphenyls and dibenzofurans, see Chapter 13.

a particular toxic exposure, the effect is said to be reversible, while permanent effects are termed irreversible. Irreversible effects of toxic exposure remain after the substance is eliminated from the body.

High levels of air pollution are associated with reduced physical growth, both prenatal and postnatal, as well as with slowed skeletal development. Since air pollution is a heterogeneous entity, it is difficult to know which component of it contributes to growth impairment. Energy, such as noise and electromagnetic fields, may also be considered as pollutants. Since xenobiotic agents like commonly used drugs can, and do, cross the placental interface, they are particularly relevant in the study of developmental toxicology (Fig. 3.3; dark ellipses).

Teratogenesis, mutagenesis and carcinogenesis

Teratogens are reproductive toxicants that cause congenital malformations and usually lead to damage to embryonic or fetal cells. Teratology is, therefore, the branch of science which deals specifically with the causes, mechanisms, manifestations and prevention of congenital defects. Congenital malformations (more generally called birth defects) are usually thought of as structural or anatomical aberrations in neonatal and postnatal offspring. It is possible that interesting myths, like the one about the Greek one-eyed giant Cyclops, originated from observations of developmental anomalies, because the ancients were not ignorant about teratological matters. For example, the earliest written expressions and attempts to understand the significance of malformations in humans date back to the Babylonian era about 2000–1000 BCE. In the ancient world it was generally felt that malformations were manifestations of divine intervention and served as an omen. The words monster (from the Latin *monstrum*, meaning warning or ill omen) and teratology (from the Greek *teras*, meaning abnormal form, and *logos*, meaning the study of) were interpreted as 'to point out' or 'to show'.

Our ancestors believed that malformations were caused by noxious occurrences during pregnancy and warned of something deleterious occurring in the environment. Malformed children were, therefore, seen to be privileged in some way because they were 'chosen' to direct attention to something that needed correction. Jews and Christians, on the other hand, taught that the malformed child was God's punishment for a grave sin committed by the parents. This interpretation resulted in an ill-fated disinterest in the role of environmental factors in the aetiology of birth defects. It took the thalidomide tragedy of the late 1950s and early 1960s for the average modern physician to be convinced that not all congenital malformations have a genetic cause.

However, not until thalidomide was shown to be directly responsible for the birth of up to 10 000 infants deformed by absent limbs or flipper-like stumps was the drug removed from the market.

In reality the aetiology of human malformations includes both genetic and epigenetic factors, as well as a large category labelled unknown. For instance, the aetiology of 20–25% of human congenital abnormalities at birth is unknown because the majority of common disorders, such as heart disease, diabetes and cancer, are caused by a combination of genetic and epigenetic factors conveniently referred to as multifactorial or polygenetic inheritances. Behavioural genetic teratology entails an interaction among genes, teratogens and behaviour. Thus, the science of teratology embraces less obvious physiological, functional, immunological or behavioural defects. For example, a teratogen may broadly include any toxicant that induces structural malformations, metabolic or physiological dysfunction, or psychological/behavioural deficits in the offspring, either at birth or in any defined postnatal period.

It is common knowledge that the process of development starts in the ovaries and testes of the parents where the cells destined to become the future gametes are first differentiated as a distinct germ-line and, on fertilization, forge the generational link between parent and offspring. Mutagens, which act on genes by altering the DNA coding sequence in the differentiating oocyte or sperm, may induce inheritable traits. Put another way, mutations (that is, exchange, addition or deletion of molecules in sex cell DNA) may result in chromosomal anomalies, which in turn may alter vital processes (synthesis of an enzyme or hormone, for example), modifying the identity of the future conceptus. Such germ-cell mutations can, thereafter, be passed on to the progeny of subsequent generations. Mutations in the genes of an individual's body or somatic cell, on the other hand, are not passed on genetically to the offspring of future generations. Cancers, for instance, are caused by somatic gene mutations, but a genetic predisposition to cancer can be passed on to members of the next generation. The underlying mechanisms of carcinogenesis and mutagenesis are similar in that DNA damage in the sex cells may predispose the subsequent offspring to an increased risk of developing particular types of cancer or birth defects. Thus, mutagens which cause birth defects are also teratogens. Mutagenesis, teratogenesis and carcinogenesis are related phenomena of major toxicological concern.

Prepregnancy care is the physical and behavioural preparation for childbearing by both parents well before conception. The next two chapters integrate biological mechanisms initiated by social events, such as drug abuse or inappropriate sexual behaviour, effectual in the appearance of serious congenital abnormalities in the offspring.

Principles of bioscience ethics for discussion

- Do changing views about genes, teratogens and extragenomic modes of inheritance have any relevance to the study of bioethics? Rationalize your point of view.
- Behavioural, dietary and other adverse epigenetic effects on development might permanently impose a vulnerability to mental and physical illnesses in the offspring even to a second generation. Explain how heritable alterations in gene expression may occur in the absence of changes in DNA sequence.
- The genetic makeup of an individual is a crucial factor in the study of teratogenic outcome so it must be taken into account when formulating behavioural guidelines. Do you agree or disagree?

4

Substance abuse and parenthood: biological mechanisms – bioethical responsibilities

> My starting point is the intuition that caring is ethically important. Caring expresses ethically significant ways in which we matter to each other, transforming interpersonal relatedness into something beyond ontological necessity or brute survival.[1]

Prepregnancy care is the physical and behavioural preparation for childbearing by both parents well before conception. This and the next chapter integrate biological mechanisms initiated by social events, such as stressful life episodes, drug abuse or inappropriate sexual behaviour, resulting in the generation of serious congenital abnormalities in the offspring. The importance of increased biological understanding and bioethical awareness in reducing haphazard pregnancies is emphasized – when reproduction is considered a privilege, not a right, the chance of a good outcome is significantly elevated.

Introductory background

The aetiology of abnormal development is a combination of genetic and epigenetic factors, as well as a large category labelled unknown. A significant proportion of congenital malformations of unknown aetiology are polygenic or multifactorial in origin. The term 'multifactorial causation' is used when the combination of environmental insult(s) and a particularly susceptible genome in the conceptus is required for adverse effects to be apparent. Research identifying functional interactions between specific gene

---

[1] Bowden, P. (1997). *Caring: Gender-Sensitive Ethics.* London: Routledge, p. 1.

polymorphisms that contribute to genetic vulnerabilities is recent and falls within the new field of ecogenetics. Malformations with an increased recurrent risk such as cleft lip/palate, anencephaly (congenital absence of major portions of the brain), spina bifida, congenital heart disease, pyloric stenosis and congenital dislocation of the hip, fit the criteria for polygenic inherited or multifactorial diseases. Ecogenetics reinforces the urgent need to upgrade more vigorously social, economic and political responsibilities.

For practical purposes, the mechanisms of teratogenesis fall into two broad interrelated categories based on their aetiologies as follows:

- Errors in genetic programming derived from deviations in the genotype of the embryo
- Epigenetic or environmental factors, such as drugs, chemical pollutants, radiation, hyperthermia, infections, abnormal maternal metabolic states or mechanical aspects that interact with an embryo/fetus during the period of development

There are four recognized manifestations of disrupted development. These are malformation, growth retardation, embryo lethality and functional impairment, including neurobehavioural. Since stress, by its very definition, is a disturbance of the normal physiology, it is highly probable that stress is the common factor in the aetiology of many developmental defects in gametes, embryos and fetuses. In laboratory animals, the glucocorticoids – or stress hormones – are almost without exception potent teratogens. Since maternal stress is generally associated with an increase in blood glucocorticoids, a recurring malformation, such as cleft lip/palate for example, may be related to stressful life events. In humans, stress has a variety of causes and is manifested in many ways on the different target organs. Common stressful conditions that have been shown to cause disrupted development follow.

1. Age and germinal mutagenesis, which is the subject of Chapter 5.
2. Infection – maternal infections where some bacteria and viruses, in particular, can gain access to the fetal circulation and have severe consequences for the fetus. The rubella (German measles) virus is such an example. If the fetus is exposed to rubella during the first trimester of pregnancy, a variety of defects related to the central nervous system (CNS), including congenital cataracts, deafness and anomalies of the heart and brain, can be caused. Other important virus infections are HIV/AIDS, herpes simplex type II, measles, chicken pox and influenza viruses.

3. Hyperthermia – temperatures elevated a couple of degrees beyond the physiological level of 36.8 ± 0.7°C induce malformations in nearly all animal species (usually the offspring exhibit some type of neural tube malformation if exposed during the critical period for CNS development). Maternal hyperthermia, regardless of cause (sauna, exercise, fever), can be regarded as a confounding factor in the developmental toxicity of other kinds of agents (such as viruses or non-ionizing radiation).

4. Chronic non-infectious disease such as hypertension, diabetes mellitus, heart disease, chronic renal insufficiency and severe anaemias, include confounding factors that are caused by the use of pharmacological agents for treatment of the maternal disease state. Preeclampsia, for example, is an abnormal condition of pregnancy that affects 5–8% of all pregnancies and is characterized by the onset of acute hypertension during middle to late gestation. Complications include premature separation of the placenta, fetal malnutrition and lowered birthweight. Healthy living conditions, including a diet high in protein, calories and essential nutritional elements, rest and exercise are associated with a decreased incidence of preeclampsia.

5. Nutrition – deficiencies and excesses have been shown to be teratogenic. It is obvious that optimal fetal growth and development in utero depends on a steady supply of nutrients from the mother to the fetus. It is generally recognized that malnutrition can impair the function of the human reproductive processes. The effect is strongest and most evident during famine and starvation, when both fecundity and fertility are reduced significantly. The incidence of fetal malnutrition varies from approximately 3 to 10% of live births in developed societies. For example, zinc deficiency is implicated in lowered fertility (especially in males) and poor pregnancy outcome; endemic cretinism is caused by severe hypothyroidism in iodine-poor areas; and folate deficiency is implicated in gross malformations, particularly neural tube defects and orofacial clefts. Mild nutritional deficiency states may be equally as critical as severe malnutrition in producing adverse effects. These deficiencies may not cause physical abnormalities, but may challenge innate programming of developmental and metabolic parameters, with consequent functional deficits throughout the course of postnatal life. Should these deficits occur in the brain, they may have critical consequences where functional impairments result in behavioural aberrations or learning difficulties.

6. Environmental pollution, where we are involuntarily exposed to a bewildering array of chemicals in the home, occupationally and in the environment proper (Chapter 13).

7. Drug abuse; the remainder of this chapter deals with preventable drug-induced disability across the generations. It is expected that increased biological awareness will enhance reproductive responsibility geared toward safeguarding the wellbeing of children and grandchildren.

Behavioural variables – biological consequences

Abuse of substances by parents is an escalating public health problem. Preconceptional and prenatal exposure to legal/illegal chemicals has been clearly implicated in fetal and postnatal abnormalities. However, because of the multiple, interrelated health problems associated with a drug-abusing lifestyle, many developmental anomalies are still not well understood. That uncertainty persists is normal because a particular type of anomaly – cleft palate, for example – can be caused by diverse agents and mechanisms, and a particular pathogenesis can result in very different outcomes depending on factors such as dose, duration of exposure, embryonic/fetal age and genetic susceptibility. Polydrug use, poor parental health, lack of prenatal medical care and low socioeconomic status are foremost among confounding variables. For example, the interaction of cocaine and alcohol in utero results in a physiologically active compound – cocaethylene – with putative adverse, long-term effects on the offspring. There is also the added complication of silent neurotoxicity, where exposure to certain chemicals during brain development causes subtle morphological/biochemical changes that are not apparent until the individual grows, matures or is exposed to additional epigenetic challenges. The harmful effects of exposure to alcohol and tobacco during pregnancy have been well documented, while the effects of marijuana, opiates and cocaine have been established more recently. Exposure of eggs and sperm to drugs prior to fertilization is also deleterious but less well publicized.

The present review may disturb many readers but must be balanced against the duty of care. In all free societies citizens enjoy a right of informed consent; it follows, therefore, that potential parents have the right to access information – to be informed how best to balance risk/benefit equations when planning to have children. If specialists in toxicology and teratology fail to inform the public adequately, they would be irresponsible and failing in their duty of care. Professionals have a duty, not only to provide scholarship, but also to share information in a practical, non-judgemental way, so parents and society can work together in solving common social problems.

The preconceptional period: male-mediated effects

The extent to which fathers can transmit debilitating effects to their offspring needs to be publicized widely. This is because the majority of investigations into drug effects have involved female exposure before and during pregnancy, while male exposure has received only limited attention. There is, of course, no a-priori reason to believe that male genetic material is more resistant to cytotoxic insult than female genetic material, and the continuous production of sperm, from stem cell spermatogonia, heightens their sensitivity to environmental variables. Consequently, sperm cells are easy targets for chemical mutagens which may be present in the circulatory system. The realization that spermatogenesis can be readily disrupted during maturational processes important for normal fertility is now reflected in the rapidly growing scientific literature.

The impact on the conceptus following exposure of sperm to a developmental toxicant is usually assessed as an increase in pregnancy loss, malformations or alterations in growth. These effects may be a consequence of any one or a combination of factors such as mutated DNA sequence, changed chromatin packaging or epigenetic modification of DNA expression patterns that adversely impact on early embryonic development. The extent to which paternal exposure contributes to infertility and adverse progeny outcome is not known; however, since sperm cells are particularly vulnerable to genetic damage, birth defects in children appear to be more often linked with paternal than with maternal DNA damage. Therefore, heightened public health measures to inform potential fathers of known and suspected risks associated with drug-induced chromosomal damage are urgently required. Equally critical is the urgent need to familiarize the scientifically untrained with fundamental reproductive principles so that it can be clearly understood what responsible reproduction demands.

Specifics

Male reproductive function can be altered by chronic exposure to bioactive compounds capable of crossing the Sertoli cell barrier following systemic absorption. Components in tobacco smoke, alcoholic beverages, selected 'recreational' drugs and narcotics (including marijuana, cocaine, heroin/methadone, amphetamines and caffeine) have a detrimental effect on male reproductive hormones and on semen quality. It is well established that smoking is positively correlated with the frequency of abnormal sperm and inversely correlated with sperm density (number), motility and ability to fertilize ova successfully. Independent of parental age and social class, the frequency of severe malformations is doubled in children of non-smoking mothers whose partners smoke more than 10 cigarettes per day. Some childhood cancers are also significantly more common among children whose fathers smoked at the time of conception. A National Institute of Environmental Health study found that leukaemia and cancer of the lymph nodes were twice as common and brain cancer 40% more common among the children of men who had smoked in the year before their children were born. As expected, paternal smoking has also been associated with a significant, dose-dependent delivery of small-for-gestational age infants who, being born with low birthweight, also risk associated long-term health consequences.

The effects of cigarette smoking on the male reproductive system are many and are not necessarily caused by a single mutagenic component, but rather may be the combined effects of many chemicals, including nicotine, carbon monoxide and polycyclic aromatic hydrocarbons, to name just a few. Much of the damage done by smoking is caused by oxidizing compounds (free radicals) in cigarette smoke which are chemically reactive and damage DNA. In normal circumstances, enzymes repair most of the damage but when the total oxidation damage outstrips the body's natural repair mechanisms, sperm DNA is irreversibly altered.

The damaging effects of paternal drinking on the offspring have been documented by many epidemiological analyses. The relationship, as for nicotine, depends on alcohol-induced decreased quality of sperm and is related to its mutagenic properties. Acute and chronic alcoholism is associated with decreased synthesis of testosterone, testicular atrophy (shrinkage), decreased sperm number and motility, and increased appearance of abnormal sperm forms. One study found a 137-g reduction in birthweight among infants whose fathers drank regularly (average of two or more drinks daily or binge drinking) in the month before conception. The effect was independent of maternal alcohol or other drug use. This and similar studies help to emphasize the importance of including paternal drinking and drug-use habits in all research related to pregnancy outcomes, rather than concentrating exclusively on in-utero events.

Unlike cigarette and alcohol consumption, human data on the impacts of marijuana use on reproduction and development is more limited. This is despite the historic use of the chemical Δ-9-tetrahydrocannabinol or THC (the principal psychoactive component in marijuana) to bring on a 'high' through altered mood and perception. Chronic heavy marijuana use is associated with a significant decline in sperm concentration, motility and fertilizability, thereby jeopardizing fertility, and the children of dope-smoking fathers suffer an increased risk of being born with a low birthweight. The strong correlation between marijuana/cocaine use, alcohol consumption and cigarette smoking in men makes independent effects of marijuana/cocaine use on development difficult to decipher. There is also a strong correlation between mothers' and fathers' use of drugs, and it is unfortunate for the next generation that common detrimental lifestyle factors are often duplicated, with both parents placing genetic and epigenetic burdens on the development of their fetuses.

Cocaine abuse has increased dramatically since the mid 1980s, partly owing to the easy accessibility of a cheap, highly addictive, smokable form called 'crack'. As for most toxicants, cocaine decreases sperm count and motility, and increases the number of abnormal forms. Because cocaine binds specifically to sperm, embryopathy may also result from a combination of potentially damaged sperm transporting cocaine into the ovum at fertilization. Thus, drug-contaminated seminal fluid may represent another possible mechanism of paternally mediated teratogenesis.

A relationship between paternal caffeine exposure and adverse pregnancy outcome has long been known. Caffeine is not teratogenic in the range of human consumption, but chemical stresses are cumulative and a synergistic effect of caffeine consumption, cigarette smoking and alcohol intake on semen quality has been demonstrated. The combination of smoking and drinking more than four cups of coffee a day significantly decreases sperm motility, reduces sperm density and increases the percentage of dead sperm. Importantly, genetic and epigenetic influences have profound lasting effects on progeny outcome and either drug-exposed parent can influence pregnancy loss, alterations in growth, malformations and overall wellbeing that ultimately identified the conceptus, newborn infant and adult.

The preconceptional period: female-mediated effects

Few studies have provided direct evidence between preconceptional maternal drug exposure and the long-term health prospects of the subsequent child. While it is evident that adverse preconceptional effects differ in fundamental respects from those documented for prenatal (in utero) drug exposure, practically speaking, it is extremely difficult to distinguish preconceptional from prenatal effects in women. A dose-dependent caffeine effect on fertility has been established, and delayed conception and infertility associated with heavy smoking is not a new concept. However, the good news for women who quit before conception is that their fertility appears no different from that of non-smokers, and ex-smokers' pregnancies seem to be as successful as those of non-smokers.

Due to nicotine's addictive qualities, maternal smoking prior to pregnancy is correlated with maternal smoking during pregnancy, though women tend to decrease their smoking during the first trimester. However, drug-dependent human fertility studies, typically, do not differentiate between preconceptional and prenatal drug intake. Therefore, such epidemiological studies cannot reveal whether drug-induced subfecundity (defined as prolonged time to conception) is the result of anovulatory menstrual cycles, faulty fertilizations, an increased incidence of unrecognized spontaneous losses of preimplantation defective pregnancies and/or a combination of all of these. For these reasons, animal-based studies provide a deeper appreciation of the significance of female drugs exposure preconceptionally and during post-conceptional development. Such experiments have demonstrated that drugs administered prior to fertilization can seriously affect the subsequent development of the embryo. By highlighting the preconceptional period as being vulnerable to the effects of drugs, this should provide a strong rationale for parents to limit their drug consumption when planning to have a child.

Drug-induced infertility

Assisted reproductive technology (ART) has become the standard of care for the treatment of many types of infertility. About one-third of all patients referred for fertility treatment have a significant history of drug exposure, reinforcing the view that drug exposure is an important consideration in all at-risk groups. Since the medical professions' social requirement is to treat infertility, ART is considered as a potential solution for most infertility problems regardless of aetiology, including self-inflicted infertility. ART has certainly offered hope to those whose fertility has been compromised by the excessive use of recreational drugs, although the technology itself may, in some cases, further compromise the reproductive outcome. The uses of more invasive technologies for treating severe male-mediated infertility (sperm micromanipulation or assisted fertilization) are being increasingly employed, but their long-term effects on the offspring are unknown. According to the Australian Institute of Health and Welfare's 2002 National Perinatal Statistics Unit, ART babies now account for nearly 3% of all babies born in Australia, and this figure is in agreement with global trends. Running parallel with expanding fertility treatment options, attention has turned to the potential risks of these procedures on the offspring's long-term health prospects.

Evidence is emerging which suggests that some ARTs are associated with low birthweight, preterm birth, increased risk of certain kinds of congenital malformations, and rare imprinting disorders such as Beckwith–Wiedemann syndrome and Angelman syndrome, when compared with the expected frequency in the general population. Worrying statistics have been confirmed from many sources, but long-term follow-up studies are needed. More reassuring, however, are other studies which find no deleterious long-term effects of reproductive technologies when a child was conceived by donor insemination, in vitro fertilization (IVF), or gamete intrafallopian transfer (GIFT). Poor IVF prognosis in the offspring may well be a contributing factor in a subpopulation suffering from drug-induced infertility rather than the infertile population at large. To this end, a precautionary approach would be to assist pregnancy with the least invasive technology possible. It is undeniable that great progress has been made since Louise Brown, the world's first IVF baby, was born in 1978, and now the possibility of a wider spectrum of ART-related complications needs to be recognized. (Chapter 9 provides a detailed description of the various ARTs.)

The prenatal and neonatal periods

Scientific evidence substantiating the teratogenic potential of mind-altering drugs (especially alcohol, opiates, nicotine, marijuana and cocaine) is steadily accumulating. These drugs of abuse cause growth abnormalities, physical malformations and neurobehavioural effects in children. However, as already pointed out, the association between drug consumption during pregnancy and increased risk of any single congenital abnormality in the offspring cannot be assessed accurately. This is due to the heterogeneity of the risk factors and of the innate genetic strengths or weaknesses of the drug-exposed fetus. Given that many drug-generated disabilities are not treatable, education ensuring that children maintain, as far as possible, their full genetic potential in order to maximize their quality-of-life capabilities, is overriding. Importantly, prevention rests on early drug awareness education so that potential parents can make socially responsible decisions to protect the health of their children. Drug addiction is not only destroying individual lives but also overburdening obstetric and paediatric facilities, adding to the ever-mounting cost of health care. These effects ripple onwards as drug-affected children with special needs grow up and enter the educational system.

Nicotine

Cigarette smoking has emerged as the single most important preventable cause of poor health, disease and death in the industrialized world. Fortunately, people are increasingly aware of the dangers to the adult of tobacco use and the associated adverse outcomes of reproductive function. It has been estimated that smoking is responsible for 20–35% of all low birthweights, and a decrease in perinatal mortality of 10% could be expected if all women stopped smoking during pregnancy. It is important to understand that low birthweight (2500 g or less) is associated with infant mortality, with most deaths occurring in the neonatal period. Women who smoke cigarettes during pregnancy deliver babies weighing 200 g less, on average, than babies of non-smokers. This finding has been confirmed in numerous well-designed studies conducted in many countries. The frequency of low birthweight is approximately doubled among smokers. Women who stop smoking before conception have babies similar in average size and risk of low birthweight to non-smokers. The effect of stopping smoking after conception depends on when cessation occurred and on how much was smoked.

The biological causes of smoking-associated growth retardation are several, with direct and indirect biological effects implicated. Direct biological effects are unavoidable because tobacco smoke contains thousands of deleterious compounds, with carbon monoxide being a primary constituent. Cigarette smoking provides a physiological dose of nicotine; one puff of a cigarette equals the exposure of approximately an intravenous injection of 0.1 mg of nicotine. Nicotine stimulates the release from the adrenal glands of stress hormones such as adrenaline (epinephrine) and cortisol, both of which reduce uteroplacental blood flow because of constriction of blood vessels. Since nicotine freely crosses the placenta and equilibrates rapidly between the mother and the fetus, it also acts directly to increase fetal blood pressure and respiratory rate. Growth-inhibiting poisons such as cyanide, lead and cadmium are found in cigarette smoke. Smoking may also affect fetal growth indirectly by damaging the placenta or by causing a smoking-induced reduction in maternal appetite, lowering her food intake and weight gain during pregnancy.

In addition to low birthweight, maternal tobacco use has been strongly implicated in other adverse outcomes of reproductive function. Specific abnormalities, or birth defects, noted in the offspring born to smoking mothers are cardiovascular, urogenital, microcephalus (small head size), neural tube defect, cleft lip/palate and finger/toe deformities. A correlation between the number of cigarettes smoked during pregnancy and cancer risk in the child is statistically established; smoking doubles the risk of non-Hodgkin's lymphoma, acute lymphoblastic leukaemia and Wilm's tumour. In 1998, scientists first identified a potent cancer-causing substance (4-methylnitrosamino-1-(3-pyridyl)-1-butanone) from tobacco in newborn infants' urine, conclusively demonstrating that the fetus absorbs carcinogens. More recently, genetic analyses of fetal cells obtained from amniocentesis have identified that smoking during pregnancy damages chromosomes, especially at the break-point localities in the fetal genome containing a number of leukaemia genes. Negative effects of smoking on various aspects of intellectual development have long been known. For example, a significant causal link exists between disruptive behavioural disorders in toddlers of mothers who smoked during pregnancy compared to non-exposed infants. Whether the antisocial behaviour is symptomatic of attention-deficit hyperactivity disorder (ADHD), also associated with maternal smoking, is not clear. The extent of the damage done – as calculated by the average antisocial behaviour and ADHD scores – is directly proportional to the number of cigarettes smoked.

Sudden infant death syndrome (SIDS)

The deleterious effects of smoking also extend into the neonatal period because it significantly influences lactation. Epidemiological studies have established reduced milk production with lower fat concentration in smoking mothers, which strongly correlated with decreased weight gain in the suckled babies. For these unfortunate babies, the nicotine-contaminated, nutritive-deficient breast milk continues the stunting effect already commenced in utero and may explain the documented relationship between smoking during pregnancy and sudden infant death syndrome (SIDS). The risk of SIDS also increases with increasing numbers of cigarette smokers surrounding the already growth-restricted infant.

Strong postnatal breathing activity in the neonate is closely related to the degree of functional maturation of the brain's neuronal mechanisms regulating the respiratory system. A term infant can quickly establish the necessary respiratory pattern changes required for extrauterine life. However, when fetal growth is inadequate, the immaturity of the infant's respiratory system may result in recurrent episodes of apnea (cessation of breathing) and chronic hypoxia (oxygen deprivation). SIDS is defined as 'the sudden death of any infant or young child which is unexplained by history and in which thorough post-mortem examination fails to demonstrate an adequate cause for death'. Typically, however, infants at risk of SIDS may carry functional aberrations not readily identifiable by post-mortem examinations.

Biblical references exist, indicating SIDS awareness since antiquity, but despite this awareness, there have been many misconceptions about the causes and associated risk factors. The incidence of SIDS in western countries is between 1 and 4 per 1000 live births, and the highest risk is in boys between the ages of 2 and 4 months; overall, it is the single most common cause of death in infants less than 12 months old. Recent research has identified several factors which put infants at a higher risk of death from SIDS, ranging from genetic predisposition to environmental, social and socioeconomic factors. Environmental factors include those to which the fetus is exposed during pregnancy, as well as those that are introduced postnatally.

Passive smoking

Exposure to tobacco smoke significantly increases the incidence of SIDS, with the risk being proportional to the extent of passive smoking. The fact that smoking and other addictive drugs are often responsible for prenatal growth restriction, and that SIDS is more common in low birthweight infants, provides a unifying lifestyle correlation. Other effects of passive smoking are also well documented; children whose parents smoke suffer more upper and lower respiratory tract diseases than children whose parents do not smoke and, as with adult non-smokers living in the company of smokers, exhibit an increased risk of both fatal and non-fatal cardiac events and cancer of the lungs. Other studies have confirmed that passive smoking is equally damaging to a woman's fertility as smoking first hand. Further, pregnant women exposed to others' cigarette smoke are also more likely to deliver a low birthweight infant, reinforcing the precarious nature of the period spanning prenatal and postnatal life.

Attention-deficit hyperactivity disorder (ADHD)

Maternal smoking during pregnancy has been identified as a risk factor for attention-deficit hyperactivity disorder (ADHD) in children. ADHD is the latest term designating a chronic disorder that begins early in childhood and is manifested by problems of awareness, difficulty with attention, excessive motor activity (hyperactivity) and poor impulse control (impulsiveness). It is among the most common causes of behavioural disturbances, estimated to affect 3–5% of school-age children, with the highest risk in boys.

Symptoms associated with ADHD (although not called this at the time) were first described in 1902 by British paediatrician George Still. Still, correctly, suggested that behaviours he had observed amongst certain children in his practice were not caused by bad parenting but by a subtle unidentified brain injury. Recent evidence points to a brain-based biological disorder where a possible genetic predisposition is activated by stressful environmental factors. Environmental factors such as hypoxia, prenatal, perinatal and postnatal trauma have been implicated, as has exposure to toxic substances such as alcohol, cocaine, nicotine, marijuana and lead. Individuals with ADHD have lower than normal levels of selected neurotransmitters, dopamine in particular, which means that the brain will metabolize more slowly. Neurotransmitters are chemical messengers relaying information between neurons, and dopaminergic neurotransmission is highly sensitive to fetal/neonatal circulatory insufficiency and is thought to underlie the chemical pathology of ADHD. This concept is reinforced by the qualified success of stimulation therapy in children with ADHD. Drugs such as ritalin, for example, act by stimulating the CNS and increase the amount of dopamine available to the brain. There are side effects associated with this treatment, however, including growth retardation, insomnia, decreased appetite and nervous spasms. Therefore, medicating young people is controversial, especially in the absence of evidence that treatment may risk long-term expression of more severe mood disorders. Nevertheless, comprehensive drug and behavioural therapies are recognized as being an effective way to treat this disorder, with the general consensus being that side effects are minimal when compared with the positive results obtained.

Ethanol (alcohol)

The problem of alcohol abuse in present-day society has reached alarming proportions. Inappropriately managed alcohol consumption places a heavy burden on society; immediately obvious are productivity losses, traffic deaths and morbidity, violent crime and alcohol-related illnesses. Less obvious are the reproductive burdens associated with alcohol consumption, which may be of even greater magnitude because excessive drinking among men and women rarely renders them incapable of conceiving. Alcohol is a potent teratogen that impairs fetal growth and development in a number of ways. For example, maternal liver disease increases the time taken for alcohol and other toxicants to be detoxified and eliminated from the body. The resulting increased concentration of toxic metabolites in the circulation is an additional burden for the fetus, whose immature liver is unable to metabolize these substances. There are several critical periods during pregnancy when the fetus is particularly susceptible to alcoholic insult. Animal research suggests that consumption of a large quantity of alcohol at one time (binge drinking) is more detrimental than the regular intake of a drink/day. However, it is also argued that since no safe level of alcohol intake has been established, women should abstain completely from drinking whilst attempting to conceive, as well as during pregnancy.

Alcohol-induced effects, in addition to those on the CNS, are not unlike those described for nicotine, and include reduced fertility, miscarriage, fetal growth retardation and developmental defects linked to immune deficits, and increased frequencies of malignancies. Alcohol's most profound effect, however, is exercised on the developing CNS during the fetal period.

Fetal alcohol syndrome (FAS)

Fetal alcohol syndrome (FAS) describes a variety of features common to babies born to mothers who were alcohol abusers and/or who drank heavily during pregnancy. Fetal alcohol spectrum disorders (FASDs), including FAS, depend on the maternal and fetal genotypes interacting with ethanol to produce significant damage in some fetuses and not so obvious effects in others. Stated simply, the range of responses to developmental toxicants such as alcohol is caused by differences in inherent susceptibility of the conceptus and/ or differences in maternal physiology and drug pharmacokinetics, including biotransformation and disposition kinetics.

The teratogenic effects of FAS include, but are not confined to, prenatal and postnatal growth deficiencies, microcephaly, distinct FAS facial features, cardiac defects, limb deformities, while genitourinary and musculoskeletal abnormalities may also be present. Common behavioural effects are ADHD, learning difficulties, delays in psychomotor and language development, poor visual memory and psychosocial maladjustment. Of all the characteristics of FAS, intellectual disability is the most damaging and consistent consequence; it is now the leading non-genetic cause of mental disability in the western world. This preventable deformation of an infant's genetic potential continues despite the fact that the detrimental consequences of alcohol consumption during pregnancy have been known for centuries. Aristotle warned that 'women drunkards' often gave birth to abnormal children and the consumption of alcoholic beverages by young married couples was prohibited in ancient Greek and Old Testament writings. A depressing aspect is that nothing was done systematically about understanding and publicizing the syndrome until 1968 when Lemoine and colleagues in France attributed a pattern, now termed fetal alcohol syndrome, of morphological and developmental effects in

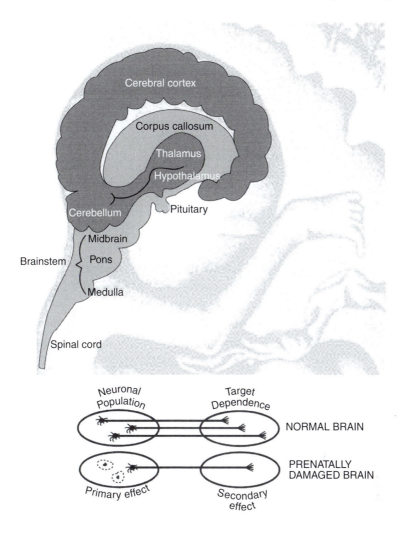

Figure 4.1 Lateral view of the structurally complete fetal brain at the third trimester, a period when the brain undergoes rapid neurological organization and differentiation, especially of the cerebral cortex. Behavioural competence continues to increase, forming a continuum from prenatal to postnatal life. Many CNS-targeting teratogens exert their toxic effects by initially killing dividing cells – the primary or direct effect – resulting in reduced neuronal populations in the mature brain. The loss of primary neuronal numbers may give rise, during postnatal life, to a cascade of secondary effects, with reduced competency in a variety of target systems.

children to alcoholism and alcohol abuse. The average IQ of the FAS children is about 70, with the severity of mental retardation being related to the degree of alcohol exposure in utero.

As described in Chapter 3, human brain development is exceptional and multiphasic, and there is not one but many critical periods during which neuroteratogens can exert their deleterious effects. Brain-targeting teratogens, like alcohol, cause primary damage during prenatal life; this can be amplified by a cascade of secondary effects after birth (Fig. 4.1). Neurotoxic exposure of multiplying neuronal cell populations during the structural phase of brain development can result in localized lesions. The primary consequence is microcephaly or a permanent reduction in the total number of cells present in the mature brain. In postnatal life, further brain damage continues during the phase of neurological organization. Primary reduction of nerve cell density correspondingly reduces the normal network of possible synaptic transmissions connecting other target-dependent areas of the brain. Further, abnormal neurotransmitter concentration at synaptic transmission sites can initiate a cascade of secondary effects. In ADHD, for example, sub-threshold dopamine levels are responsible for a cascade of multiple, heterogeneous secondary effects in fine-tuning of functions scattered throughout the cerebral cortex. Thus, as a result of primary prenatal growth restriction, a self-reinforcing cycle of secondary injury is initiated in one or more target-dependent systems controlling cognition, behaviour, somatic sensation, vision and movement, in children originally genetically robust but drug damaged. Of course, parents have, since time immemorial, randomly genetically engineered their own kids through preventable congenital disorders. The 'dice syndrome' describes the random exposure of any individual to unsuspected disturbing influences of environmental origin. Exposure of the fetus to drugs and its resulting damage may well be considered to be an example of the random fall of the parental dice.

Other factors which frequently accompany alcoholism may contribute to FAS; in particular, multiple or polydrug abuse which usually includes cigarettes, marijuana and cocaine reinforced by poor nutrition. Postnatal growth and neuroanatomical development is also adversely affected by exposure to alcohol-contaminated breast milk. Growth deficiency continues over the period of breastfeeding owing to a combination of nutritional deficit and toxic drug effects.

Cocaine

According to recent surveys, the age group most likely to abuse cocaine is the 20–25-year-old group, with women cocaine users having an average age of 25 years, coinciding with peak reproductive years. Prenatal cocaine is associated with a variety of obstetric complications. These include increased incidence of spontaneous abortion, intrauterine growth retardation (IUGR), placental abruption, stillbirths, premature birth and precipitous labour. Infants exposed to cocaine prenatally are at increased risk for a number of problems, including retarded physical growth, significant cognitive deficits and other neuropsychological abnormalities (cocaine exerts a vasoconstrictive effect on fetal vasculature, decreasing fetal cerebral blood flow and risking oxygen depletion), withdrawal symptoms, cardiorespiratory anomalies and increased incidence of SIDS. Cocaine babies suffer particularly severe drug withdrawal symptoms that include tremulousness, irritability, jitteriness, high-pitched cry, vomiting, abnormal sleep pattern and convulsions. Some long-term neurobehavioural problems include ADHD, short attention span, short-term memory loss, abnormal motor performance and play patterns, uniformly flat, apathetic moods and discomfort in new situations.

Since the 1980s, the United States has witnessed an acute crack cocaine epidemic that has disproportionately compromised the section of the population which is of reproductive age, and consequently has placed at risk a sizable cohort of cocaine-exposed infants who are more likely to experience adverse birth and growth complications, and whose long-term physical and cognitive health prognoses remain undetermined. With alcohol and heroin addiction, the maternal instinct does often overpower the drug craving, enabling these women to remain clean throughout pregnancy. This is less the case with crack – cocaine's cheap and highly addictive derivative, where the women are more likely to continue their abuse throughout pregnancy. A confounding effect of maternal cocaine use is that the drug is not only associated with, but may even advance, the abuse of other drugs. Cocaine withdrawal is associated with a number of unpleasant side effects (agitation, unhappiness, paranoia), so users may take other drugs to reduce these discomforts. Limited availability of data makes it difficult to ascertain the effects of numerous other street drugs used singly or in combination; consequently, the neurological damage of low-dose exposure to drugs such as cocaine, alcohol and nicotine might be of considerably greater concern as drug effects are typically synergistic, rather than additive.

Marijuana

After alcohol and tobacco, marijuana (or cannabis) is the most popular psychoactive substance used during pregnancy. Studies of the consequences of prenatal marijuana use have reported effects predominantly on the behavioural and cognitive development of the children. Prenatal marijuana exposure is associated with impaired executive functions that require impulse control, visual mapping and analysis/hypothesis testing. Specifically, prenatal marijuana exposure in the first and third trimesters significantly increases hyperactivity, inattention and impulsivity symptoms in affected children, which might explain increased behavioural problems and delinquency. A more recent epidemiological study using functional magnetic resonance imaging (fMRI) established long-lasting damage resulting from in utero exposure to marijuana. Some studies have reported a correlation between marijuana use during pregnancy and smaller infant size at birth; others, however, have claimed that gestational marijuana exposure causes differential effects on neonatal body proportionality, such that body fat is unaffected, while arm circumference measures indicate significant decreases in lean body mass. A relationship between regular maternal dope smoking and fetal cannabis syndrome, which resembles fetal alcohol syndrome, has also been reported.

Narcotics

The terms opiate and opioid refer to a group of natural and synthetic narcotic, analgesic substances with morphine-like effects. Methadone was first synthesized in the 1940s and was widely used in the treatment of heroin addiction by the late 1960s. Opiate-exposed infants show high rates of IUGR, preterm delivery and several neonatal withdrawal symptoms. Among the reported neonatal problems associated with narcotic substance abuse in pregnancy are changes in sleeping breathing patterns and an increased incidence of SIDS. There are no documented structural anomalies in exposed offspring, in spite of concerns over chromosomal damage. Other measures of growth deficiency, including head circumference and postnatal growth, have not been conclusively linked to opiate use during pregnancy; however, long-term studies have found that prenatal exposure to heroin could result in alterations of physiological patterning, behaviour, developmental lags and learning impairment.

The substitution of methadone for heroin is of particular concern as the reproductive outcome for those infants born to women in methadone maintenance programmes is no better than following heroin addiction. The risk of postnatal environmental injury added to prenatal biological insult appears to be particularly acute for low birthweight or preterm infants who have been exposed to narcotics in utero.

Caffeine

Caffeine, a trimethylxanthine alkaloid, is the most widely consumed psychophysiologically active substance in the world. It is readily available in coffee, tea, some cola beverages, cocoa, chocolate, as well as preservatives, analgesics and other pharmaceutical preparations. The drug's popularity is also reflected in the number of children consuming caffeine-containing substances. Caffeine is a powerful CNS stimulant and, because of its structural similarity to DNA, it may interact chemically with DNA within the rapidly dividing embryonic and fetal cells. This characteristic may explain why caffeine has a variety of teratogenic effects even at a moderate level of intake. Women drinking the equivalent of three or more cups of brewed coffee per day during the first trimester have an increased risk of miscarriage, and caffeine consumption prior to and during pregnancy is associated with prematurity, fetal IUGR and neonatal withdrawal symptoms after delivery. Neonatal withdrawal symptoms are a result of the drug's addictive properties and may also be a potentiating factor in neonatal apnea and SIDS. Because caffeine has not been studied as extensively as nicotine or ethanol, the drug's effects on human development are not fully known. It is clear, however, that caffeine is a strong potentiator of adverse reproductive effects when co-administered with other drugs and exacerbates the toxic effects of nicotine and ethanol.

Behavioural variables – bioethical challenges

The previous sections have reviewed adverse alterations in reproductive potential associated with exposure to a number of widely consumed recreational drugs. Since, by their very nature, drugs are xenobiotics which alter biological processes, the potential for harm is almost always present. It follows, therefore, that if we are to engage proactively in bioethical discourse effective in generating a relevant behavioural response, bioscience ethics has to guarantee an availability of suitable scientific understanding. By being forewarned, we may now confront the bioethical challenge and participate in the prevention of known risks to children associated with certain lifestyles. Successful interruption of the drug-propagated cycle of transgenerational ill health requires major social and personal intervention. The realization that significant biological aspects of adult health are laid down well before birth has set a new agenda for urgent action into the common social causes of preventable disability.

Socioeconomic factors

It is a matter of pride that the neonatal mortality rate in affluent societies has dropped substantially since the late 1970s. The Australian national average is typical for western societies; about 7% of babies are born with low birthweight and about 4% with some form of congenital abnormality visible at birth. The risk of major malformation is increased to 8–9% when delayed developmental abnormalities such as mental disability, behavioural anomalies and childhood cancers in the post-neonatal period are included. These burdens are not, however, evenly distributed among the population as there are social and demographic differences in infant mortality and morbidity, with exceptionally high reproductive dysfunction being associated with poor living conditions.

Biosocial interactions between physical growth and maturation in children and socioeconomic status have long been appreciated and formally documented. Put another way, the socioeconomic class of children, youth and adults powerfully influences body stature and composition (fatness, muscularity), and rate of emotional development. In late- eighteenth- century Europe it was shown that sons of the nobility were, on average, taller than sons of bourgeois families, while in the United States, measurements of 24 500 schoolchildren from the Boston area revealed that children of working class parents were significantly smaller in height and weight than the children from non-labouring upper middle classes. What is important here is the realization that the standard of living or the economic wellbeing of individuals and families can be considered to be a proxy for more direct influences on growth, such as nutrition, health care, physical labour and psychological stimulation among children.

More recently, interest has focused on the origin and development of lifestyle diseases according to race as a social, not biological, construct. Overall, significant relationships exist between ethnicity/race and failing health and, conversely, health-promoting behaviour is inversely associated with self-reported racism. It is patently obvious that, if we are to address the combination of risks attributable to persistent developmental problems and socioeconomic disadvantage, experiences from preconception to birth through to adulthood have to be taken into account. The following specifics relate to the indigenous peoples of contemporary Australia but at the same time also expose its universality.

Many Indigenous Australians experience levels of disadvantage and ill health akin to the poorest nations on Earth. Entrenched poverty, welfare dependence, social breakdown and unacceptably high rates of morbidity and mortality are reflected in intergenerational disparities in socioeconomic wellbeing, lifestyle and access to health and other services. The current reprehensible situation is not only consequent on past inequities but also on present marginalization and neglect. Since European arrival, Aboriginals have been systematically dispossessed of their land, separated from their children and disconnected from their culture, all of which has had dramatic impacts on Indigenous health, wellbeing and reproductive resilience.

From the Australian Bureau of Statistics (www.abs.gov.au) we can access the following figures. Fifteen per cent of households with Indigenous person(s) are considered overcrowded, requiring at least one extra bedroom, compared to 4% of other households. The level of infant mortality in the Indigenous population is three times the national average. Babies weighing less than 2500 g at birth are classified as being of low birthweight; in 2001, babies of Indigenous mothers were twice as likely to be of low birthweight (13% of births) than babies of non-Indigenous mothers (6%). Aboriginal children under the age of 2 years are 80 times more likely to suffer from diseases such as pneumonia, septicaemia and meningitis than non-Indigenous children, while the risk of dying from SIDS in Aboriginal infants living in outback Australia is nearly four times that of non-Aboriginal infants. In early-to-middle age, diseases of adaptation such as ischaemic heart disease, hypertension, diabetes and depression (legacies of intrauterine and postnatal deprivation) have disturbingly higher prevalence among Australian Indigenous people when compared to the rest of the population. In the United States of America, socioenvironmental factors are similarly responsible for the significantly higher than average prevalence of low birthweight and birth defects among offspring born to black women younger than 35 years of age.

Many of the persistent health problems within the Aboriginal communities relate to alcoholism, other drug dependencies, and depression. The Australian population, like many western societies, most commonly uses and abuses legal drugs, particularly alcohol and tobacco; these drugs are associated with more chronic illness, disease, accidents, social problems, unemployment and days off work than all other drugs together. Aboriginal Australians also mainly use legally obtainable substances: alcohol, tobacco, analgesics, solvents and kava, although illegal drug abuse among urban Aboriginals has also been reported. In remote bush communities, availability narrows the range of substances used; however, alcohol, tobacco, inhalants (particularly petrol), kava and methylated spirits are regularly available.

It is no surprise, given existing conditions, that the average life expectancy for Aboriginals is 15–20 years below that of the general population. A comparative perspective shows that a person from Nigeria or Bangladesh can expect to live about 10 years longer than an Indigenous Australian, or that a present-day Indigenous person has about the same life expectancy at birth as the whole Australian population had in the early 1920s. Deaths from external causes such as accidents, suicide, homicide and assault account for one in every six registered Indigenous deaths and this astonishingly high rate is considered a conservative estimate because of substantial under-identification. Scandalously, suicide is 2–3 times more common among the Aboriginal and Torres Strait Islander peoples and 5–6 times more prevalent among Indigenous youths compared to non-Indigenous youths. Although Indigenous people constitute only 2% of Australia's population, they account for 20% of the prison population. It is not uncommon for young offenders to move through the depressing cycle from juvenile correctional services to imprisonment only to re-offend on release. The Royal Commission's recommendations into 'Black deaths in custody' have helped to reduce suicide rates of Aboriginals under arrest; however, the striking imbalance of incarceration remains unchanged.

Indigenous peoples all over the industrialized world receive worse treatment for services, are considered ignorant, and are patronizingly told what they are doing wrong rather than being consulted about what needs improvement and ways of achieving these improvements. Thus, economic, political and cultural systems act to differentially allocate the benefits and risks for growth between socioeconomic groups. Epidemiologists refer to this process as 'risk-focusing'. Surely in affluent societies such as Australia and the United States, justice should insist that all children have an equal share in the environmental opportunities for growth and development.

Parental drug abuse resulting in a compromised offspring is definitely not consistent with respect for human life, but discrimination has social implications extending far beyond the welfare of the poor. The view that it is a moral crime (against the unfortunate offspring as well as against society) to bring a child into existence without fair prospects needs to be widely publicized. However, instead of confronting the 'child abusers' (often themselves victims), official attention has to be focused on correcting the root problems responsible for the generations of compromised children. A supportive society can nurture respect and concomitant behavioural change by removing the major causes of grief and providing a model for the younger generations. These younger generations, in their turn, would then naturally accept that respect for their unborn is their foremost responsibility, which can be gained by healthy biological behaviour. Parents would value the concept that a fundamental right of their children is the expression of a full genetic potential free from preventable harm; a win-win situation in which 'damage control' care is secondary to preventative measures. Sickness-driven medicine is costly and will not improve overall health standards.

There have, however, been many encouraging developments. These have coincided with changed popular sensitivities and political thinking, and have led to considerable advances in Indigenous health and pregnancy education. Training in culture-specific health care has been particularly helpful. Culture-specific health care is where traditional medicine is acknowledged as a complementary and fundamental part of health care. Teaching of traditional knowledge alongside western insights is now a routine procedure in the training of Aboriginal health and community workers at all Australian tertiary institutions. Another valuable development has been culture-specific trialling programmes called the 'circle court' alternative means of sentencing. The circle court, designed for serious repeat offenders, is a court overseen by a magistrate but supervised by community elders, and aims at involving the whole community in the sentencing and rehabilitation processes. The aim of the court is twofold: to set a sentence plan for the offender and to address the underlying causes for the offence. The facts of the case are presented to the circle by the crown, followed by the defence, after which the whole circle is opened up for a comprehensive discussion. Importantly, the offender must also address the circle, perhaps after a statement by the victim about the impact of the crime is made. The bringing of offender and victim face-to-face has several beneficial effects, not least increasing the programme's success rate. The circle then examines what must be done to help the victim and the offender and, more broadly, underlying issues in the community that are causing serious problems and ways of addressing them. At the end of these deliberations, bail conditions are set for the offender such as curfew, work programmes, abstention from alcohol, cognitive behavioural therapy, anger management and any other penalty deemed appropriate, not excluding imprisonment. The immediate good news is that circle sentencing has slashed recidivism rates in all locations since the scheme was first introduced in 2002. The strength of the circle court is the close kinship between the elders and the accused where the circle is built on trust and respect. Within the circle context it is understood that to break the law you break the law of the traditional owners of the land as well as the Australian court. The excellent outcome reinforces the fact that the crime rate is not contingent on ethnicity but on socioeconomic disadvantage and lack of control in one's life. Lasting transgenerational change has to be forged out of the entire life–death and renewal cycle, not from short-term fixes.

An ecologically based model of preventative care – government and citizens in equal partnership

The differential allocation of risks and benefits for growth between differing socioeconomic groups is central to addressing transgenerational equity issues. We know that children who have experienced a good prenatal environment and were well nurtured in their early years have better outcomes throughout their lives. They do better in school, have higher self-esteem, fewer social, health and behavioural problems, and are less likely to become teenage parents, abuse drugs or be involved in crime. We also know that lack of control over one's life engages harmful dynamics symptomatic of marginalization, alienation, resentment, depression and environmental deterioration, and that these harmful dynamics are self-perpetuating across generations. Persistent powerlessness in marginalized populations is a shameful consequence of the failure of political, religious, health and legal institutions to bridge the gap between knowledge and effective action. Many lines of research have made the connection between unwanted births and the offspring's greater than expected risk of criminality, and that domestic violence and abuse is a strong motivation among women seeking an abortion.

Given scientific acumen and good will, it is possible to choose to prevent, postpone or skilfully control the worst consequences of poverty, depression, child neglect and drug dependence. The uneven distribution of common bio-logical rights has serious psychological, social and economic implications for nations as a whole. We have the scientific evidence – what is required is the emotional intelligence to understand social and ecological systems compassionately. It is time to translate biological imperatives into ethical action and demand individual and collective commitment in eradicating the worst consequences of poverty. Public acceptance that health begins well before conception and that each of us is custodian of the next and subsequent generations would be a good start in the development of effective bioscience-bioethics education programmes. Given a just standard of living, preconceptional care should significantly reduce the social and health risks to future generations of children. Governments must give special attention to the education of young people so that they can exercise a responsible attitude to themselves and their children. It is imperative that we as a nation develop a practical and satisfactory scientific framework activating the acceptance of reproduction as a privilege, rather than a right, a right which is all too often trivialized.

Importantly, the allocation of health and educational resources should be on the basis of need, and disadvantaged minority groups, whether Indigenous or other, must be involved in designing and implementing the solutions. Muting the Indigenous voice is counterproductive, since self-reliance is the key to good health and wellbeing (Chapter 7). All societies provide special rights to specific groups to ensure equal outcomes for all. That is why we have wheelchair access and designated parking for disabled people and diesel fuel subsidies for farmers. Health and living standards of neglected peoples around the world are in need of special measures that require addressing the underlying causes of severe deprivation. In order to tackle inequality there must be a 'fair go' for all. Reconciliation is possible only when people make it their concern and actively work for it. In particular, biomedical issues concerning health and wellbeing of parents and children need to be addressed, and provision of health and health education expanded for all.

The emotional brain and the biology of addiction

The emotional, or limbic, brain is central to working memory, depression and also serves as the prime target for consciousness-changing/mood-altering substances. From Figure 4.2 it can be seen that the functional compartments of the limbic brain include the thalamus, hippocampus, amygdala, hypothalamus and pituitary gland. The thalamus processes incoming information from the senses (eyes, ears, nose, touch, etc.) and outgoing information from the brain, acting as a relay station where information is appraised and decisions are made. The hippocampus, central to the operations of memory consolidation and learning, is where the thalamus's information is sorted and significant emotional memories are adapted for long-term storage in the frontal region of the limbic system. Situated in the front portion of the hippocampus and intimately connected to the hypothalamus is the amygdala, which is involved with emotional experience and reactions. The amygdala – originally thought to play a central role in the acquisition and processing of fear, anger, flight and defence – is now known to be crucial in processing emotions indispensable for social communication. The hypothalamus, together with other brain circuits, is involved with motivation and reward mechanisms. Through the endocrine system it controls most of the body's housekeeping needs such as brain clocks, temperature regulation, appetites for food, sex, aggression and pleasure. Attached to the hypothalamus is the pituitary gland, which orchestrates the messenger hormones influencing the homeostatic stability of every organ in the body, including the brain itself.

The highly complicated brain circuitry described above synchronizes the differing levels of the fight/flight and reward systems. Importantly, the emotional brain is richly connected to other brain centres/circuits, particularly the

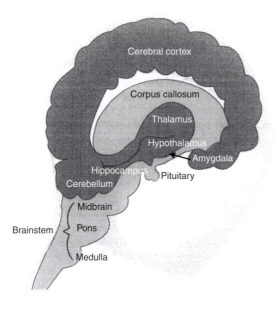

Figure 4.2 The functional compartments of the limbic, or emotional, brain are the thalamus, hippocampus, hypothalamus, amygdala and pituitary gland. Embedded within the brain are other major anatomical divisions. The limbic brain is central to memory, depression and also serves as the prime target for consciousness-changing/mood-altering substances.

cerebral cortex, or higher brain centres of the mind, which, in total, make up the processing mechanisms by which human beings regulate their behaviour in conformity with social convention and in pursuit of chosen goals. Under healthy conditions, they help to generate a holistic and adaptive response to changing environmental conditions.

An ecological approach to ethics recognizes that substance abuse is part of a dynamic in human behaviour that can be altered through addressing the many problems which lead to transgenerational poverty, alienation and addiction. Many chemically dependent women are also survivors of childhood sexual abuse, which is a main contributing factor in women seeking counselling for problems related to substance abuse, family violence, rape and destructive relationships. Similarly, men are more likely to seek help for the consequences of sexual abuse (depression, alcoholism) than for the abuse itself. It may be that survivors of sexual abuse are uncomfortable discussing these matters, or do not view their current drug problems as connected to earlier abuse. Of course, drug abuse is a very complex phenomenon, reflecting a multiplicity of environmental and genetic factors. The aetiology, however, does not matter;

what matters is that the drug of choice effectively 'fixes' a basic, often deeply embedded, need for an emotional transformation.

The phenomenon of drug addiction can be seen as the perfect integration of biological and behavioural factors. Scientists have long understood the common neurobiological mechanisms of addiction, and how it can be converted into compulsive drug-taking behaviour. Each drug has its own mechanism of action(s), resulting in the distinctive drug experience. In addition, many drugs of potential abuse such as nicotine, marijuana, alcohol, cocaine and heroin, have a common effect on the dopaminergic pathways, causing a rise in the neurochemical dopamine. Dopamine, serotonin and noradrenaline (norepinephrine) are the emotional brain's three principal neurotransmitters that balance the chemistry of mood. Dopamine is involved in the control of numerous functions, including the normal experience of pleasure and it is thought that the drug-induced dopamine surge plays a central role in addiction – perhaps by training the brain to associate a drug with pleasure.

Apart from being the brain's reward system, dopamine also functions as a main neurohormone, mediating neural interactions with the pituitary gland which controls metabolism, growth and reproduction. Dopamine has been dubbed the courier of addiction because the drug-stimulated spike of its release fades in response to repeated use. The brain has to maintain stability in the face of challenge, so accommodates to the artificial stimulus by changing function in fundamental ways. For instance, prolonged cocaine or heroin use lowers the brain's homeostatic set points and manner in which dopamine is effectively utilized. This changed function can persist for up to two years after an addict has stopped taking the drug. The most significant homeostatic change, as far as addictive behaviour is concerned, is that the initial high dopamine spike gradually becomes lower and lower, forcing addicts to keep bingeing in an effort to 'normalize' their neurotransmitter levels. Specifically, repeated drug intake, while initially stimulating the desired rush, provokes the brain to accommodate to the prevailing conditions by decreasing its previous baseline level which, in turn, forces the addict to increase the drug intake in an effort to bring back previous working dopamine levels within the brain. It is the brain's attenuated neurotransmitter concentration which continues the craving long after drug use ceases.

The extant debate of whether addiction should be viewed as a brain disease or a matter of personal choice is far from being resolved. Those who argue for the disease model quote recent insights from neuroscience that suggest that addicted individuals have substantially impaired cognitive control of behaviour and ask the question as to what extent can society justly hold addicted individuals responsible for their actions. Evidence for the disease model, however, does not resolve the problem of voluntary control because drug seeking and drug taking involves a series of voluntary planning activities. Since there remains much to learn about the pathophysiology of addiction, understanding the causes of alcoholism, drug addiction, poverty and ignorance is more caring than being judgemental about specific adverse reproductive outcomes. That the opportunity for high-quality education and health is a right rather than a privilege is more in tune with an ecological model of care. By integrating contemporary biological insights into matters of bioethics, bioscience ethics teaches us that parents and their children have common interests, and that the most challenging decision anyone ever faces is whether or not to become a parent. The bioethical principle of beneficence is respected when caring communities promote that all individuals – women, men and children – have a right to substance-abuse education, treatment and, as adults, good preconceptional/prenatal care.

Issues of stress reduction, environmental quality, housing and workplace safety, and educational reform do not need to be uniform; rather the framework should incorporate regional diversity and pluralistic problem-solving in tune with ethnically diverse populations. Part and parcel of consciousness raising is that all voices are heard, acknowledged and valued. It seems fitting, therefore, to close with the words of one such voice: 'with respect comes attitude'.[2]

Principles of bioscience ethics for discussion

- Because body chemistry can fluctuate within certain limits, homeostasis is often described as dynamic equilibrium. This ability of the body to support life by keeping the internal environment constant within a variable range of values is considered adaptive, as it allows humans to live in a variety of conditions such as deserts or the tropics. Is drug abuse an unadaptive option possible only because it exploits the body's ability to survive under difficult conditions or, since drug use has been a constant characteristic of human evolution, can it have unidentified survival values?
- Stresses which impair growth and development during critical periods in fetal life or infancy can lead to long-term, even permanent, abnormalities in adult function. Thus, fetuses that were growth-restricted in

---

[2] *Tackling Crime in Aboriginal Communities.* Australian Broadcasting Corporation Law Report June 2006 [http://www.abc.net.au/rn/lawreport/stories/2006/1655030.htm].

utero are at greater risk of morbidity and mortality during the peri-natal period, and risk an inability to perform some or all of the tasks of daily life. If information brings responsibility, does the burden of proof have to demonstrate lack of harm before remedial action is necessary?

- Carbon monoxide is a colourless, odourless gas which binds to haemoglobin 200 times more tightly than oxygen, resulting in impaired delivery of oxygen to the tissues. Cigarette smoke contains carbon monoxide, which is delivered directly to non-smokers nearby. In your opinion, does the addictive quality of nicotine justify an acceptance to passively do harm?

- Do you think that society has the right to direct its citizens to lead a healthy lifestyle, or ought encouragement and support be sufficient?

5

Fertility awareness: the ovulatory method of birth control, ageing gametes and congenital malformation in children

Procreation in our species is so haphazard that only in the last few decades [have] people started to pay attention to the intact and potentially perfect survival of the offspring. Previously, it was considered an Act of God that carried off a large number of the infants born alive and left many of the rest permanently damaged. Only in this century have people started to question such a fatalistic approach and look to ways of reducing perinatal mortality and morbidity.[1]

The previous two chapters reviewed common biological mechanisms linking stressful lifestyles, drug abuse and significant increased risk of serious structural and/or functional anomalies in the offspring. It was also emphasized that drug abuse, being predominantly a consequence of poverty, social alienation and biological ignorance, is a matter of personal and collective responsibility. A judgemental attitude is not an effective method of reducing preventable disability in children – raising standards of living and providing the empowering qualities of high-calibre education is much more effective. The present chapter provides information about fertility and ageing gametes, and promotes increased awareness about possible relationships between 'natural family planning' methods of contraception and pregnancy outcomes.

Fertility awareness is far more than just the accumulated basics of the reproductive process. Fertility awareness involves being knowledgeable about

---

[1] Chamberlain, G. & Lumley, J. (eds) (1986). *Prepregnancy Care: A Manual for Practice.* Chichester, UK; John Wiley & Son, p. 1.

the physiology of reproduction, applying that knowledge to oneself and one's partner, and then making informed decisions concerning the timing of intercourse and understanding how each contraceptive method interrupts fertility and how that method may fail if not used correctly. Fertility awareness information is necessary both to plan pregnancies as well as to avoid them. Couples who plan their pregnancies, as compared with unplanned conceptions, have fewer complications during pregnancy and better pregnancy outcomes. This reinforces a social obligation to officially promote sex and relationship education in the school curriculum. All citizens, but especially the young, should be appropriately educated about reproductive processes and protected from misinformation. In this context, however, there are many important social, cultural and religious taboos which effectively prevent the acquisition of significant biological information that sustains universal reproductive health needs. Alarmingly, the revision of bioethical discourse is more often obstructed when the discussion revolves around human sexuality and reproduction, seriously threatening this area of health education. From the ethical perspective, inappropriate behavioural directives may be understood as a transgression of the duty of care. Bioscience ethics affirms the human right of access to comprehensive, high-quality and updated scientific information so that knowledge may be applied under varying social conditions. However, before an analysis of common behavioural directives in matters of sexuality is undertaken, a brief precis of basic principles of genetics may be useful.

The laws of inheritance

The adult human body is made up of more than one hundred trillion (10^{14}) different cells which perform specific functions, and the genes provide instructions for how each cell should effectively operate. As described in Chapter 2, genes and epigenetic variables provide the basis of growth and development; that is, from fertilization through to adulthood and death, the information necessary for the daily maintenance and functioning of our bodies is organized. All cells typically contain a full set of genes; however, within any particular cell type it is only those genes which are relevant to performing the cell's specific task that are expressed, or switched on.

Genes are sections of DNA (deoxyribonucleic acid) which are contained in the chromosomes passed on from our parents at conception. Typically, human somatic cells have two sets, or 23 homologous pairs, of chromosomes, making 46 in total. These 46 chromosomes contain two sets of genes; one set inherited from our biological mother and the other from our biological father. The germ cells are exceptional in that they develop into gametes, either sperm or eggs, each carrying only one set of 23 chromosomes in total. The single set of chromosomes in the egg or sperm cell is a unique recombination of maternal and paternal genetic material. Recombination, or the process of crossing over, is a key event that involves physical exchanges between chromosome pairs and provides the mechanism that promotes genetic diversity among the resulting gametes. At fertilization the full complement of 46 chromosomes is restored, resulting in an equal contribution of genetic material from each parent except for the pair of sex chromosomes. All eggs carry an X chromosome (one of the mother's two X chromosomes), but a sperm cell may carry either an X or a Y chromosome. Since the mother always passes on an X chromosome, the sex of the child is determined by the father. At fertilization, a sperm bearing an X chromosome makes XX or a girl, and a sperm bearing a Y chromosome makes XY or a boy.

The intricate mechanism that copies the genetic material in preparation for cell division is mitosis, which produces exact copies of the nucleus. A drawback of mitotic (asexual) reproduction is its very uniformity as it leads to the production of a clone of genetically identical progeny. Although the clone may be well adapted to its existing environment, it may be at real risk should conditions change. In contrast, organisms that produce genetically different offspring are more successful when the environment varies unpredictably in time and space – at least some of their genetically diverse offspring may be able to meet the challenges of a changing environment. Diversity is fostered by sexual reproduction; that is, by the production of gametes containing a single set of chromosomes. The mechanism for nuclear division, which reduces the chromosome number and ensures genetic diversity among the products, is called meiosis. When meiosis is complete, it is very unlikely that any two human gametes will have the same combination of homologous chromosomes.

The DNA molecule consists of a double-stranded helix with each strand held together by a bonding between pairs of four possible nitrogenous bases called adenine, thymine, cytosine and guanine (abbreviated A, T, C and G). The information content of DNA is given by the order in which these bases occur along the DNA molecule. Genetic information, as passed through the generations of cells, is complex and sophisticated, but an often-used analogy to illustrate the relationship between genes, DNA and chromosomes has proved helpful. A chromosome can be compared to an audiocassette, DNA to the tape inside the cassette, and genes to the songs on the tape. Genes are not separate from DNA but are an integral part of it just as the song is an indivisible part of the tape.

Human fecundity

As we have seen in Chapters 3 and 4, genetic information can be passed on to the next generation erroneously, resulting in faulty, mutated genes. The majority of common disorders, such as heart disease, diabetes and cancer, however, are caused by a combination of genetic and environmental factors, and are said to be multifactorial in origin. A variety of stresses, including ageing, may cause mutations either early during the division and differentiation of germ cells or later in development. Mutations can occur where one or more entire chromosomes or parts of chromosomal material are either lacking or present in excess, a condition known as aneuploidy. Aneuploidy usually results in a specific malformation and/or severely restricted overall growth of the fetus. Children with Down's syndrome, for example, have an extra copy of chromosome 21. At birth, approximately 5% of humans have a significant or serious congenital abnormality. Half of these defects involve chromosome imbalances; the other half involve complex congenital abnormalities and common diseases caused by single-gene defects. Despite their importance from the clinical, economic and social perspectives, these surviving cases represent just a small fraction of those present in early developmental stages. The truth is that the human fecundity rate (that is, the probability of achieving a clinically recognized pregnancy within any given menstrual cycle) is about 25%, and high levels of fertilization failure or early developmental death are the norm. This high attrition rate is due to abnormalities in the gametes and faulty development, leading to embryo death prior to implantation.

Scientists arrive at fertility estimates by studying large cohorts of fertile women who are attempting to conceive, and from these studies it is clear that humans are unique in the very high frequency of chromosome abnormalities and consequent early embryo wastage. Clinically recognized pregnancy loss, on the other hand, is usually quoted as 15–20%. It is this clinical fraction of failed pregnancies that has been extensively studied cytogenetically and in which a chromosome abnormality rate of at least 50% has been established. This contrasts markedly with a 5% chromosome abnormality rate found in stillbirths, illustrating clearly the natural in utero selection process that eliminates 95% of chromosomally unbalanced conceptions. Figure 5.1 assigns categories of known and unknown human anomalies at birth. It can be seen that 50-60% of developmental anomalies at birth are of unknown aetiology, while known causes can be assorted into chromosomal aberrations, mutant genes and environmental factors. Of the known categories, 20–25% are

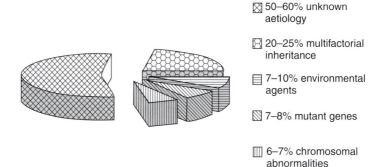

50–60% unknown
aetiology

20–25% multifactorial
inheritance

7–10% environmental
agents

7–8% mutant genes

6–7% chromosomal
abnormalities

Figure 5.1 Causes of human congenital abnormalities at birth. (Reproduced from Pollard, I. (2006). Lifestyle and fertility. In D. Macer (ed.) *A Cross-Cultural Introduction to Bioethics*. Christchurch, New Zealand: Eubios Ethics Institute, Fig. 1, p. 193, with permission.)

multifactorial inheritances. Prenatal diagnosis such as amniocentesis, chorionic villus sampling and preimplantation genetic diagnosis (which may result in voluntary pregnancy termination), can thus be seen as a medical extension of this natural process.

Female libido: procreational versus recreational sex

The human is an extraordinary species, with freedom to deviate from strict stereotypical behaviours, especially sexual. Most mammals are sexually receptive only when fertile, whereas the human female's potential for sexual arousal and orgasm at all times in the menstrual cycle is no secret. To achieve sexual independence from fertility, however, Nature had to invent a new strategy. The solution was to transfer the physiological control of libido from the female sex hormones (estrogens and progesterone) involved in ovulation and pregnancy, to another set of hormones, in this case the androgens testosterone and androstenedione. A woman's complement of androgens, derived from her ovaries and adrenal glands, keep her sexual drive active throughout the menstrual cycle. The advantages of retaining sexual receptivity at all times, including those when conception is not a physiological option, is obvious. Such a strategy clearly helps to maintain long-term relationships. It is an evolutionary device to maximize parental care of the young and provide sexual pleasure and comfort for the highly sexed human being. Early human societies throughout the world understood this and developed many ways of thoughtfully preventing unwanted conceptions.

Since we have evolved into an extremely socialized species, sexual intercourse has a greater significance than the mere transmission of the genotype. As already alluded to above, sexual pleasure is particularly important, but continued sexual receptivity favours pair bonding, essential for the maintenance of long-term relationships and the raising of offspring. Cooperative living reinforces self-sufficiency and wellbeing and for that reason helps in raising the offspring. Other aspects can also be identified; sexual behaviour may be used to establish dominance in relationships, express hostility or be used for material gain. It is clear that the sociobiological functions of human sexuality go far beyond reproduction and pair bonding. They influence the shaping and linking of groups of individuals into communities and communities into societies; that is, in anthropological terms, the humanizing of biological relationships. Procreational sex, in becoming recreational sex, also became the glue of society. Nature has taken care of our ongoing fitness by providing behavioural flexibility. So, who are we – especially in our present state of biological ignorance – to ethically question the logic of our evolutionary heritage? Certainly we cannot pontificate about what is 'natural' and what is not, before we have become a good deal more knowledgeable about our uniquely human heredity.

Principles of reproductive ageing

In a system where sex can be separated in time from ovulation, aged/defective sperm, eggs and conceptuses are a natural byproduct. Flexible sexual behaviour results in genetic wastage, which is adaptive and balances evolutionary-directed change in behaviour. Nature's solution is to provide high-quality fertility by an excess of potential with the intention that only a small proportion of that potential will ever be realized. Because of the ease in achieving fertilizations (as demonstrated by in vitro fertilization technology), embryo wastage is high in humans; however, severe chromosomal abnormality in the conceptus ensures the natural discontinuance of such pregnancies. Specifically, spontaneous abortion is Nature's way to counter environmental factors which exert an important influence on ageing processes of gametes and conceptuses. This explains the low percentage of all human fertilizations which survive to birth, with a large majority of these lost in the very early stages of pregnancy. Similar reasoning can also be applied to fertility; that is, gamete wastage prior to fertilization. In fertile men, the sperm concentration varies between 60 and 80 million active sperm per millilitre of semen in an ejaculate volume of approximately 2.5–3.5 ml. Despite the fact that each active sperm (given the chance) is a potential person, the turning point between fertile and infertile sperm number is approximately 20 million active sperm per millilitre (Chapter 9).

Ageing can be defined as the decline in body functions with time associated with a reduced capacity to maintain control of the body's basic stability, or homeostasis. Many theories have been developed to explain the causes of ageing, but it is doubtful that any one theory is adequate to explain the entire ageing phenomenon. Investigators do agree, however, that the genome has a major role in determining the maximum length of the lifespan, with environmental factors exerting an ongoing influence on ageing processes. In women, cyclic and orderly changes in ovarian function during the normal menstrual cycle are closely timed and regulated by the actions of the brain, particularly the hypothalamus and the pituitary gland. In turn, steroid hormones (estradiol and progesterone) produced by the ovary modulate hypothalamic and pituitary function through feedback mechanisms. Follicular growth and steroid hormone secretion are controlled by the two pituitary gonadotrophins – follicle stimulating hormone (FSH) and luteinizing hormone (LH). FSH stimulates follicle development, growth and estrogen synthesis, while LH stimulates progesterone secretion and prepares the dominant follicle for ovulation. Thus, at mid-cycle, the preovulatory LH surge is followed, about 38 hours after its onset, by ovulation. At least this is the simplified textbook story. Recently, ultrasound scans have demonstrated that women may ovulate more than once per menstrual cycle, which may result in ovulation on separate days. They may experience two and three follicular growth waves per menstrual cycle with any, or none, resulting in ovulation. It has been estimated that double ovulations separated in time may account for 10% of fraternal twinning.

As with all complicated physiological functions, oocyte maturation during peak LH levels consists of a series of events occurring between 4 and 38 hours after the onset of the LH surge. After ovulation, also under LH action, the ruptured follicle is luteinized to form a corpus luteum which secretes hormones preparing the uterine endometrium for implantation of the embryo. The period between ovulation and fertilization, likewise, consists of important temporal maturational and ageing processes. Following fertilization and implantation, human chorionic gonadotrophin (hCG) produced from early placental tissue prevents the corpus luteum from regression so that pregnancy can be established. However, if implantation is not successful, menstruation occurs and the cycle is repeated.

The average age at which a woman goes through the menopause is 49–52 years, and the most dramatic event associated with the menopause is the loss of cyclic ovarian function and cessation of menstrual cycles. The number of follicles in the ovaries of a healthy young woman is estimated to be 400 000, but only an estimated 0.1% is actually involved in ovulatory function, while the remainder degenerate during the reproductive years.

Ageing in men is subtler than in women, as men often remain fertile into old age, but there is a parallel reproductive decline in testicular function with age. Testosterone secretion and spermatogenesis decreases. While sperm number may remain relatively high in healthy older men, degenerative changes are observed in the germinal tubular membrane, due to sclerosis and closing of the tubular lumen. Consequently, there is an age-related reduction in the daily production of sperm, the number of normal sperm and the conception rate. Most de novo mutations causing inherited disease are paternal in origin. Sperm vulnerability is thought to be related to fundamental differences between spermatogenesis and oogenesis. Early in gametogenesis (the production of gametes), the numbers of primordial germ cells increase by mitosis. In the female, this mitotic expansion continues until late in gestation when the germ cells (oogonia) enter meiosis and remain arrested (now primary oocytes) until years later when ovulation occurs and the oocytes are stimulated to resume meiosis. It is significant that this pool of non-growing primary oocytes represents the sole source of unfertilized eggs in the sexually mature female and is the link with the next generation. In the male, mitotic division of germ cells (spermatogonia) begins at puberty and continues actively throughout life. Thus the risk of replication errors preceding spermatogenesis increases with advancing age.

It is important to note that paternal-mediated contributions to birth defects (as demonstrated by fetal death rates and genetic abnormalities in offspring) increases sharply with paternal age. Fathers above 39 years of age have an elevated risk of having a Down's syndrome offspring, with a strong effect from the age of 41. One of the most comprehensive studies in this field is from the French Medical Research Agency, using coordinated data from 22 fertility clinics across the nation. This calculated the percentages of babies with Down's syndrome according to the age of the sperm donors. The results showed that 0.14% of the children born to fathers under 35 had Down's syndrome compared with 0.23% of babies born to men aged between 35 and 39, and 0.41% born to men over 39 – an almost threefold increase over those in the youngest age group. Other investigations have revealed a strong correlation between paternal age and increased risk for neurodevelopmental anomalies such as schizophrenia and autistic spectrum disorders. Fathers aged between 45 and 49 years were twice as likely to sire a child with schizophrenia and three times as likely if over 50 years of age. Since a male biological clock definitely exists, some sperm banks cut off donations at the 35th birthday, while others cut off sperm donations at the 30th birthday. The above data, equating advanced paternal age with increased risk of genetic disorders, reinforces the view that fathers have a very personal responsibility toward their unborn children.

There is a risk, however, that too much emphasis is placed on genetic explanations for illnesses so that we begin to see ourselves simply as the sum of our genes. This attitude is known as genetic determinism and is dangerous, as an overemphasis on genetic explanations can undermine the assumption of personal responsibility for our actions. It may even be used to justify antisocial or unhealthy behaviour (belief in a 'master' race, for example). Congenital anomaly is not determined solely by genetic factors, but by a complex interaction of genes, teratogens, environmental and behavioural variables.

Ageing gametes and ovulatory method of birth control

Culture is a potent factor affecting our biology, just as biological factors put constraints on culture. During the hunting and gathering phase of human history there existed millions of years of equilibrium between a nomadic, small community lifestyle and continuity in terms of a balanced interaction with the environment. With the domestication of plants and animals in the Neolithic era (beginning around 10 000 BCE), however, came a radical change in subsistence activities and a more restricted interaction developed between humans and their environment. Social aggregations of people brought about by farming and the manufacture of technologically advanced stone implements made it imperative to invent new restrictions and laws. Increased social regulation had to follow increasing sedentism and the aggregation of larger populations which were now at greater risk of poorer hygiene and disease. Thus, new sociobiological rules developed to make the sedentary, village lifestyle more manageable and healthier. Since the scientific revolution, however, human knowledge has expanded and it is again a good time to reassess our social mores adaptively. Taking into consideration new scientific insights, we may be able to keep what is biologically relevant and makes adaptive common sense, and modify what is not – in other words, respond to the objectives of bioscience ethical thinking.

There has always been a need to control human fertility. Prevention of unwanted pregnancy dates back over 4000 years with successive ancient civilizations recording recipes for abortifacients, vaginal pastes and medical tampons. Modern insights connecting sex and sexually transmitted disease probably dates from the use of the linen sheath in 1564 as protection against syphilis. Now, as never before, because of population expansion, diseases such as AIDS and widespread poverty, human society needs ready access to safe, effective, reversible and affordable methods of contraception. Modern contraceptives provide personal empowerment, whether this is for the protection of health or family planning by number and spacing of children. However, countless women still needlessly die every year, or suffer from debilitating ill health as a result of complications of pregnancy, with the majority – but not exclusively – in the overpopulated developing world. Effective contraception also reduces the incidence of high-risk, unsafe abortions and what this means in terms of human suffering. As we have learned earlier, all methods of contraception are natural in the biological sense since all humans can do is to embellish the sexual benefits already inherent in Nature's creativity.

Contraceptive approaches that rely on coital technique, rather than on the use of technical or pharmaceutical aids, are generally referred to, in common parlance, as 'natural' methods. To the lay person, the ovulatory method of birth control (or natural family planning if you like) equates with the 'rhythm' method and relies on periodic abstinence intended to coincide with the time surrounding ovulation. To be effective, the ovulatory method of birth control depends on the woman being able to detect her fertile time. This is done by estimating the number of days from the commencement of menstruation to the beginning of fertility or, more accurately, by measuring her basal body temperature (a small rise in basal body temperature of 0.2–0.6°C occurs post-ovulation), examining the consistency of her cervical mucus, or by variable combinations of all these methods.

Ovulation detection by measuring basal body temperature is a retrospective approach and will only be safe if the woman's cycle is sufficiently constant from month to month. Given the menstrual cycle's susceptibility to emotional or stressful disturbances, it often is not. Under the grip of intense emotion, it is also possible for ovulation to be induced by intercourse, as has been demonstrated in rape victims. Other difficulties of the rhythm method are the requirement for high motivation and cooperation by both partners. In summary, therefore, 'safe period' predictions are unreliable, as confirmed by the rhythm method's failure rate of between 2 and 24% in the first year (some 20-fold less effective than oral contraceptives at their worst). To improve on this method's effectiveness, sexual intercourse should be avoided through much of the first part of the cycle; this takes into consideration the potential life of spermatozoa in the cervix (of several days) and a 24–36-hour life of the oocyte(s), which may not necessarily arrive at the expected time. Given these cycle variables, conceptions resulting in unwanted pregnancies are realistic options and are, presumably, considered as acceptable 'chance' failures.

Because of the rhythm method's cheapness, there has been increasing pressure since the 1990s to make it a suitable contraceptive choice in the developing, overpopulated world, where natural family planning is the sole method of fertility control for some of the world's poorest couples. It is true that natural family planning allows couples to avoid, or achieve, pregnancy. Those wishing to achieve a pregnancy will have extremely high pregnancy rates, while those strongly motivated and understanding the practicalities underpinning the method can enjoy extremely low pregnancy rates. However, it is in the interest of couples, and the society in which they are living, to be educated and unambiguously informed about the relative risks and benefits of competing artificial contraceptives relative to natural family planning. Major concerns are unwanted pregnancies, fertilizations with aged gametes resulting in possible genetic defects and growth anomalies, and exposure to sexually transmitted diseases. Individuals and couples deserve to be provided with the latest available scientific information if they are to make informed decisions about their sexuality.

In the event that natural family planning is chosen, then the women concerned should expect to be given clear guidelines as to how to recognize indirect symptoms of ovulation accurately, so that the possibility of becoming pregnant is minimized. The cervical mucus test (or Billing's method) is effective but not infallible. Cervical mucus changes its consistency according to the hormonal balance between estradiol and progesterone. Under estrogen domination, around the time of ovulation, cervical mucus is composed of parallel chains of fibrils with sufficient space between them to permit the passage of sperm. At other times, cervical mucus is thicker and lacks the micellar structure, making it an effective barrier to the entry of sperm and bacteria. However, as for all bodily functions, the physiological changes are not abrupt but progress gradually according to a predetermined series of events. Thus, as the estrogen levels begin to rise, driving the approaching ovulation, sperm passage may no longer be completely blocked, allowing some to shelter in storage crypts at the upper end of the cervix where they are sealed in by a mucus plug. Just before ovulation the mucus plug dissolves, releasing the trapped sperm from the cervical crypts, facilitating their further passage towards conception.

With the development of new technology to both predict and to detect ovulation, 'fertility awareness' contraceptive methods may become more reliable in the future. The already marketed but expensive *Persona* is a small hand-held electronic computer and urine testing device. The idea is that the device attempts to predict ovulation by initially measuring the sharp rise of estrone-3-glucuronide, a urinary metabolite of estradiol, to establish a personal menstrual profile. Then, in subsequent cycles, the device warns the woman, through a red light, that she is entering her predicted fertile period. From the main European clinical trial the failure rate among consistent users was 6% in any one year – not an encouraging result.

The gametopathy hypothesis and congenital anomalies

It was back in the 1970s when Piet Jongbloet and colleagues first published data demonstrating that the incidence of Down's syndrome amongst Roman Catholic women living in Western Australia was more than double that in all other religious groups. During the same decade, the Dutch Ministry of Health reported a similar difference in Down's syndrome incidence between Catholic and other religious groups from every province in the Netherlands. Work from other countries, similarly, described a Catholic over-representation in a variety of congenital anomalies, including oral cleft lip–palate defect, spina bifida, anencephaly, low birthweight and psychological/neurological abnormalities. These findings raised concern about method failures associated with natural family planning, where conceptions due to intercourse before the fertile period could arise from aged sperm, and conceptions after the fertile period could occur with a post-ovulatory aged ovum. This was of particular interest since the 'ovulation' method of birth control had been encouraged among the Catholics in Australia where there was a strong correlation between contraceptive practice and religious affiliation. It was also reported that women delivering an oral cleft infant were three times as likely to have used the rhythm method for contraceptive purposes at the time of conception, compared with women delivering healthy babies. That corticosteroids and their chemical byproducts are incompatible with good reproduction has been known for a long time and, evidently, an unwanted pregnancy is a stressful life event. It has also been known for a long time that the primary defect induced by excess concentrations of circulating corticosteroids is cleft lip-palate, demonstrable in all species. Since the publication of Jongbloet's early reports, the identification of reproductive dysfunction has widened to include a range of abnormalities of the placental unit as well as the embryo. Placental anomalies may lead to pregnancy and birth complications, while the embryonic anomalies may be observed as developmental abnormalities.

The above, initially perplexing, observations have now been defined in biological terms, as follows. During irregular menstrual cycles when spontaneous ovulation occurs earlier or later than estimated, the prescribed sexual abstinence does not precisely coincide with peak fertility; that is, the synchronous presence of fresh gametes at the fertilization site. Desynchronized ovulation and fertilization may facilitate the union of over-ripe ova, surviving aged sperm, or a combination of both. That is, in the case of an unplanned conception, the rhythm method prolonged the post-ovulatory delay beyond the optimum before fertilization took place, compared with instances of continuing intercourse during the mid-cycle. Nevertheless, risk estimates derived from unconfirmed studies must be interpreted with caution as there is always the problem of ascertaining whether a conception arose from aged gametes or other confounding effects. There is also the potential for bias in maternal recall. However, the gametopathy hypothesis is supported by animal experimentation, where delayed ovulation and fertilization increases the risk of a continuum of anomalies; some are developmental, while others are associated with chromosomal aberrations and mutations. Delayed fertilization in the rat and rabbit, for example, is associated with intrauterine growth retardation (IUGR), developmental abnormalities and increased embryo mortality in post-implantation conceptuses, clearly demonstrating that non-optimum fertilization is one source of reproductive wastage.

Ovopathy and spermopathy may be evoked by a series of physiological disturbances of the ovulation and fertilization system, not all connected with a failure of the rhythm method of contraception. Such conditions may include advanced parental age, poverty and decreased frequency of sexual intercourse. It is worth noting, however, that the suggested causal relationship between contraception failure and the birth of infants with pathological conditions, especially cleft malformations, has decreased in industrial societies following the use of modern, effective contraceptives which result in reduced numbers of unplanned pregnancies. Since its early documentation and as new evidence has accumulated, the gametopathy concept has gained credibility in reproductive biology, and is currently being integrated into standard manuals of obstetrics. With this in mind, the present is an opportune time to extend the scientific ethical engagement by debating bioethical concerns in relation to currently acceptable norms of human sexual behaviour.

As described above, human beings are unique in the very high frequency of chromosomal abnormalities and embryo wastage. Of the 50–60% unexplained developmental anomalies (see Fig. 5.1), it is entirely possible that a proportion of these represent fertilization of old, past their 'due date' gametes. It follows, therefore, that influencing human sexual behaviour through health care programmes for avoiding non-optimum conceptions can prevent many pathological conceptions. If the public were to be given better information about the ovulatory cycle and contraceptive methods, the conception of wanted children would occur under optimum physiological conditions. Such health care programmes can readily be incorporated into general education programmes and are much more humane than alternative and expensive prenatal (that is, post-conception) diagnoses, such as amniocentesis that may lead, in the event of a positive identification of genetic abnormality, to the necessity for traumatic parental decisions to be made.

It may be appropriate at this point of the discussion to quote from contemporary Catholic aspirations: 'In order for the kind of openness to life described by Humanae Vitae to cut through the contraceptive mentality that permeates American culture, many experts agree that more medical professionals must be brought to see NFP (natural family planning) as at least a valid, if not preferable, alternative to artificial birth control.'[2] From the biological perspective, however, can the rhythm method of contraception be accepted as being more natural than the use of alternative forms of birth control? It is certain, in this instance, that the medical profession has to be vigilant not to succumb to influences which may violate the doctor's ethical obligation not to cause harm.

For millions of people, in particular those living in poverty in overpopulated developing countries, the promotion of the Catholic Church's teaching is an important part of their life's work. At the same time, women in those corresponding developing countries suffer considerable morbidity and mortality because of their inability to control their own fertility. Maternal mortality related to pregnancy or delivery is now estimated to be around 529 000 each year, with an estimated further 10 million women a year suffering from related complications.[3] Unsafe abortions account for between 25 and 40% of the mortality, with an overall two-thirds of the deaths being preventable, if contraceptives were provided and family planning services dealt comprehensively with women's health issues. There can be no ethical defence of the systematic denial of the right of freedom from excess fertility, condemning so many innocent women and their children to a life of illness and poverty, and often death. Yet these horrendous figures serve to highlight the failure of political, religious, health and legal institutions to address the most fundamental injustice of our time. Women must urgently be given the responsibility to decide whether, how and when to have children, and the right to information and services necessary to exercise that responsibility. To do less is a gross denial of the freedom from excess fertility, referred to in free societies as the fifth freedom, developed along the lines of the other four fundamental freedoms; that is, freedom of speech, freedom of worship, freedom from want and freedom from fear.

[2] 30 years after *Humanae Vitae*. (1998). *Catholic World Report*, **8**, 55.

[3] Maternal mortality – estimates developed by WHO, UNICEF and UNFPA. See http://www. who.int/reproductive-health/publications/maternal mortality 2005/index.html..

Men are also not getting just treatment. Potential fathers are often excluded from reproductive health care and, typically, are not sufficiently informed about the menstrual cycle and the need for conception to occur under optimal physiological conditions to maximize the probability of the offspring expressing its full genetic potential. For example, there are not many parenting workshops for men, and even fewer on male sexuality and probably none on male responsibility, the last especially being pressing as women do not make sexual/reproductive decisions on their own. Without the involvement of couples and without a revolution of openness in considerations of sexuality, society cannot expect to overcome the health challenges and conquer the population crisis.

How can it be then, from the point of view of one of the world's most powerful religions, that the rate of reform is so disconcertingly slow? The path of directives, as they move from the actual encyclical, through the bishops, to the diocesan marriage preparation programmes, to the natural family planning teachers, to the priests and seminarians and, finally, ending with the individual married couples, is twisted and long. Given this tortuous path, it is appropriate to ask how biological teaching and understanding is preserved. The Church states that periodic continence shows due respect for the Church's moral law, but does the denial of responsible control over one's own reproductive and sexual health accord due respect for biological law, and does it justify the additional risk borne by the next generation of children? In civil societies, each individual is expected to be responsible for matters of conscience and, in turn, society has a responsibility to protect and teach its citizens that the creation of new individuals is a privilege. Thus, parental sexual behaviour, as well as other lifestyle variables such as drug consumption, should be part of the continuing educational process. It is ethically unacceptable for us to stand idly by and watch the hard-earned demographic shift of birth rate decline, caused by growing prosperity and female literacy, be ruthlessly overturned by unqualified directives.

Family planning education in a number of developing countries has become an underground movement as a result of Church leaders inveighing against contraception, and inspiring fear among politicians who may want to, contrary to the religious demands, promote individual choice in matters of reproduction. The Philippines, for example, has a fertility rate of 3.05 children per woman (2007 estimate) and an estimated one-fifth of 15–24-year-old girls have had an illegal abortion; or every year about 750 000 women undergo an induced abortion in illegal clinics scattered all over the country. Since the Catholic Church forbids the use of barrier methods of contraception, how does it wrestle with unwanted pregnancies and related responsibility in sexually transmitted disease awareness promotion? The global summary of the AIDS epidemic informs us that 4.3 million people were infected with HIV in 2006 where 530 000 were children under 15 years of age. In Africa and Latin America, strict obedience to the Church's teachings remains strong, so it is reasonable to assume that by failing to use condoms hundreds of thousands of new cases of HIV/AIDS infections each year are officially sanctioned by the Church's contraception policy. In 2003 there were an alarming 29.4 million HIV/AIDS sufferers living in sub-Saharan Africa, with the total figure predicted to double by 2010. No wonder that limited use of condoms (as the 'lesser' evil in the fight against AIDS) is allowed by some more liberal African and Latin American clergy. Nevertheless, the need for sexual education is urgent as HIV/AIDS and other sexually transmitted infections spread, and children are brought into a world without a just future. Making condoms more accessible, lowering their cost, promoting them more, and helping to overcome social and personal obstacles to their use would save many lives and reduce the enormous consequences and costs of sexually transmitted disease and unwanted, at-risk pregnancies.

Principles of bioscience ethics for discussion

-   Myth no. 1: that people with influence, in their present state of biological ignorance, are qualified to enunciate which methods of contraception are natural and which are not.
-   Myth no. 2: it is only a woman's age that matters; men can have healthy children well into their old age.
-   Not a myth: the United Nations statistics for 2006 revealed that a total of 39.5 million adults and children were living with the human immunodeficiency virus (HIV) and a total of 2.9 million adults and children died of AIDS that year. Ninety per cent of new infections occur in the developing countries where ready access to condoms may be restricted and post-infection treatment is minimal or non-existent.
-   Can institutionalized denial of responsible control over one's own reproductive and sexual health justify the addition of serious health risks borne by the next generation of children? How may we best annul long-held belief systems which are biologically impertinent and inhumane?

6

Understanding child abuse
and its biological consequences

Her early childhood memories seemed entirely focused on punishment, whether it was with beatings, or being given away to strangers, or being made to do other awful things she didn't specify but which felt bad, hurt, tasted bad, smelled bad or whatever, all of these terrible memories dominated . . .[1]

The above quote typifies the recurring theme of Mary Bell's life story who, at age 11 years, strangled two little boys aged 3 and 4. What happened to Mary Bell from the moment of her birth and which influenced her maturing awareness, can only be guessed at. A life of unrelenting abuse is, however, the sad lot of numerous, potentially normal, healthy children whose personal experience with violence leads, as in the above example, to an exceptional form of retaliatory behaviour. According to the author Gitta Sereny, the 11-year-old Mary was not a murderess but a severely damaged child whom no one helped in her despair and who was unable to realize her intrinsic potential. However, it must be said that Sereny's point of view is grounded in the belief of the innate goodness of all human beings, a belief which is open to challenge. In instances of unwitnessed murder, where no one knows what really transpired, there cannot be clearcut explanations. It is possible that Mary Bell's adult memory was distorted and questionable as to detail. We must also be aware that by placing the violator centre stage we, by inference, deny the victim's full significance and may be committing an ethical breach of justice.

This chapter is concerned with the everyday nature of the senseless acts of cruelty and violence committed by adults against children but avoids an

---

[1] Sereny, G. (1998). *Cries Unheard: The Story of Mary Bell.* London: Macmillan, pp. 336-7.

overconcentration on criminality and issues of law. Senseless acts of cruelty are, seemingly, tolerated within families and their communities; it is therefore appropriate that the more recent scientific insights into the origins and consequences of violence are reviewed in the hope of raising general awareness about society's unacceptably high tolerance of child abuse. Mary's childhood experiences, for example, would have remained unnoticed if she had not committed the crimes. Failure to make sufficient connection between the crimes damaged children commit and the oftentimes horrendous environmental conditions in which a child's mental and emotional development takes place, is the measure of how society fails in the care of its children. Frequently, breaking-point behaviour follows long-term suppressed emotional pressure and outrage, and is a reaction to ongoing neglect and abuse. Retaliatory reactions may be directed towards self or others, including small animals and helpless individuals. Child suicide often follows repeated attempts at self-mutilation and, according to psychologists, represents the concluding manifestation of inwardly driven anger, frustration and despair, culminating in complete withdrawal and final extinction. The alternative response, to attack, may become increasingly serious. Exposure to violence in the home is often linked to involvement in endemic street and playground violence, bullying in school, educational failure, and exclusion from or dropping out of school, and an increased incidence of attention-deficit hyperactivity disorder.

Many of the causes of violence in the family are beyond the reach of health professionals, but official acknowledgement by society that child abuse happens but is unacceptable, is the first step towards protecting children. The same may be true for other forms of violence in the family since several forms of violence and abuse may occur in the same family with children, parents, their partners and older family members being victims or perpetrators. Children in violent households are many times more likely to be injured and abused, either directly or while trying to protect a parent or sibling. Individual responsibility needs to be impressed on adults and nurtured in the young. Perhaps parental courses should become compulsory for all couples wishing to have children. However, before looking at the root causes supporting trans-generational cycles of domestic violence and criminal behaviour, we will revisit the continuum from the single cell to the newborn child, and from the youngster to the adult.

Adaptation of the newborn to extrauterine life

The technical term, derived from the Greek and Latin terms, for the newborn is neonate and refers to the baby from birth to the end of the first month of independent life. The neonate is a curious mixture of competence and helplessness. The growing, developing embryo/fetus is far from an acquiescent entity passively accepting events taking place in its protective uterine environment. Rather, the fetus is an active, dynamic individual, increasingly engaged in the regulation of its own development. Between fertilization, when the genetic makeup is set, and birth, babies accumulate a load of experiences that will contribute to the shaping of who they are and what they can bring to their new life. Throughout gestation, a plethora of genetic–epigenetic interactions exert profound influences on physiological function, and set the preconditions that will build the individual into a social being with a sense of self. By means of fetal programming mechanisms, fetuses remember their early physiological environment in utero and prepare, under the prevailing conditions, for the future (Chapter 3). The degree of maturity at birth varies from offspring to offspring, therefore the perinatal period spans the continuum from late fetal to early postnatal development.

The significance of gestation as an experience for the mother must also not be neglected. Normally both the mother and newborn adapt easily because the relationship established during pregnancy continues to develop postnatally. Mother and child are already familiar with each other and their mutual responses to the environment. Sounds penetrate from the outside world to the fetus, and movement of the fetus is felt by the mother. Pregnant women have recurring periods of activity and periods of rest to which the fetus accommodates. Fetal activity patterns closely follow the maternal day/night activities and endocrine rhythms, which are significant in entrainment of the fetal biological clock. Thus mother and child share rhythms of sleep and wakefulness, eating and socializing. The baby's capacity for social interaction begins to develop in the 3 months before birth. By 28 weeks gestation, the fetus's hearing functions are much as they will be after birth, and the fetus hears and responds to speech, learning the rhythm before the words. The newborn actively selects and filters visual and auditory stimuli and can recognize its mother's voice, and the voices of those close to her. Experiments have shown that a 3- or 4-day-old neonate prefers a recording of its mother's voice reading a story to that of another woman reading the same story. Instinctive baby care is based on near-universal experiences – singing to, rocking, swinging, swaddling and holding babies close; these show up in all cultures in various forms. Babies are soothed by singing – the rhythm of singing is probably the way fetuses hear their mothers' voices in utero – and by being held firmly, reflecting the uterus as a tight swaddle with the contractions of pregnancy providing frequent 'hugs'. Babies are soothed by being held close to the heart, and the adult heartbeat rate of 72 beats per minute has been exploited commercially by the manufacture of teddy bears that play a recorded human heartbeat at this rate. The rocking chairs, cradles and hammocks used all over the world duplicate the soothing rock of the pelvis when the mother walked during pregnancy. Babies seem to need to be rocked or walked, which is understandable as they recently left an environment in which they had been rocked for many hours each day. Early in-utero experiences leave permanent legacies; in grief, children and adults alike may revert to a perceived time of security by rocking.

Fetuses have the most direct relationships with the mothers, and it is on mothers that fetuses have the most direct effects. However, it is not only to the mother that fetuses relate. An emotional relationship also develops with the ones close to her and the mother will often use this closeness to create a bond between the fetus and the rest of the family. It is natural for the father and siblings to reach out and feel the fetal movements and to make contact. Thus the process of socialization, which goes on for a lifetime, begins before birth. Of all senses, the sense of touch seems to be the most important for the fetus because by this the fetus can avoid obstacles and, hence, can prevent becoming entangled with the umbilical cord. Similarly, social and physical contact is vital to the neonate. Many subtle long-term influences of physical deprivation during the neonatal period have been documented. In all mammalian species, physical contact (handling) assists physiological mechanisms to function optimally, and a resulting acceleration of all parameters of growth and development is noticeable. Accelerated maturation following physical stimulation has also been reported for premature babies in intensive care. When first declaring pregnancy, the out-of-fashion term 'with child' affirms this mutual relationship far more than the contemporary term 'expecting'.

Bonding and social relations

It is easy to see how social interaction within the family could be influenced by the baby's particular characteristics. Newborns differ in their motor activity, irritability and responsiveness, but they all engage in primitive social relations. Soon after birth the infant will recognize the facial and olfactory characteristics of persons mostly in contact with him or her, especially if the most constant attendant is the mother and she is breastfeeding. A steroid molecule (a possible progenitor of 4-α-andosterone) in human sweat concentrates in the nipple/areola region and acts as a pheromone, aiding speedy mother–infant bonding. The mother's breast pheromone triggers head turning towards the nipple which helps to guide the infant to nurse. In addition, the mother's unique odour signature has natural tranquillizer properties, and assists in furthering mother–infant attachment. Socialization is aided by the effects of hormones, including pheromones, which provide the offspring with a concept of self derived from the familial smell. Experiments demonstrate that non-human primate females reared in a socially deprived environment make poor, aggressive and rejecting mothers. However, human bonding is very complex, utilizing many variables, but there are parallels linking childhood distress and substandard parental care. Simple needs for food, closeness and sucking comfort should be satisfied. Failure to satisfy these simple needs can lead to distress as the baby does not understand reasons, only needs. Learning appears to depend on the timing of reward and the repetition of the stimulus. Early learning is also linked to conditioning and may set subsequent behavioural patterns.

Crying is the most obvious method that the newborn uses to communicate with its social environment. Quite young babies display different cries depending on whether the crying is stimulated by hunger, pain or anger. Communication also occurs when a parent responds to a crying baby; for instance, the mother's breasts respond by gushing milk when her baby has given a hunger cry. The 'milk ejection response' is triggered by the hormone oxytocin – also called the 'cuddles' hormone – because it facilitates maternal behaviour and plays a role in both sexes by reducing anxiety and aggression and so facilitating long-term pair bonding and attachment. Oxytocin is thought to have evolved to regulate both sociosexual behaviours and physiological mechanisms encouraging fertilization and offspring survival. Mothers quickly learn to give their babies the stimulation to which they seem to respond. There are several effective ways to quiet a crying baby besides feeding. Most of these relate to the in-utero experience already described and include rhythmic movement, auditory stimulation and swaddling.

In summary, behaviours relating to crying, sucking, smiling, clinging, eye contact, sound and movement can be seen as important mechanisms fostering attachment. They are also mechanisms signalling the baby's genuine need for parental care. Generally the parents are the most significant people in a baby's environment, with the mother usually being the primary attachment figure. Typically, the parents' interaction with each other and with the baby will form the basis of its social, emotional and personality development. The quality of these early interpersonal interchanges is therefore crucial. By the second half of the first year of life, the infant will begin to develop an ethical system based on the world it has previously experienced – this is an integral part of psychological development, ensuring that the infant grows up to be a stable and well-rounded individual.

Unwanted birth and crime

Many lines of research make the connection between unwanted births and the offspring's greater than expected risk of criminality. Epidemiological studies clearly demonstrate that unwelcome children, born into harmful family environments, are more likely to be rejected and physically abused, and are also more likely to be delinquent. Investigations have repeatedly pointed out the connection between family size, religious denomination and the rate of delinquency, and have, interestingly, linked this to the gametopathy concept (Chapter 5). Studies in the UK have highlighted that Roman Catholics were over-represented among the prison population relative to their proportion in the population as a whole. This over-representation was not attributable to an overconcentration of Catholics among the poorer socioeconomic sectors of the community. To explain these puzzling observations, researchers put forward the hypothesis that unwanted children resulting from contraception failures are, simply, resented and more likely to suffer rejection and parental neglect.

There was a dramatic fall in the crime rate in the United States of America during the 1990s. Several hypotheses have been offered for this demographic change, but each had difficulty explaining the timing, large magnitude, persistence and widespread nature of the drop. The only hypothesis which consistently fits is that falling crime rates have, region by region, followed the legalization, roughly 20 years earlier, of abortion. Other studies support this hypothesis. In 1966, Nicolae Ceauşescu (authoritarian head of communist Romania) declared abortion illegal and children born following the abortion ban were significantly more likely to become criminals compared with children born earlier. Studies in other parts of Eastern Europe and Scandinavia from the 1930s through to the 1960s revealed a similar trend. Of the millions of women likely to have an abortion following Roe v Wade,[2] most are the poor, unmarried and teenage for whom illegal abortions had previously been too expensive, or too hard, to obtain. They are the very women whose children, if born, would have been much more likely than average to become criminals. Thus, Roe v Wade triggered, a generation later, the greatest crime drop in recorded US history. When a woman does not want a child she usually has a good reason, and many surveys suggest that domestic violence and abuse among

---

[2] A class action lawsuit that ultimately made it to the US Supreme Court. On 22 January 1973, the court ruled in favour of Ms Roe, allowing legalized abortion throughout the United States.

women is a strong motivation for seeking an abortion. The gametopathy hypothesis (reviewed in Chapter 5) highlights the consequences of the failure of political, religious, health and legal institutions to address the most fundamental injustice of our time – the inability of women to control their own fertility. Surely the evidence authenticates that social reform has to be spearheaded by reproductive health education, improved contraceptive care and the liberalization of abortion laws.

To bring a child into the world that one is not ready for and would, or might ultimately, resent, presents a huge social problem. Parents who physically and emotionally batter their children or isolate one to dominate are in need of help. Pathological feelings towards one's own child are not always effectively controlled and lead to gratuitous punishment like hitting, slapping, sulking and other forms of torment, including verbal, physical and sexual abuse. If a child is to thrive, its simple needs must be respected. These, in general, include gentle but unambiguous discipline mixed with gaiety, love and a sense of humour. Total consistency with the parent's own behaviour and what they communicate as acceptable behaviour for the child is essential for the healthy development of the sense of what is socially acceptable and what is not. To learn responsibility and a maturing familiarity with ethical judgement, children have to make conscious decisions of their own and know that those decisions have value and can be respected. This can be done very naturally because humans are able to communicate respect indirectly, and the message goes across by the way things are said. It is this non-verbal communication by body language which is so important in childhood. In order to mature, children have to be trusted. Effective maturing opportunities for kids are allowing them freedom within a protective, supportive environment and to do things on their own and with friends. In essence, to embrace responsible freedom, a child must be sufficiently loved, to feel it, and also to be able to give love.

Conditional love (that is, having to 'please' in order to 'earn' love) leaves the child confused, repressed and emotionally isolated. Common consequences of repressed development include hostility, anger, fear, cruelty and denial. An ever-present risk of thwarted emotional development is that the unhealthy aspects become the transgenerational legacy of maladjustment. For example, a mother (or surrogate) who appeals to emotional blackmail to get her way by resorting to sulking, crying or withdrawal, is dangerously manipulating the better nature of her child and violating the child's better sense of justice. The child's justified anger at invaded privacy and sense of betrayed justice may then begin to show itself in vengeful, maladjusted behaviour, such as using people for trivial advantage and escalating conflict points. Because the child feels radically powerless, he or she may develop a form of cruelty born out of helplessness, continuing feelings of guilt, worthlessness, disempowerment, isolation and grieving for lost opportunities. In extreme situations there is always the additional danger that the victims of abuse would perpetuate this ugliness when they have their own children, who become, in turn, unfit to raise a family.

When the human need to control others is extreme, we are facing a classic example of violence perpetuated. For example, some parents never let up; from the child's point of view there is no choice but to lash out violently as it is the only way in which he or she can gain some control for him- or herself – fighting aggression with aggression. Unfortunately, this originally adaptive strategy risks becoming a losing strategy as the child grows up. In the worst case scenario, the now maturing person will continue to seize control and dominate others, ending up just as dominating as the parents were. This example illustrates one of the means through which violence and fear are perpetuated from one generation to the next. It is frightening to consider how fascism, for example, profits from generations of abused children. According to psychohistorians, terrorists, dictators and dysfunctional leaders are not born but raised; thus, centuries of child abuse are reflected throughout history in recognizable patterns of institutionalized violence (Chapter 14). It is of interest to note that reliable accounts have documented that Josef Stalin, Adolf Hitler, Saddam Hussein, Slobodan Milosevic and Osama bin Laden were products of isolated and brutal rearing; all learned to hate before they learned to decide whether there was an issue to hate, and all found their recruits in the waste-land of lost childhood. Dysfunctional child rearing, however, does not have to be perpetuated into the next generation, and in most cases it is not, as a majority of abused children become exceptionally conscientious, decent adults who take care not to preserve what they have suffered.

In the above context it is interesting to note that some psychologists believe that anxiety very early in life may also prompt the child towards compassionate, intuitive behaviour. Intuition, or the ability to read others' needs and moods, is an especially valuable gift in circumstances when, instead of the mother (or surrogate) anticipating the child's needs, the child has to learn to anticipate the mother's needs. In circumstances where signals are confusing or threatening, anticipating the correct response becomes linked to survival, because not to anticipate creates even greater anxiety. The child, who is the victim of irrational, dysfunctional behaviour, tries - often unsuccessfully - to use intuition to create a sense of meaning and understanding when there is little or no evidence of either on the adult's part.

Post-traumatic stress disorder or the physical signature of unresolved trauma

Teachers and other professionals unfamiliar with traumatized children often ignore a child's tortuous thought processes and muddled words because the current system neither requires, nor provides, mechanisms for appropriate communication and training. In the event of a serious crime being committed, there is no automatic investigation into the family background and circumstances of the child, which would be admissible as evidence in mitigation. Children who appear to be properly fed and clothed and are attending school are, generally, not considered to be at risk. Such an attitude, however, abandons at-risk children because it means that unless parents are conspicuously negligent or abusive, society's preference has been for family self-rule. In recent years the Australian juvenile court system has been pro-active in matters of child justice by breaking free from family tradition of self-rule and considerably reshaping the Children Act, 1989, and the Criminal Justice Act, 1991. The courts now provide protection and psychological security to young defendants allegedly abused as proceedings are not open to the public, defendants' names cannot be disclosed, and reporting is restricted.

The brain is most plastic in early childhood and, given optimal experiences, it develops healthy, flexible and diverse capabilities. In abusive and neglectful environments, the process of normal neurodevelopment is disrupted as these children's brains are 'frozen' in a state of fear-related activation. The key neural systems activated by stress lead to adaptive changes in emotional, behavioural and cognitive functioning to promote survival in the short term; however, chronic brain activation triggers altered patterns of brain growth that may initiate the beginnings of neural pathology associated with anxiety, depression and impulsive aggression. Deep, emotional turmoil in children can be revealed by the combination of common physical symptoms of a fear state; these include hypervigilance, increased muscle tone, focus on threat-related cues, intermittent and selective stuttering, sleep walking and talking, nightmares, nervous facial and upper body ticks, nose-bleeds, high-pitched nervous laughter and bed-wetting (enuresis), including daytime incontinence. Behavioural symptoms may include expressive dirty and angry language, being loud, throwing things and having tantrums. Other not so easily recognized symptoms which may, however, signify anger or calling for help are eating disorders, somatic complaints such as irritable bowel syndrome, and post-traumatic stress disorder (see below). Chronic pain and illness is intended to make the parent (or surrogate) sorry or feel guilty when the ailing child's psychological and physical needs are not respected. Some neglected children have craved all their lives to be recognized but, owing to inappropriate behavioural responses when attention is focused on them, become still further isolated. Consequently, these insecure children may become withdrawn and unable to show their true feelings, including affection. The ongoing risk is that some of these disturbed children develop into shy, compassionless adults with low self-esteem and dangerous levels of resentment.

Exceptionally harsh treatment can trigger a 'last resort' biological reaction described as body–mind dissociation. During the aftermath of World War II, this phenomenon was documented in detail in children who had been traumatized by their experiences in Nazi concentration camps, or working as forced labourers in Germany. At the time the majority of these children were between the ages of 4 and 12. Dissociation in the worst cases was identified by a blankness of facial expression in conjunction with a degree of body self-control which could readily be interpreted as an incapacity to feel anything. Others, probably less affected, were either silent to the point of being catatonic or hyperactive, talking all day and night in their sleep. Some tolerated physical contact, others shrank into themselves at the least touch. What these children had in common was a traumatized mind which remained frozen, despite their improved situation.

Scientists have known for a long time now that life-threatening situations propel the body and mind to engage in the struggle for survival, by inactivating all non-essential activity and emotions and channelling all available energy into staying alive. This adaptation involves the stress response, the so-called 'fight or flight' mechanism, that is crucial for survival. However, when the stress response is too severe or sustained for too long, it has disastrous consequences for physical and mental health. In other words, the stress response is a good survival strategy in the short term but also carries long-term adverse effects (Chapter 7). One such long-term effect can be identified in the syndrome suffered by about 20% of individuals exposed to extreme trauma. The syndrome is termed post-traumatic stress disorder, a condition not new as it is the bane of the military, forming part of the 'collateral damage' of systematic human brutality. However, only through recent advances in neuroscience and neuroimaging technology has the condition become more identified physiologically. Normally the workings of the brain allow a gradual process of desensitization of raw emotions, allowing the victim to look back at the traumatic event with some detachment. Post-traumatic stress disorder sufferers, however, react with undiminished intensity years after the actual traumatic event. Specifically, they respond to unidentified, non-threatening environmental stimuli with flashbacks, not only of the sights and sounds but also the smells of past traumatic memories. Acutely, these flashbacks are powerfully played over and over in the present but cannot be controlled or altered. Thus, post-traumatic stress disorders generated in children can last for life and not be recognized. With advancing age and memory deterioration, the reliving of past traumas can become more frequent and sharpened.

Modern functional imaging technology has generated a dramatic increase in our understanding of the neural mechanisms underlying cognition, behaviour and moods. Mood is the consistent extension of emotion in time, while emotion is typically transient and responsive to the thoughts, activities and social situations of the day. Thus it is our mood – the state of our emotional balance – that powerfully influences the way in which we interact with and perceive the world. Emotion corresponds to an ancient signalling system that evolved millions of years ago in all mammalian species living in social groups. Emotion and emotional expression is the preverbal communication system genetically preprogrammed but shaped by life's experiences. As related above, from the very first, the newborn makes use of emotional signals of joy, sadness, anger and disgust to stimulate the parents to protect its basic needs. The free expression of these primary emotions, and their recognition, interacts to shape the quality of the bonds that develop between family members and is funda- mental to the brain's further development. Later, as the infant's brain develops, personalized configurations of brain connections expand to con- struct the mind – the individual's unique personality. Pure emotion becomes tempered with individual memories, experiences and cultural/private mean- ings. Significantly, attachment and emotional expression between parent and offspring go hand in hand with the development of the emotional self. Situations that promote intimacy, attachment and safety evoke expressions of emotional pleasure and moods of happiness; loss and threat engender the opposite. The development of the secondary emotions of shame, pride and guilt (sometimes referred to as the self-conscious emotions) rely upon the ability to make intelligent (cognitive) judgements against an acquired set of ethical standards. As mature adults, the secondary emotions dominate our social behaviour, the stability of social relationships and our personal ethical consciousness.

Intriguingly, one interesting attribute that almost all the children from the Nazi concentration camps had in common was an absolute rejection of any- thing that resembled moral value. The concepts of 'good' and 'evil' had no meaning for these children, as became apparent when attempts were made to explain the necessity of a few social rules. That adult disapproval could have no meaning is, of course, not surprising. In the older children, the experience of irrational cruelty induced a healthy scepticism for adult values, while the younger children had never had the opportunity to learn that what is agonizing for self could also be equally agonizing to others. As we now know, many genetic and environmental forces shape a child's innate level of ethical competence, its expression demands nurturing during infancy before it can be cognitively understood and practised in maturity. An infant's love relationships, for example, originate within the continuum of affection given by its carers at critical phases of brain development. Neglect can be deeply intractable, not least because it has neurological as well as psychological dimensions. Healthy development is nurtured as infants learn about the dimensions of love and affection, joy and anger, and fear. Disquietingly, we may well ask ourselves, as we see all those terrible childhoods of brutality, poverty and trauma around the world, whether these damaged children will continue to spread brutality and trauma and become the future 'militia' acting out unresolved stress.

The biology of behaviour and cognition

In human biology, the traditional approach to growth and development has been to address all kinds of physical changes in the body, from conception to death. Emotion, on the other hand, is a concept that has been largely ignored because it has to deal with feelings that are highly individual and which defy any attempt at objective biological definition. The growth process, from a single cell to some 10^{14} cells making up the adult human body, increasingly requires the interaction of genetic and environmental variables to mature the controlling networks which integrate complex structures, functions and behaviours. The most fundamental behaviours related to the maintenance of life, such as heartbeat and breathing, are involuntarily controlled by the phylogenetically older portions of the central nervous system (CNS) (the spinal cord, medulla and hypothalamus). Behaviours related to experience, on the other hand, are acquired gradually and are controlled by the newer portions of the CNS (particularly the cerebellum and cerebral cortex). As emphasized in Chapter 3 and illustrated in Figure 3.1, human brain development is exceptional and multiphasic, extending over the entire prenatal period and through the first 2–3 years of postnatal life. Almost all the neurons constituting the adult human brain are formed prenatally, mostly in the first 3 months, when neurological domains are formed. Subcortical structures controlling motor, sensory and reflex functions emerge first, followed by the development of the centres underlying instinct, emotional response and postural behaviour. These are succeeded by the cortical centres associated with higher functions involving attention, awareness and understanding. Cognition is a collective term for the psychological processes involved in the acquisition, organization and use of knowledge. It includes perception, memory, attention, problem-solving, language, thinking, judging, reappraising and imagery. Memory allows experience to become knowledge.

Emotions have an experiential component and play an essential role in growth and development, social relations, and mental and physical wellbeing. The distinction between 'physical' and 'mental' is, however, much less clearcut than previously believed, with the two continuously interacting via the neuroendocrine, immunological and other biological systems. The capability to express varying emotions appears progressively in the course of infant development, reflecting mainly genetic effects in the early stages, and psychosocial conditioning and environmental factors in later ones. Insufficient emotional stimulation and/or an excessive amount of negative stimulation in the early stages of life is likely to result in a higher risk of mental health problems down the track. On the positive side, however, the brain remains functionally plastic throughout the prenatal–neonatal periods and infancy, allowing it to adjust neurophysiologically and, increasingly, to adapt to the prevailing environment. Importantly, the brain's psychological achievements and consequent behavioural repertoire – which gradually characterize the adult personality – depend largely on the prenatal neurophysiological development and postnatal maturational accomplishments during infancy.

It is appropriate to remind the reader of the grounding information detailed in Chapter 3, where both normal and abnormal developmental processes are described. Just as brain-targeting teratogens, toxins like alcohol may cause primary damage during prenatal life which is then amplified by a cascade of secondary effects after birth, so dysfunctional family environments accompany a history of serious emotional troubles: childhood neglect and/or abuse, parental immaturity, alcoholism and a vulnerability to depression. In the present context, the long-term consequences of brain-targeting effects of parental lifestyle habits should be noted. The role of the early environment in relation to increased risk in adulthood of developing certain chronic diseases of adaptation may now be expanded to include behavioural functions susceptible to environmental manipulation at critical periods in behavioural growth and development. In this context, the importance of positive psychosocial factors during childhood cannot be overemphasized. In fact, some experts explicitly state that if society wants an effective, dynamic economy in 30 years' time, then good parenting is the key. Alternatively, how society will act 30 years down the track is what is happening to our children now. In essence, what the brain learns to feel in the early years is important for the future health of the economy and the social wellbeing of its citizens. What can be a stronger argument for universal investment in continuing parenting education?

The outcome of children raised in dysfunctional families is not completely negative. Recent studies have indicated that such children are much more resilient than previously suspected. In other words, for the child suffering extreme deprivation, the chances for recovery in an improved environment are far better than previously expected. The resilience of the human mind is powerfully illustrated by a group of children who had spent their first year in orphanages in Romania and who were adopted by nurturing British parents. When they arrived in London, the children were emaciated and psychologically deprived owing to their harsh institutionalized experiences. However, when the children were re-evaluated several years after their adoption, a majority, though not all, were similar in intellectual profile and social adjustment compared to the average British child. This was despite the fact that, when they were adopted, 78% of the orphans were delayed in fine and gross motor skills, and personal, social and language proficiency.

Psychologists tell us that there are two sensitive windows when institutionalization is especially likely to cause delays in emotional and cognitive development. These are the second half of the first year of life, and the period between 25 and 36 months when, typically, children experience the thrill and danger of moving away from their parents/providers as they search for their inner resources, strengths and independence. This crucial stage in development is best experienced in the ambiance of unconditional love.

Stress and psychosocial short stature

Good relational contact and stimulation heightens the infant's growth and survival prospects. For example, it has been known for centuries that infants confined to cold institutional environments have a very high morbidity and mortality rate. This phenomenon can be illustrated by what has become a classical study. The study compared children from two German war orphanages who, although receiving exactly the same measured amount of food, were found to show very different weight gain. The difference was identified as differing relational and emotional conditions between the staff and the inmates of the two orphanages. One orphanage treated the children kindly and they thrived; the other was run along authoritarian lines and the inmates wasted. The non-organic failure to thrive is universally recognized as a syndrome, variously called 'hospitalism', 'environmental retardation', 'maternal, emotional or psychosocial deprivation', but is best known as 'psychosocial short stature' and 'non-organic failure to thrive'. Failure to thrive in the absence of physical disease or disability is termed 'non-organic'. Recent studies of hospital records have provided substantial evidence that physical growth retardation can frequently not be attributed to any known organic factors but is instead associated with emotional problems. The condition has been found to occur in all countries, in all socioeconomic groups, and at all ages through to adolescence. The syndrome is now so widely accepted that it has become practice for conscientious paediatricians to warn parents that the failure of infants to thrive, when forced to stay in hospitals for relatively long periods of time, might be due to loneliness and emotional deprivation. As a result, many modern hospitals provide parents with domestic facilities and overnight accommodation adjacent to their children's quarters.

Non-organic failure to thrive used to be considered indicative of neglect, but it is not necessarily associated with frankly abusive or neglectful parenting. A cluster of factors that affect families seems to be important. These include single parenthood, overcrowding, low disposable income, parental ill health, dependence on social welfare, poor quality of maternal care, and parental drug and alcohol abuse. In both developed and developing countries, a similar association is found between stature and socioeconomic status, height correlating positively with wealth and privilege. Despite the fact that stress during critically sensitive periods in infancy is the crucial factor affecting growth and maturation, the condition is potentially reversible. When emotionally or physically abused children are removed from their environment, they usually start to grow at an accelerated rate. Investigations of endocrine dynamics show that psychosocial short stature children secrete very small quantities of growth hormone while living under conditions of high stress, and may not respond to therapy with exogenous growth hormone. Yet if they are removed from the abusive parent or stressful environment, there is often a rapid and spontaneous increase, to above normal levels, in their endogenous growth hormone, resulting in catch-up growth to a dramatic degree.

Future prospects

Since our future is a bid for survival, we must try not to become victims of other people's agenda. Adults who continue to abuse their children are not only passing on their responsibilities to the next generation but are opening themselves up for future litigation from their abused children. Children who have suffered throughout their lives as a result of early abuse may soon be able to prove neglect in courts of law. Scientists at McGill University (Quebec) have recently discovered important epigenetic differences between the brains of suicide victims who had experienced abuse as children and so-called normal control brains. Now energy is being directed at developing a blood DNA diagnostic test for persons suffering mental distress who may be at risk of committing suicide. The hope is that these telltale punctuated DNA marks would lead to treatments that may possibly erase them and reverse their stress-combating programme. Long-term trauma is especially acute following incest and other forms of sexual abuse, a particularly disturbing topic not specifically addressed in this review. Naturally, the sexual violation of children is a subject that strikes, in most, an immediate visceral response of disgust. Transgenerational abuse of all forms has to stop and child welfare should be factored in every public decision made.

When a child is born into an abusive community and subsequently suffers emotional problems, the fault does not, necessarily, have to lie solely with the mother, father or other family members. A large proportion of the blame has to lie at the community level, for accepting and tolerating fellow human beings living in abusive situations over which they have little or no control. Every citizen must accept some responsibility for the health and wellbeing of the children and grandchildren living within their community. All of us have an obligation to work together and find new ways to bring child raising within universally acceptable standards. If we do not, we cannot guarantee a sustainable future on this planet. The indicators of poverty (such as ill health, poor nutrition, excessive alcohol consumption, poor water and food supplies, inadequate shelter and high rates of community violence) are also, typically, indicators of a higher than expected risk of child abuse. But this is not necessarily so, since affluence too may generate its own problems with abuse. Those who maintain that large-scale infrastructural reform cannot be afforded should consider that prevention is cheaper than cure. If we juxtapose severe crowding, poverty, inequality of resource distribution (both within and between national boundaries) against the physiology of stress, then social instability and problems threatening global peace seem more understandable, and wars predictable. The critical issues here are social justice, fairness and ethics in core economics – not key issues shaping our present-day culture. We are, therefore, propelled to look ahead and do what we can to work towards a valid ethics, by reducing the plethora of preventable abuse-induced disabilities in children. A valid ethics, for starters, may entail responsible reproduction and an acceptance that the right to reproduce is also a privilege, not to be taken lightly.

Worldwide, millions of children are used as cheap factory workers or free labourers in the home. Working children enjoy little, if any, of their childhood, and are deprived of their right to a good education. Such physical and mental exploitation is unacceptable. To take a daughter or son for granted and to exploit this potentially free individual as if it were 'property' is a gross abuse of power. Adults often glamorize the idea of large families and children growing up together, but children should learn the world from adults, not solely from other children. Too frequently, children are used to bring up their younger siblings. This represents a denial of parental obligations. We should never attempt to take responsibility for more children than we can give adequate attention to. If there are too many mouths to feed, too many to support spiritually and financially, parents become overwhelmed and unable to give enough. The children then begin to compete with each other for the adult's time and resources, and some may also begin the cycle of real or perceived neglect. It may be appropriate at this stage to quote Erica Jong: 'We would do well to baby each other instead of making all these unwanted babies that no one has time to nurture or to love' (from *Fear of Fifty*, p. 352).

Principles of bioscience ethics for discussion

- A 2004 study found that one in eight soldiers returning from Iraq reported symptoms of post-traumatic stress disorder. A 2007 study found that inhibiting the activity of a molecule in the brain called Cdk5 helps to eliminate fears learned in traumatic contexts. By applying this knowledge, it is now possible to provide an anxiety-reducing drug when traumatic times are predictable. In your view, should soldiers be given memory-blunting agents on the eve of combat to fortify memory extinction of unwanted memories? Might not therapeutic forgetting desensitize combatants, or terrorists, to commit repugnant acts which, if constrained by shame and guilt, they would never think of doing? On the other hand, when society demands that soldiers participate in the horrors of warfare, does it also carry the responsibility to help those soldiers get through the aftermath of having been part of that horror?
- A major research effort is being directed to the development of memory-enhancing drugs. The effort is primarily aimed at finding treatments for dementia (such as for Alzheimer's disease), but includes developments that could enhance normal memory, particularly in middle and older age when a degree of increased forgetfulness is normal. Memory-enhancing drugs target the molecular mechanisms involved in memory consolidation and exploit the stress-driven adrenergic system that spontaneously becomes overactive in those suffering from anxiety disorders. Give reasons why a precautionary approach is critical when memories are manipulated to alter their emotional content. Are there any ethical implications?

- Scientists have drawn attention to the need for parental responsibility to commence well before the child is born. Should the quest for 'good parenting' shift from individual to shared concern? Some activists have argued that an effectual step towards protecting children is by adopting an enforceable child protection policy. Do you agree or disagree and why?
- In order to develop a mature conscience capable of responsible ethical judgement, the child has to be sufficiently loved. Does this statement seem sound to you and, if so, can current biological knowledge be used to enhance the value of human love? Discuss the distinction between practical and pathological love.

7

The state of wellbeing: basic principles, coping strategies and individual mastery

A life course approach says that the management of adult chronic disease cannot be separated from the management of women in pregnancy and children.[1]

Modern technological advances have offered humans, especially those living in industrialized communities, innumerable opportunities to enjoy a more comfortable, healthier and proficient lifestyle. The rapid expansion of scientific knowledge and medical skills has provided options that could not have been anticipated by those living one or two generations ago. This newfound knowledge has, in general, reinvigorated interest in 'the meaning of life' issues and stimulated vigorous debates, ranging from right-to-procreation to right-to-die concerns. Unfortunately, our unprecedented medical successes and 'wonder' cures have effectively encouraged health service providers in the belief that, given time, science will successfully meet all health challenges. In turn, this attitude has generated a mental passivity or confidence that biomedical technology can, indeed, take care of all our health problems. As we enjoy the advantages of the modern biomedical revolution, it is opportune to reassess modern and ancient insights with a view to integrating the essentials of healing and wellbeing. In biological terms, health and ill health are not alternative states; rather they are part of the same continuum. This concept is well expressed in an old Filipino saying: 'Ang sakit ng kalingkingan ay sakit ng buong katawan' or 'a pain in the little finger is something the whole body

[1] Dr Tarun Weeranmanthri on 'Mastering the Control Factor'. ABC Radio National – The Health Report transcript 30 November 1998, p. 12 (http://www.abc.net.au/rn/talks).

suffers' (Leonardo Castro, personal communication). Traditional wisdom, as in the quote above, is also supported by a rapidly growing research-based literature, particularly that of stress physiology. Since the early 1950s, researchers have identified key factors in the generation and maintenance of physical, psychological and social wellbeing, the most notable being that a sense of control over our lives promotes wellbeing more powerfully than an appropriate command of behaviours such as smoking, diet and exercise.

Health, as defined in the Constitution of the World Health Organization (WHO), is a state of 'complete physical, mental and social wellbeing, not merely the absence of disease or infirmity'. A disease, disorder or injury, according to WHO, produces impairment. Impairment implies a change in the normal structure or function of the body or part of the body which may lead to disability or a reduction/loss of the ability to perform certain activities. The above WHO classifications are consistent with modern ethical principles in medicine as they reflect issues surrounding responsible empowerment over patient health, such as adherence to informed patient consent, respect for patient confidentiality, frankness about medical uncertainties and justice. They are also consistent with the various international bodies of human rights law; such as the United Nations Committee on Economic, Social and Cultural Rights issued in 2000, which treat health as a human right and proclaim 'the right of everyone to the enjoyment of the highest attainable standard of physical and mental health' and obligates state parties to respect that right by providing appropriate health care in the event of sickness. While personal mastery is becoming a top priority in sickness, disappointingly, its practical implications in the maintenance of the continuum of wellness derived from the holistic context of life have been neglected.

Embedded within the concept of wellbeing are the psychobiological mechanisms related to stress physiology that explain why some of us become ill while others, in seemingly similar circumstances, stay well. The stress response occurs whenever an individual is faced with a challenge; however, the health effects depend on the combination of demand and recovery necessary to rebalance the body's adaptive systems. Physical variables, such as serum cholesterol baseline levels, blood pressure and lifestyle factors like smoking, are significant but need to be understood within the holistic context of empowerment. To reduce the risk of succumbing to acute or chronic disease states, psychobiological variables that lower the body's resilience to environmental challenges need to be understood and factored into the equation. Therefore, lifestyle diseases such as atherosclerosis, hypertension, diabetes, cancer and disorders such as post-traumatic stress syndrome and depression must be taken within the context of life in the family, the community, socioeconomic status and important incidents in childhood. The importance of the dynamics, and often precarious interactions between genetic and epigenetic factors in the maintenance of long-term health, cannot be overemphasized. Previous chapters emphasized how stresses, which impair growth and development during critical periods in fetal life or infancy, can significantly elevate the risk of disease in the adult. The present chapter builds on this understanding by focusing on ways in which wellbeing can be improved through self-sustaining behaviour, advanced by heightened personal empowerment. Key aspects in the control of health and ill health are identified and ways that individuals can best determine the limits of their inner resilience are explored.

The link between population density and reproduction

A key factor affecting our physical health relates to our psychosocial way of being in the world. Pioneering work in the 1950s by Calhoun demonstrated that rats placed in a confined space with shelter and unlimited food and allowed to breed freely, curtailed their breeding in response to the reduction in space rather than the availability of food. Subsequently, Christian's groundbreaking research demonstrated a direct link between population increase, adrenocortical activation (or heightened stress levels), immune deficiency and reduced fertility. Scientists have given much thought over the nature of 'space', which prevents social creatures, such as humans and rats, from expressing their full reproductive potential. We now know that the population density of a given animal species in a particular environment is rarely dependent on its breeding potential. Rather, densities fluctuate, sometimes widely, but tend to return to a relatively narrow range known as the carrying capacity. The mechanisms underlying this tendency are inbuilt into the species' physiology and confer survival value.

Increased circulating levels of the stress hormones, cortisol in particular, adaptively re-set the body's equilibrium by adjusting the neuroendocrine control mechanisms of practically every physiological system. Homeostatic control and physiological fine-tuning work because the stress response is directed via neuroendocrine signals generated during social interactions. The inverse relationship between crowding stress and fertility is just one example illustrating the many psychosocial adaptive responses simultaneously at work. If a population continues to breed, exceeding the limit that can be sustained by the resources in the habitat, the subsequent generation will have its resources (particularly food) seriously depleted. A well-directed stress response achieves group fitness by increasing the odds on survival of the species, albeit at the expense of the individual. Group survival is an adaptive evolutionary strategy which has served us well (group selection is described in Chapter 1). Although the same micro-evolutionary processes regulating animal populations are operational across all species, humans might seem to be an exception. Nevertheless, we do not live outside Nature's laws; it is just that we are skilled at transforming the world around us and clever in ways that our populations are organized. Nature's means evolved to curb non-adaptive high fertility rates and modern developments in assisted conception/contraception devices (Chapter 9) have up till now bought us precious time.

Stress – the General Adaptation Syndrome (GAS), allostasis and disease

The physiological basis of stress was further interpreted and refined by Hans Selye, whose many contributions culminated in the description of the General Adaptation Syndrome, or GAS. The GAS (also known as 'reactive homeostasis' or the 'fight or flight' response) emphasizes the role of the hypothalamic–pituitary–adrenal axis in the adaptation to stress. Selye borrowed the engineering term 'stress', signifying fatigue in metal under strain, to describe the body's adaptive response to any challenge placed on it. 'Allostasis', so critical for survival, describes the mechanisms which enable the body to withstand challenge. The word allostasis is derived from the Greek '*allo*', meaning 'variable', and '*stasis*', meaning 'stability', and literally means 'achieving stability through change'. Allostatic systems, in particular the nervous, hormonal and immune complexes, protect the body by adapting to the ever-changing internal and external demands made on it. Allostatic load refers to the price of adaptation; that is, the accumulated wear and tear from chronic over- or under-activity of the allostatic systems. The allostatic load concept explains an apparent paradox of stress physiology; namely, why the protective mechanisms activated by stress increase resistance to stress in the short term, while chronic allostatic activation during prolonged stress damages and weakens the allostatic complex. Acute stress is an essential function that protects our bodies against demanding life events and can actually boost wellbeing, as it increases arousal and attention. Acute stress also enhances our immunity. Chronic stress, whether physical or psychological, depresses our immune system function through an over-production of the stress hormones.

Current psychoneuroendocrine advances in the biology of stress are predominantly driven by social scientists, as it is they who are resolving the apparent paradoxes underlying the different roles of adaptation and their relation to the concept of wellbeing. Questions such as 'how does stress influence the pathogenesis of disease', and 'what accounts for the variation in vulnerability to stress-related diseases among people with similar life experiences', have to be understood before there can be further medical progress in the maintenance of the continuum of wellbeing. The findings of the multifaceted longitudinal studies by Michael Marmot (University College, London) and an extensive team of scientists have been crucial in providing answers to questions such as those posed above. These many-faceted investigations, collectively identified as the Whitehall Studies, meticulously recorded the lives of cohorts of British civil servants from different socioeconomic hierarchies. A highly significant finding was that morbidity and mortality rates mirrored the social gradient (that is, the employment level), with a fourfold difference in disease rate, top to bottom. As expected, the individuals at the top, consisting of senior executives and heads of the British Civil Service agencies, were the healthiest. What was unexpected, however, was the shape of the social gradient, with those at step 2 (professionals, executives, doctors and lawyers) suffering a disease rate twice as high as those at the very top. A similar stepwise illness gradient has now been established for virtually every disease studied and seems to be the norm for industrialized nations.

While none of the civil servants in the Whitehall Studies could be considered as being poor, we can accept that individuals at the very bottom of the social scale generally suffer higher rates of morbidity because of their relative deprivation owing to lower income, lower education, poorer medical care and poorer housing. The critical factor explaining the unexpected findings at step 2 of the social hierarchy was identified as insufficient self-control of one's working life. The lower down a person is in social standing, the less opportunity and training that person has to influence the events that impinge on his or her life. Consequently, it is not the high-powered executive who succumbs to stress-related disease, but the person below who has been instructed in what he or she has to achieve, with very little flexibility in decision-making and ways of achieving set work targets. The resultant feeling of impotency describes people who have very high work demands placed on them, but little latitude or discretion for dealing with these demands. It is these people who suffer the highest rates of disease. 'Demand latitude' describes the degree of flexibility in dealing with work and/or social situations.

Laboratory experiments have corroborated these human findings. When an experimental animal is subjected to a trauma it has no control over, the motivation to escape to avoid this ordeal significantly diminishes. Dogs, for example, when given an inescapable electric shock, typically develop what psychologists term 'learned helplessness'; that is, rapidly giving up any attempt to escape, even when the possibility of escape becomes available.

When an individual learns that an outcome is independent of his or her reaction, it has profound emotional and physical effects. The loss of control over external events in some circumstances may also produce an overall powerlessness or learned helplessness. Ironically, the belief that one has lost control over one's fate and is in a helpless situation all together may be more imagined than real. There are distinctions in the ways individuals view uncontrollable distressing events – some believe that life's rewards are to be found internally and through their own efforts and abilities, while others rely more on external events or chance happenings. Self-trust is empowering. It provides confidence from the freedom of knowing how to construct solutions suitable for life's challenges. Mastery over one's life is not really a question of intelligence; rather it is the confidence that one is empowered to respond adaptively to environmental challenges by virtue of training and experience. Paradoxically, however, powerless people often achieve less because lack of power itself erodes cognitive functioning. Therefore, mastery of day-to-day encounters should definitely be a skill taught early in any child's life. Families where children are encouraged in creative ways of managing their destiny soon enjoy the follow-on benefits in social harmony, thus highlighting the importance of 'empowering' early in life to stimulate the full expression of innate cognitive abilities.

In the consideration of health, two sets of interrelated relationships need to be identified. The first set of relationships includes physical or lifestyle risk factors such as elevated serum cholesterol levels, high blood pressure or smoking which are linked, albeit imperfectly, to the occurrence of disease (imperfectly because all known risk factors for, for example, heart disease combined may account for only 25–35% of the disease gradient). Risk factors by themselves are useful, but not necessarily predictive of disease because the disease risk of people with equivalent levels of smoking, blood pressure and plasma cholesterol is still powerfully related to position in the social hierarchy.

The second set of risk factors is psychosocial relationships. For example, how much control have you in the workplace: are you part of an integrated social network; do you live in a situation of interpersonal conflict, or in a dangerous neighbourhood? All of the above may, potentially, produce a chronic state of anxiety and/or vigilance. So it can be seen that social factors dramatically control an individual's behaviour. Smoking, for example, may be a behavioural way of reducing anxiety which, in turn, affects the body's defence systems, increasing the risk of diseases of adaptation such as arteriosclerosis.

Psychoneuroimmunology investigates how loss of personal control adversely modifies hormonal secretory profiles, causing a cascade of secondary ill health effects. An individual's inability to cope with the environment creates a

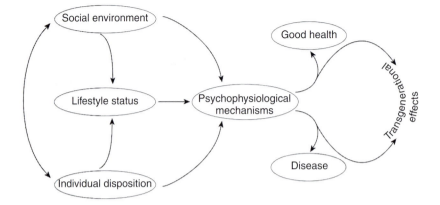

Figure 7.1 An overview of the broad domains of variables affecting health and wellbeing or the onset of disease. (Reproduced from Pollard, I. (2005). Bioscience-bioethics and life factors affecting reproduction with special reference to the Indigenous Australian population. *Reproduction* **129**, Fig. 4, p. 399, with permission.)

physiological situation which leads to the gradual degeneration of the body. Children who have chronically high allostatic loads are at increased risk of developing insulin-dependent diabetes and other serious lifestyle diseases.

Since the body's defence system is compromised by stressful social variables that affect quality-of-life issues, it is appropriate to agitate for social improvements that allow communities to become familiar with necessary healing mechanisms. Dry, factual health information alone is unproductive unless the information is supported by additional survival skills. This is not a criticism of the medical profession who, in industrialized nations in particular, have succeeded in significantly reducing major risk factors, such as smoking, in the adult population. Nevertheless, children in these same nations are taking up smoking at an alarmingly increasing rate. Surveys of young smokers have unequivocally demonstrated that they intellectually understand the health risks involved, but smoke anyhow. This brings us back full circle, emphasizing that the ability to control decisions depends on changed behaviour, which requires relevant information within the context of empowerment. If children with a sense of mastery over their lives are provided with the information they need, they will use their mastery to advantage and structure their own decisions in light of the best information available. Since behavioural change is mostly ineffectual by 'top-down' proclamations, parents and professionals need to empower children so that they can participate fully in the events that impinge on their own lives across the generations. Figure 7.1 provides an overview of the broad domains of variable genetic and epigenetic interactions that shape the social health gradient. It can be seen how psychophysiological mechanisms may either weaken individual genetic susceptibilities to disease or elicit a strong positive response influencing health and wellbeing. We know that children who have experienced a good prenatal environment and were well nurtured in their early years have better outcomes throughout their lives. We also know that lack of control over one's life engages harmful dynamics symptomatic of disempowerment, depression and environmental deterioration, and that these harmful dynamics may self-perpetuate across subsequent generations.

Adaptive strategies

To summarize, an individual's inability to cope effectively with life's challenges creates a mental state which, in turn, creates a physiological situation predisposing to the gradual degeneration of the body. But what can best be done? There are a number of counteracting strategies which can assist us to cope more effectively with our allostatic load, or even bring the body back to full homeostatic balance. Health is balance – balancing the yin and yang of life, so to speak. We know that isolation is harmful because it increases allostatic load, while social support and expressing one's emotions and anxieties reduces allostatic load which, in turn, increases survival by moderating the pattern of stress hormone secretion. It is interesting to note that during the great depression of the 1930s suicide was a rare phenomenon yet since the 1980s, in Australia, one of the most privileged societies in the world, its rate has climbed significantly. During the depression everyone was in a similarly disheartening situation and the recognition of a level playing field helped in coping with hardship.

Another insight comes from the realization that individuals who use humour to cope with stress have a more resilient immune system and age more gracefully. Laughter involves a unique form of consciousness that operates within a cultural context and provides a therapeutic respite from the everyday clutter of thought. Thus, humour – as it enables us to experience pleasure even when faced with adversity – is the perfect antidote to stress. Researchers have long identified that laughter can lower cortisol levels and thereby protect our immune system. More recently, by means of functional magnetic resonance imaging technology, researchers have established that positive sounds, such as laughter, trigger a strong response in the listener's premotor cortical region of the brain that primes the muscles in the face for laughing. By actively interacting and mirroring the behaviour of others in one's group, we are promoting social bonding that assists feelings of security and wellbeing. Moreover, psychoimmunologists have confirmed what we all know instinctively, that the immune system is boosted by helping others and even just hearing about other people's good work appears to boost our immunity. The scientific evidence again confirms the point that not only are we physiologically constructed to need others, we are also constructed to want to be needed. During critical periods in our evolution, *Homo sapiens'* social drive for personal survival became interdependent with our collective survival (Chapter 1). Put in anthropomorphic terms 'our immune system knows that helping others ultimately helps our own wellbeing'. The same insight is common to all religious faiths, whether Hindu, Muslim, Christian, Jewish, Buddhist or any other. In all cases, religious faith is preoccupied with rendering service to the Deity and fellow human beings. To quote from the Bhagavad-Gita '. . . every living being is constantly engaged in rendering service to another living being. A living being serves other living beings in various capacities. By doing so, the living entity enjoys life', and 'In this way we can see that no living being is exempt from rendering service to other living beings, and therefore we can safely conclude that service is the constant companion of the living being and that the rendering of service is the eternal religion of the living being'.[2]

Forms of contemplative practice, such as meditation, are also effective in overcoming and treating stress-related states. The contemplative customs practised in many cultures evoke decreases in heart rate, breathing and blood pressure. Compared to controls, individuals who meditate enjoy significantly increased alpha brainwave activity (low frequency brainwaves that occur during relaxation), increased orderliness of brain activity, and a unique form of consciousness different from relaxation states. Meditation also has a positive health effect in cancer treatment, with a notable study showing tumour cell growth rates to be significantly decreased in prostate cancer patients who practise Zen Buddhist meditation. One of several possible mechanisms by which meditation may relieve the physiological symptoms of stress is through the release of nitric oxide. Nitric oxide is an antagonist of the stress hormone noradrenaline released in preparation for the fight or flight response. Nitric oxide dilates noradrenaline-constricted vessels and restores efficient blood flow. Nitric oxide is also linked to the release of endorphins – our natural body opiates that counter pain and produce feelings of wellbeing. The new concordance between science and spiritual practice is timely because, in order to survive adaptively, present-day culture is more and more dependent on our ability to cope with new possibilities requiring emotional flexibility. In an age

[2] Bhaktivedanta Swami Prabhupāda, A. C. (1998). *Bhagavad-Gita: As it is*. Mumbai, India: The Phaktivedanta Book Trust, p. 19.

of rapid technological advances, intelligent flexibility makes evolutionary sense. However, to access a level of new-found freedom and wellbeing, we may also have to break with outmoded belief systems and constraints, even if this means losing or reworking some aspects of our valued heritage.

The most important advantage arising from advancements in medical neuroscience is the realization that we are not totally passive recipients of our mental states but possess powerful mechanisms that bring about changes in the underlying chemistry of how our brains function. The strength of this realization carries bioscience ethical significance as it touches on personal responsibility and treatment of sociopsychological problems affecting community health and wellbeing. Simply, by focusing the mind, as in forms of contemplative practice, we can now demonstrate scientifically that our minds have the power – or neuroplasticity – to affect our thoughts in adaptive ways. This knowledge provides us with a means of changing the inner wiring of our brains in ways that could promote cultural change touching on quality-of-life issues.

A key future health objective must be the promotion of wellbeing. This includes development of a positive sense of fulfilment, capability and pleasure in life as well as strategies to cope with loss and depression. A relatively recent social challenge, attributable to the biomedical revolution, is that a smaller percentage of individuals have to progressively support and nurture a growing ageing population. Support for the old is particularly pertinent to the industrialized world, where it is feared that the infrastructure supporting education, childcare, single parent allowance, sickness and disability pay will be eroded. It is also feared that an unhealthy generational top-heaviness may result in unpleasant political confrontation between the young and old, generating social instability. Since it was new medical knowledge which has given the ageing – but now not so old – innumerable opportunities to enjoy better health, it is now time for ageing but savvy elders to challenge social change wisely by contributing more fully.

The search for meaning is a natural and ordinary part of human nature. Indigenous cultures all over the world have always known what psychoimmunological research has recently demonstrated empirically. There is no indigenous culture without its spiritual tradition – whether it be the rite of passage into adulthood involving greater responsibility, or initiation rituals conferring the status of 'wise elder' commanding a deeper service to the clan. In this context, several hypotheses exist regarding the evolutionary advantage of the menopause apart from the obvious reproductive ones. From the social perspective, the menopause may have an adaptive advantage enabling some older women to pass on acquired wisdom and skills. By eliminating the special hazards of late childbirth, there was an improved chance of women living on and some of these becoming wise to the benefit of their tribe and clan. For our hunter–gatherer ancestors, the only means of passing on knowledge was by example, demonstration or word of mouth, and elders of a tribe were given special status in return for knowledge and advice. This still holds true for many Indigenous peoples, including the Australian Indigenous population.

In the modern context, our elders may well design new 'businesses' with the focus not wholly on making money but on returning something on a sustainable basis. Such a mutualistic approach may well assist in breaking down traditional boundaries between giving and taking, between dependence on charity and reciprocity. The section on 'Fundamental symbiosis' in Chapter 12 describes how, in Nature, it is the rule for two or more organisms to evolve together for mutual benefit, and that symbiotic associations are the fundamental ecological processes of life. Healthy elderly citizens may well profit from creative, sustainable endeavours which are part love, part business, part education, part recreation, and part whatever seems personally authentic. Renewed access to creativity, heightened motivation and vision will, in turn, free up the ageing brain and lead to more satisfying living. Survival in our present-day culture increasingly depends on the ability to cope with new possibilities, rather than stability which used to be equated with emotional survival. Stability encourages resistance to change – not a good evolutionary strategy in an age of rapid technological advances. Breaking from conditioned beliefs, whether they be age constraints or other valued traditions, may help each one of us to access a level of new-found freedom and wellbeing. After all is said and done, the perception of stress is very personal so it is not so much what one changes but how one changes.

Principles of bioscience ethics for discussion

- The feeling of control over our lives promotes wellbeing more powerfully than appropriate command over behaviours such as smoking, diet and exercise. So why is it that, while personal mastery becomes a top priority in sickness, so little emphasis is placed on the continuum of wellness?
- Helping others augments the efficiency of our immune system and, amazingly, just hearing about other people's good works appears to also boost our immunity. Reflect on the adaptive value of this biological characteristic.
- Health and ill health are deeply dependent on the conditions under which we live and the ways in which we behave. How may bioscience ethics assist in deciding the kinds of societies we want to live in and how to achieve these goals?

8

The state of wellbeing: on the end-of-life care and euthanasia

> Caring control takes place when medical professionals or public health authorities refuse to act according to the patient's wishes, or they restrict the patient's freedom or in other ways attempt to influence the patient's behavior, allegedly in the patient's own best interest.[1]

The previous chapter focused on the biological basis of happiness and wellbeing; this chapter focuses on justice and freedom when the process of dying has already begun. Freedom can be seen as the ability to decide for ourselves what happens in our lives without excessive constraints; that is, being in control. Of course, as social creatures, we are never totally free, even when we are not actively hindered from doing what we wish to do. The defining attributes of freedom have always collided with age-old debates on the meaning and value of human life which, in the contemporary context, have fuelled passionate discourse about the significance of abortion and euthanasia. Many contend that it is morally wrong to terminate an unwanted pregnancy or to give a lethal injection to a terminally ill patient who wishes to die expeditiously and without excessive pain. In the latter context, the act of euthanasia is understood as termination of life on request. Pro-life proponents see euthanasia as violating the principle of the sanctity of human life. Others maintain that such an inflexible stance is socially destabilizing because it is based on doubtful ethical principles and inaccurate understanding of the power of modern medicine. Most of us genuinely believe that human life has special value and that it is wrong to destroy it wantonly except, evidently, in

---

[1] Hayry, H. (1998). *Individual Liberty and Medical Control*. Aldershot, UK: Ashgate, p. 14.

specific circumstances, such as killing in battle which is considered by many as a 'sacred act' (Chapter 14).

The sanctity of life principle is recognized in the prohibition of unlawful homicide, which retains its absolute force irrespective of the quantity or kind of life in question. In this respect, all human life is absolutely inviolable and equally valuable. It follows, therefore, that doctors must never take life but are duty-bound to protect and prolong it whenever and however they can. By contrast, an alternative principle recognizes extenuating circumstances and maintains that sophisticated high-tech medicine needs to be balanced by imaginative insight, compassion and acceptance that conscious adjustment to awesome technological capabilities is inevitable. As a result, social, scientific and judicial preoccupations have moved away from an emphasis on preservation of life at any cost, favouring the inclusion of quality-of-life considerations. Consequently, in particularly difficult clinical situations, the medical profession has come to a form of consensus by supporting the ethical rights of doctors and others in the caring professions, not to undertake treatment which is contrary to their conscience. To this effect, 'do not resuscitate' orders are routinely utilized.

Life's balance sheet

All organisms have finite lifespans where the core issue in ageing is to resolve environmental effects and endogenous ageing processes – to be alive means to be mortal. The seeds of individual ageing are found before birth and reflect genetically programmed regulatory systems which evolved hundreds of millions of years ago. These systems determine the level of molecular and cellular repair mechanisms in specific tissues and organs. Statistics show us that arterial disease and cancer are the main causes of death across ageing human populations yet are low until after 35 years of age, which was approximately the life expectancy in most human populations before the nineteenth century. Ageing increases the load of oxidative damage in DNA, lipids and proteins; for example, accumulation of oxidized lipids in the aorta and other central arteries begins during prenatal life and marks the beginning of arterial ageing which progresses to a greater or lesser extent depending on circumstance (Chapter 3). The main causes of early death are extrinsic risks such as infections, malnutrition and trauma. These extrinsic risks, until very recently, allowed just a minority of humans to survive to older ages.

In the course of the death process, nervous, endocrine and cognitive functions, in particular, display marked declines. Gerontologists refer to this phenomenon as 'terminal drop'. The terminal drop may linger for weeks or years and is the critical period where the impending future, distant past and heavy present coalesce. It is a time for appraising the ideals of independence, participation, care, self-fulfilment, dignity and for gaining, hopefully, peace of mind. However, for the contemporary citizen living with limitless developments of modern technologies, the question is asked 'who should take responsibility for determining death?'

End-of-life care, advanced directives and 'do not resuscitate' orders

There are valid reasons behind the search for new criteria which define the beginning and the end of a meaningful human life. Two such criteria can be found by focusing on consciousness, and by measuring the value of individual lives through directly consulting the individual concerned. Consciousness, generally regarded as the hallmark of a true existence, represents the ability to choose and decide to take action and assess reaction. Many argue that it is against this notion of conscious ability that quality of life should be measured. In essence, quality of life reflects an elusive individual perception about one's position in life within specific cultural and ethical contexts, and relates to one's personal goals, expectations, standards and level of awareness – it can be known only by the individual concerned. However, there is also total agreement that one of the most difficult issues in biomedical ethics today is the question of killing or letting people die.

While modern medicine has increased its capacity to cure and to prolong life, it has also generated serious bioethical difficulties. Scientific advances, including treatments for the extremely low birthweight infant, for example, are achieving cures or amelioration of many afflictions which in the past resulted in death or severe handicap. Assisted by complex life-supporting technologies, such as mechanical ventilators and dialysers, the functions of most failing organs can be maintained for prolonged periods of time. As a result, the previously incurably ill now have a chance of survival. There can be no doubt that modern high-tech equipment together with skilled surgery has significantly increased the survival rate and quality of life of the seriously ill, including neonates and infants with severe malformations. However, there are still many for whom modern technology achieves little more than delaying death or averting it at the cost of permanent ill health, unhappiness and lifelong handicap. Such case histories have magnified concerns, as demonstrated by the plethora of existing discussion papers on withholding and withdrawing life-prolonging treatments and do not resuscitate (CPR or cardiopulmonary resuscitation) orders. A 'do not resuscitate' (DNR) order is a written order from a doctor that resuscitation should not be attempted in the event of a cardiac or respiratory arrest. The withholding or withdrawing of artificial life support is practised in situations where, despite all care, there is little or no hope of recovery; this includes patients in whom the quality of life is unacceptably poor, where the dying process is prolonged, causing severe distress, or where the patient is in a permanent vegetative state. In all of the above cases, reaching a satisfactory outcome involves addressing a number of difficult ethical and legal issues, including issues of over- or under-treatment towards the end of life.

It goes without saying that when life-support treatment is withdrawn, palliative care to relieve pain and distress is essential. Analgesics and sedatives are routinely given, even though they may coincidentally shorten life. On the other hand, despite technological capabilities to prolong life well beyond what is considered to be the limits of the natural term of life, physicians are still trying, in the Hippocratic spirit, to preserve human life whenever possible. This is in the face of a growing suspicion concerning the quality, or value, of the life counterbalanced against the procedures used to maintain bodily functions. Life-support systems are complicated and usually cause pain, sometimes to such an extent that patients openly express their wish to die rather than continue living under such extraordinary circumstances. Some physicians have been reluctant to come to terms with the validity of the patient's wish to die, but many patients label this intransigence as medical paternalism. Medical paternalism is characterized by an attitude that the patient's wishes may be ignored or not respected because patients, unlike the supervising physician, cannot know what is best for them. Particular criticism, however, is reserved for the indiscriminate use of medical technology on severely handicapped and dying neonates. Some critics have even maintained that the practice of indiscriminately treating and repeatedly operating on nonviable infants amounts to human experimentation and child abuse. The death of an infant is a devastating experience for the parents, made even more difficult by the burden of guilt associated with having to decide whether extreme medical intervention is appropriate for their critically ill baby. In a climate of accusation and counter-accusation, it becomes particularly difficult for all well-meaning physicians who, to protect themselves from prosecution, cannot risk forgoing reckless treatments. Doctors have a duty to give priority to patients on the basis of clinical need, while seeking to make the best use of resources using up-to-date evidence about the clinical efficacy of treatments. Doctors must also take care not to allow their views about particulars, such as a patient's age, disability, gender, race, colour, culture, belief, sexuality, social or economic status and lifestyle, to prejudice the choices of treatment offered or the general standard of care provided.

Because of the complexities of modern medicine, the sick, the frail or those in advanced old age are experiencing significant additional anxiety as they wonder whether they have lost the right to an earlier easier death, in harmony with human dignity. As a consequence, advanced directives, or living wills, have gained popularity among those who wish to maintain control over their lives. Advanced directives inform your doctor as to the kind of medical care you would like to have in the event that you are unable to make these decisions yourself. Living wills are one type of advanced directive. Living wills are legal documents by which individuals may direct in writing that they do not wish to receive treatment by extraordinary means, if in the future they become terminally ill or severely impaired. A durable power of attorney for health care is another kind of advanced directive, which states whom you have chosen to make health care decisions on your behalf and may include directions requiring that life-sustaining treatments be withheld or withdrawn. It becomes active any time the person responsible loses consciousness or is unable to make medical decisions directly. The concept of advanced directives first received legal acceptance in the 1976 Californian Natural Death Act, which was passed as a consequence of a number of right-to-die cases, such as the Karen Ann Quinlan decision. Ever since their inception, more formal legalistic documents have been developed, but, in essence, all advanced health directives are formal documents through which an adult may give directions about their future health care (both general health and special health care matters) and may appoint one or more individuals (an attorney or attorneys) to make decisions on their behalf. Advanced directives may be changed or cancelled at any time as long as the individual concerned is considered of sound mind. Evidently, such a document raises wider socioethical and legal problems relating to 'good medical practice' such as issues of limits on the operation of advanced health directives, protection for health providers relying on potentially invalid advanced health directives, validated copies of advanced health care directives, and the requirement to provide futile treatments in the absence of consent to withhold or withdraw life-sustaining measures. As if these dilemmas are not sufficient, recent research has suggested that, while a significant majority of terminally ill patients suffering unremitting pain supported euthanasia and physician-assisted suicide, only a minority of these patients considered these options for themselves.

In summary, the issues raised so far generally fall into two categories. The first deals with listing and defining the values that are challenged when human quality of life becomes the target of intervention and conflict. The second seeks to provide a social and political process that can mediate among those involved. The belief that it is permissible to withhold treatment and allow a patient to die passively while it is never permissible to take direct action designed to kill the patient is endorsed by a majority of nations and accepted by their respective Medical Associations. This distinction, however, has been extensively challenged on the grounds that if one simply withholds treatment of a dying patient (or malformed infant), it may possibly take the patient/infant longer to die and so prolong the suffering. Is it as unethical to inflict unwanted pain and suffering on an ill and dying person as it is on a healthy living one? If so, active intervention may become the preferred humane course of action. If euthanasia is to make it possible for people to live together in reasonable security and peace of mind, medical technology has to work for and not against the ill. Death is not always avoided in the patient's best interests.

Euthanasia, an evolving concept

One of the nagging ironies of modern medicine is that while it has enormously extended life spans, it has also stretched out the dying process.[2]

Traditionally, death was recognized 'on the cessation of blood circulation, respiration, pulsation, and other essential vital functions of the body'; that is, the irreversible cessation of function. Only in modern times has the concept of brain-death become central in biomedical discussions. A human being is brain dead if, and only if, the activity of his or her central nervous system has irreversibly ceased. The stimulus to redefine death in terms of brain activity emanated from the practice of organ transplantation. Evidently, if the patient were defined to be alive as long as the heart beats, organ transplantation would mean killing one patient to provide another one with the functioning organ. In ancient times euthanasia meant a 'good death' without severe suffering. Today one no longer thinks of this original meaning, but rather of some medical intervention whereby the sufferings of sickness, or of the final torment, are reduced; that is, the modern understanding of euthanasia is more akin to mercy killing for the purposes of putting an end to prolonged or extreme suffering which could impose too heavy a burden on the patient, the family or on society. Therefore, euthanasia in its modern terms of reference has its defining characteristic in the methods utilized. The distinctions which have become crucial in current medical ethics are 'active' or 'passive', 'voluntary' or 'involuntary' as described below:

---

[2] Horgan, J. (1997). Seeking a better way to die. *Scientific American* **5**, p. 74.

- Active euthanasia refers to an act by another person intended to cause the death of a patient and may entail, for example, administering a larger-than-usual dose of an analgesic drug.
- Passive euthanasia generally refers to the act of letting someone die by withdrawing life-sustaining treatment or not implementing treatment in the first instance.
- Voluntary euthanasia refers to euthanasia that involves the fully informed consent of a competent person.
- Non-voluntary euthanasia involves a person who is not competent to give informed consent (for example, infants, the unconscious or senile) or one whose wishes are not, or cannot be, known.
- Involuntary euthanasia is the act of killing or allowing to die of a competent patient without the person's consent.

To the above can be added concepts like 'assisted suicide' which can occur when a fatal hypodermic syringe is left within easy reach of a patient who self-injects and subsequently dies, or 'indirect death', the necessary administration of drugs (painkillers, for example) that have the indirect effect of hastening the patient's death.

As defined above, active, voluntary euthanasia is the deliberate hastening of death, on request, of a competent person. Vigilance, however, is strongly advised in order to distinguish consensual euthanasia from active, involuntary euthanasia, in which patients' lives may be ended against their will. Opponents of euthanasia have expressed concern about the latter scenario, particularly in relation to the Netherlands where an increase in non-voluntary and involuntary euthanasia, following legal tolerance of the voluntary consensual form, has been claimed. They warn us against the 'slippery slope' into moral abuse, an argument that relies on the notion that allowing something in one situation opens the way for the same action to be used unacceptably in another different situation. It is in this context that a clear definition of the circumstances under which a sentient individual might be allowed to make the final decision concerning his or her own life is required. According to the standard medical interpretation, individuals should not be granted the right to full self-determination if they are very young, very old or are severely disabled mentally. Furthermore, individuals should not be given a decisive say in matters which have to do with their wellbeing if they lack sufficient psychological control over their choices owing to temporary emotional disturbances, lack of knowledge or undue coercion by other people. Admittedly, testing for full competency raises serious medico-ethical difficulties because the very act of testing implies the suspicion that the individual is incompetent, which is itself a violation of the assumption of competency. The assumption of competency depends on understanding what is involved in making an autonomous informed decision. At the same time, health professionals are expected to protect those who are unable to make medical decisions in their own best interests – a difficult ask.

Restrictions of sentient individuals from full self-determination may be justified by reference to the needs of others, like those whose lives depend, directly or indirectly, on the person's actions. In these cases, the harm inflicted on self may harm others in the shared social environment, usually children or grandchildren, to an unacceptable degree. Otherwise, fully conscientious and autonomous beings should be allowed to determine the limits of their inner freedom on the basis of their own experiences and beliefs.

Chapter 7 reviewed modern insights into the essentials of healing and wellbeing. It was emphasized that, in biological terms, health and disease are not alternative states; rather they are part of the same continuum. This applies equally to the continuum of life and death. The urge to be in charge of one's destiny motivates those who hope to improve the quality of their dying by actively participating in a traditional, or physician-assisted, death far removed from the impersonal hyperactivity of hospital or nursing home. Increasingly, it is the hospice which is ministering to the needs of the terminally ill, either at the centre or at home. The modern hospice is a multidisciplinary system of family-centred supervision, designed to assist the terminally ill person through the phases of dying. Hospice care includes home visits, professional health care, education, emotional support for the family and physical care of the patient. A major landmark in society's increasing perceptiveness of the true nature of death was the publication of the book *On Death and Dying* by Elisabeth Kübler-Ross. Following her lead, a general awareness, including our bioethical responsibility to the dying, has matured. Prior to that time, death was the sole province of the priest, since doctors were expected to concentrate on the living. It is for this reason that modern medical education must ensure that physicians are trained in the art and science of improved terminal care of dying patients. An important goal in modern palliative medicine and hospice care is to promote an acceptance of death and gratitude for being allowed to live and transcend the present self.

The practice of 'protecting patients' best interests' against their expressed wishes or preferences, and rationalizing these unwelcome interventions on medical grounds, is often encountered. However, owing to changing ethical demands, these and similar medical attitudes are rapidly disappearing. In essence, the central requirement of professional medical ethics is that physicians, nurses and others in the caring business must, under all circumstances, regard their patient's best interest as paramount. Unwarranted restrictive controls, such as the refusal to sterilize women with children who request it, are numerous, so a challenging request for euthanasia is even more likely to be refused. It is self-evident that when we act according to our inner directed principles we may not always be free from harming others, whose personal beliefs differ from our own. In respect of another's point-of-view or judgement, however, it may help to recall the three basic principles of bioethics: namely, the principle of autonomy or liberty, the principle of beneficence or responsible tolerance of difference, and the principle of justice, taking into consideration democratic decision-making. We respect autonomy when we refrain from interfering with people's opportunities to control their own lives and when we accept as worthy of respect the existence of individual values we do not share. In the modern medical context a physician's obligation to preserve life may conflict with the obligation to do no harm or to do good. It may also conflict with the patient's liberty; by refusing a request to end a suffering patient's life, the doctor is overriding the patient's right to choose death.

Ethical dilemmas such as the above cause justified unease; however, with the doctrine of individual autonomy replacing earlier medical authority, there is a stronger emphasis on patients' self-reliance and empowerment (refer back to Chapter 7 on wellbeing). Because of this biological association between self-empowerment and wellbeing, unacceptable restraint on the fully informed cannot be justified by appealing to the beneficiary's best interests. It is impossible to better the best interests of competent persons by violating their autonomy. Significantly, the principle of autonomy is closely related to self-determination, which states that persons should have the right to make their own decisions about the course of their own lives whenever they can. As reviewed in this chapter, self-determination – autonomy – over the important events in our life's choices and actions is a necessary pre-condition of genuine wellbeing. Therefore, there is only one sure-fire defence to unacceptable intrusion; that is, to include the dying individual in the final decision of his or her life.

Principles of bioscience ethics for discussion

- In biological terms, life and death are not alternative states; rather they are part of the same continuum. Do you agree or disagree?
- Death is caused not only by injuries and pathological conditions, but also by programmed intracellular and extracellular signals. Therefore,

individual death is not a negative process; rather it is the natural process of adjustment to change. Discuss.

-   Most individuals are appreciative of living longer, especially if modern medicine can treat the illnesses traditionally associated with old age. However, as a society have we seriously examined how we feel about longevity, and its local and global consequences? Discuss ethical solutions to the problem/blessing of increasing longevity. Do you think that older citizens are an asset or a drain on society?

Current reproductive technologies: achievements and desired goals

A woman shall not be provided with treatment services unless account has been taken of the welfare of any child who may be born as a result of the treatment (including the need of that child for a father) and of any child who may be affected by the birth.[1]

Lifestyle, fertility and the Assisted Reproductive Technologies (ARTs)

Modern developments in assisted conception and contraception have reinforced the idea that reproduction is largely a matter of choice. We are able to decide whether or not we wish to have children and, if so, under what circumstances. In many instances, having children is not necessarily the result of a conscious decision-making process. Social pressure, ambivalence, conflicting needs and simple socioeconomic disadvantage interfere with or confuse reproductive choice. Importantly, however, modern developments in technical control over the reproductive processes have increased reproductive options. These options have led to a new and unique therapeutic relationship in which important reproductive decisions are transferred to the medical scientists. Consequently, these physicians are called upon to assume a greater share of the responsibilities regarding reproductive matters. In turn, our own increased expectations have fuelled an escalating reliance on medical manipulations, which impact on ethical and social concerns. Reproductive choice should not be taken casually, as the main themes of Chapters 3 to 6 have tried to justify.

---

[1] The UK Human Fertilization and Embryology Act. (1990). S13, 5.

The origin of certain aspects of human fertility, development and offspring wellbeing centres on parental lifestyle and behavioural factors, while others are unexplained or attributable to changing environmental conditions. What is certain, however, is that 'bearing a child' means a lot more than just generating a child, and requires many skills. Love and parental care go well beyond questions of fertility and, where assisted conception is involved, the best interest of the potential child should always be the overpowering consideration. Since the overall social consequences of reproductive choice are fundamentally a mix of personal, medical and political concerns, choice needs to be firmly anchored in ethical notions of autonomy, freedom of action, responsibility, interdependence and regard of consequence.

Bioethical discussion of the Assisted Reproductive Technologies (ARTs) has been extensive, controversial and confusing – confusing because these technologies are complex and require a sound grasp of human reproductive physiology for their comprehension. In dealing with clinically assisted reproduction, full and accurate biological comprehension has to be a fundamental part of the bioethical debate if responsible judgements are to be made. Since biological understanding is bioscience ethics' major goal, the foremost discussions in this chapter and Chapters 10 and 11 deal with the necessary biological foundations. It is my hope that these chapters will generate informed ethical debate regarding the procreative technologies.

Fertility control – the evolutionary perspective

The idea of contraception (literally, against conception) is not new. People have tried to prevent unwanted pregnancy for thousands of years. In early times, a naturally high mortality rate, augmented by abortion, infanticide and sometimes human sacrifice, usually controlled population size. Yet the concept of preventing unwanted pregnancy was advantageous and drove reproductive technology very early in humankind's evolution. Throughout the ancient world, as our ancestors learned more about bodily functions, they developed various behavioural and biological means of controlling fertility in their societies. Methods such as prolonged lactation, delayed marriage, celibacy, withdrawal, periodic abstinence or natural medicinal treatments were all techniques used to prevent unwanted pregnancies. Plants and animals are responsible for a variety of useful medications (approximately 40% of all prescriptions written today are composed from the natural compounds of different species). Our ancestors also relied on medicaments ritually delivered by medicine men and women, on fertility-altering diets, and 'magic' root potions. Our ancestors' desire to reproduce responsibly can be easily verified from many ancient documents. For example, a surviving Chinese medical text written around 2700 BCE contains a prescription for an abortifacient. Prescriptions for contraceptives have also been discovered in ancient Egyptian medical papyri. The Kahun Papyrus, dating back to about 1850 BCE, provides recipes for various acidic vaginal pastes and menses-inducing tampons. The Ebers Papyrus (~1550 BCE) is particularly interesting as it describes a spermicide made from ground acacia, a plant containing gum arabic that ferments, releasing lactic acid. Indian Sanskrit medical writings likewise refer to medicated tampons, vaginal pastes and abstinence. Some later cultures used fish and goat bladders as forms of condoms. Knowledge and practice of separating sex from conception has been with us for a long time. In evolutionary terms, the human female, by retaining sexual receptivity at all times, has freed the species behaviourally to use sex for pleasure, recreation, bonding, competition and aggression, as well as procreation (Chapter 1).

The present-day medicalization of reproduction is a naturally evolving and integral part of our human heritage as it is derived from our intellect, consciousness and the desire to heal, improve and manipulate. Reproduction is healthy only when it is ecologically sustainable; unregulated population growth is the thoughtless 'plague' strategy driving its own destruction. By appropriating all available resources for ourselves, we are witnessing the last desperate struggle for survival of the unique Quaternary fauna and flora. The Quaternary period was characterized by the flourishing of an astonishing diversity of life, including the appearance of *Homo sapiens*. Given this diversity, it seems natural that human procreation has to function within acceptable norms and values, giving due dignity to all creatures and environmental justice to future generations. Population growth will be forcefully controlled if we do not ourselves choose to control our natural birth rate, intelligently matching it with our power over the natural death rate. Unsustainable growth is the root cause of social dislocation, accelerating conflict and rising rates of infertility.

If the scientific revolution is to be sustained, our technological power has to become an integral part of bioethics and make our planet a fairer and better place for our fellow travellers and ourselves. The technologies, by which we can ethically manage optimum population growth, have long been available. Nevertheless, millions of women worldwide are, by circumstances, forced to bear more children than they want, or can care for. Choice, or being in charge of one's destiny, is empowering and heightens personal wellbeing, while individuals with very little flexibility in decision-making easily succumb to disease (Chapter 7). Now, more than ever before, knowledge gained from research which gave us the reproductive technologies is also offering us a plethora of lifestyle choices. This is true for both sexes. The following sections deal with the biological principles underlying the new, potentially liberating, technologies loosely referred to as physician-assisted conception; that is, the ARTs where 'assisted' means 'technologically assisted'.

Infertility – the price of excess fecundity

Fertility is a very sensitive indicator of health status and can be impaired by a modest failure in physiological homeostasis. Paradoxically, one of the biological consequences of unregulated fertility is infertility; humans are not exempt. For example, a survey by the US Office of Technology and Assessment found that the rate of infertility among women aged 20–24 years rose significantly, from 3.6% in 1965 to 10.6% in 1982, and the number of couples with primary infertility doubled, increasing from 500 000 in 1965 to 1 million in 1988. A comparable British study suggested that subfertility was also on the rise since 20–35% of pregnancies take more than 1 year to be established. Pregnancy provides the best basis for assessing a couple's fecundity, and a couple is considered infertile if conception has not been achieved after 12 months or more of unprotected intercourse of average frequency. Infertility due to primary gonadal failure, such as a permanent inability to produce sperm (azoospermia) or the congenital absence of ovaries, is described as sterility.

Human infertility is hard to assess accurately, but there is medical consensus that about 15% of couples in developed countries are involuntarily infertile, with a much higher percentage in developing countries (30–40% of women in parts of tropical Africa). The main causes of infertility in developing countries are sexually transmitted diseases (principally gonorrhoea and chlamydia) and repeated pregnancies coupled with poor hygiene at the time of childbirth, abortion or miscarriage causing secondary infertility. In the absence of disease, female infertility is normally age-dependent and increases from 30 years of age to the menopause; the age-related rise in male infertility is more gradual, and sperm number and quality steadily decline between the third and fifth decades of life. On average, pregnancy attempts are 70% more likely to fail when the man is age 40 or older than if he is younger than 30, regardless of his wife or partner's age. Since the 1970s, an increasing number of couples, mainly from industrialized societies, have been seeking medical treatment for infertility. This may have been encouraged by increased acceptance of the improving reproductive technologies, or it may reflect a genuine increased rate of infertility. Most disturbing are reports documenting changes in human semen quality such as the meta-analysis, which identified a significant decline in average sperm concentration, from 113×10^6/ml in 1940 to 66×10^6/ml in 1990. In general, lower sperm count is also associated with decreased sperm nuclear DNA integrity, a necessary prerequisite for the completion of fertilization and subsequent embryo development. Since the 1970s, increased incidences of testicular abnormalities (including undescended testicles or cryptorchidism), moderate to severe penile anomalies with the urethral opening displaced from the tip of the glans penis (hypospadias) and testicular cancers have also been reported.

There is the strong suspicion that increased male-mediated infertility may result from, among other things, exposure to low concentrations of a range of toxins. Thousands of potential toxins are continually released into the environment, the great majority of which have never been studied for their effects on mammalian reproduction. Some scientists link rising estrogen levels in the environment with the male reproductive anomalies described above. Some environmental pollutants such as polychlorinated biphenyls (PCBs), organochloride insecticides and detergents exhibit estrogenic activity and may affect normal differentiation of male fetuses (Chapters 2 and 12). Other common causes of male infertility can be categorized as lifestyle choices. For example, associations between tobacco, marijuana and other substance abuse, and teratozoospermia (sperm morphology less than 50% normal) have repeatedly been documented (Chapter 3).

According to WHO's estimates, fertility problems warranting ARTs have been linked to male infertility in 40% of cases and female problems in 40% of cases, with the remaining 20% due to problems in both partners. In as many as 35% of couples, the infertility may have multiple origins. According to the Australian Institute of Health and Welfare's 2002 National Perinatal Statistics Unit, ART babies now account for nearly 3% of all babies born in Australia, with nearly comparable statistics for the UK and the United States. The tragedy is that, while scientists are good at monitoring and investigating possible causes of infertility, human nature is hopelessly slow in accepting that serious problems exist which may need urgent attention. Time-wasting strategies and lengthy controversies as to the data's authenticity, causes and implications, have effectively obstructed remedial action. If reproductive health is genuinely deteriorating, then the longer we dither, the greater the consequences, with the stress of uncertainty further adversely affecting fertility. Much of the available data is open to criticism – such as being retrospective, collected in different countries, at different times, using different methods of recruitment and laboratory methodology, and more in-depth evidence is needed. Nevertheless, difficulties of data collection should not induce a paralysis of mind and thus ignore the big potential problem because 'we may never be able to resolve the issue with certainty'. Trends such as population increase or semen quality decline have an inbuilt inertia and, consequently, things will get worse before any remedial action kicks in to improve the situation.

Unwelcome interference over a couple's right to choose the most suitable contraceptive is still tolerated, in direct violation of the bioethical imperative of responsible autonomy and despite our awareness of the desperate consequences of overpopulation (Chapter 5). Denying a couple's right of freedom from excess fertility by reducing reproductive options is unethical as it encourages irresponsible procreation. Surely, in the age of almost unlimited medical options, we have advanced sufficiently to overcome cultural inertia and the wish to dominate human sexuality and procreation. The most probable legacy of unregulated population growth coupled with progressive environmental deterioration would be infertility on a mass scale. The future cost for the present excess fecundity is too high, especially when we also factor in the suffering of those millions of infertile couples living a lifelong loss. Large-scale surveys demonstrate that over 50% of women considered being unable to achieve pregnancy more traumatic than losing a sister or brother or divorce. Those who advocate authoritarian tactics that interfere with reproductive rights might well recall an age-old piece of wisdom 'to treat others as we would like to be treated in similar circumstances'.

Assisted reproduction: social considerations

To beat infertility, increasing numbers of couples are seeking medical treatment and, as familiarity with the available technology broadens, so does its acceptance, generating further demands for medical intervention. Among infertile couples seeking medical treatment, 50% will achieve a viable pregnancy, but the great majority of these will be the result of conventional therapy. Because the more complex 'extracorporeal' methods, generically known as in vitro fertilization technology, involve extensive intervention, a counselling component of ART is of primary importance. A genuinely informed consent from the commissioning couple can only be obtained after issues relating to procedural methodology, scientific uncertainties, biological risk factors and psychosocial needs or requirements in the offspring have been clearly acknowledged. The signing of the consent forms implies that the parents have understood, as far as possible, the broader biological implications of ART and given due thought to possible risk factors and valid alternatives.

ART procedures, especially the more recent developments, should still be viewed as experimental until such time as long-term outcomes are known and properly informed risk assessments can be made (see section on Epigenetics,

p. 163). A precautionary approach is not intended to curtail present trends in clinical practice, but to ensure that collection and maintenance of records is universally thorough, and that any adverse long-term outcomes are promptly publicized. To do this effectively, international collaboration in short-term data collection and long-term follow-up studies through childhood, puberty, mid-life and post-menopause years are required. We are a long-lived species so there is a need for caution; potential drawbacks should be fairly balanced against the advantages given to the ART children who are much loved, cared for and paid for – all contributing factors in guaranteeing good prospects. Safety and efficacy are the primary concerns of the reproductive biologists who are only too aware that it is not just a simple matter of claiming that the end (a live take-home baby) justifies the means; that is, they not only serve a couple's wish to procreate but also have a duty of care toward the resulting progeny. The infertile couple, probably more than any other, appreciates that repro-duction is indeed a privilege and not a right.

When donor material has been used it is particularly significant that the progeny should be allowed access to their identifying heritage. Therefore, issues connected with access are a major aspect of prenatal ART counselling services. Knowing one's origins (especially in cases of adoption) provides emotional security in terms of identity and belonging, and in terms of medical history, genetic knowledge is sometimes indispensable. In most western democracies, parents are now expected to plan to tell their children the truth about their origins, preferably before the child reaches the age of consent. The importance of access to information applies equally whether the child is the result of donor gametes, donor embryos, some variant of surrogacy or just technological support. Parents and their communities have a responsibility to protect the ART children's interests since such children had no say about the method of their conception. Detailed record-keeping, whether through legis-lation, regulation or comprehensive reports, is one good way of demonstrating caring. The near universal acceptance of medically controlled donor insemin-ation (DI) services following the AIDS pandemic in the early 1980s also heralded increasing acceptance of other key ARTs. In turn, the growing number of fer-tility clinics has changed public attitudes in favour of openness and information sharing, allowing the resulting children to eventually learn about their mode of conception. This attitude is in stark contrast to the former secrecy which sur-rounded donor gamete programmes and related technologies.

Nowadays, many facilities recruit only identifiable gamete providers; that is, those willing to be identified to their offspring in the future. Sweden, in 1985, was the first country to legislate that semen providers must register and so facilitate future requests as to parentage from children born by DI. At the time, it was argued that semen providers would be unwilling to come forward if they could be identified, although Australian surveys do not support this. A majority (56%) of Australian men supported the idea of a national register of names and addresses of providers and recipients; 68% would not mind if identifying information to trace the provider were given to DI offspring at age 18, and 73% would still provide semen if they could be traced.

Irrespective of what technology is used, the key elements minimizing long-term physiological and psychological risk are: adequate donor screening to ensure freedom from inheritable and communicable diseases, comprehensive counselling of prospective parents and clarification of the legal status of ART children. The central issues in reproductive and sexual health, as in other health areas, are the rights to responsible autonomy in making sexual and reproductive decisions, and the assurance from health care providers that safety, efficacy and informed consent are paramount and that confidentiality in relation to health services is protected.

Assisted reproduction: technological considerations

Fertility, often in the form of a goddess or phallic symbol, has been worshipped since ancient times because the 'barren woman' caused much concern. The etiologies of female infertility are similar to those for the male, although some kinds of treatment for infertile women has always been available. Since the early 1960s, however, important breakthroughs, such as ovulation-inducing drugs and gynaecological microsurgery, have resulted in more women being successfully treated than their partners. Female infertility can be classified under the following broad categories: endocrine (hormonal) causes, including anovulation and other menstrual dysfunction, abnormal growths (fibroids), endometriosis and hostile cervical mucus, immunological causes and infections. Both men and women can develop antisperm antibodies, with some evidence that women infected with sexually transmitted disease are more likely to develop antibodies against sperm because sperm contact the immune system through genital lesions.

Miscarriage is quite common in all pregnancies (15–20% of all human embryos die in the early stages of development), but is significantly higher in communities with substandard hygiene, poor nutrition and a high rate of disease. Subfertility and infertility caused by obsessive psychological demands, such as excessive physical activity, food restriction and abnormal eating behaviour (as in obesity and anorexia nervosa) have been well documented. The caloric regulation of fertility is complex, involving hormones, neuro-transmitters and neuropeptides which are modulated by environmental, behavioural, psychogenic and physiological requirements. Since the body saves energy when moving from the fertile to the infertile, situations of chronic energy imbalance (a sustained decrease in total calorie intake or sustained increase in total calorie expenditure) result in decreased fertility.

Many opportunistic infections may be introduced during coitus, especially if the immune system and the cervix are compromised by miscarriage, abortion, cervical surgery, intrauterine contraceptive devices and/or primary infections such as *Neisseria gonorrhoea* and *Chlamydia trachomatis*. A major cause of infection in women is pelvic inflammatory disease (PID). It has been estimated that between 30 and 50% of all cases of female infertility and ectopic pregnancy are caused by PID-related tubal adhesions. Complete or partial tubal occlusion may be diagnosed by hysterosalpingography, which involves introducing radio-opaque dye through the uterus into the Fallopian tubes under X-ray fluoro-scopy visualization. When the dye moves into the Fallopian tubes, occlusions or other abnormalities can be identified: if the Fallopian tube is open, the dye fills the tube and spills into the abdominal cavity. If the hysterosalpingogram is abnormal, laparoscopy allows direct visualization of the pelvic organs through an endoscope. Complete or partial tubal blockage and adhesions can sometimes be corrected by microsurgery.

Sexually transmitted diseases underlie an estimated 75% of all cases of PID, but infection after backstreet abortion and genital mutilation in teenage girls at circumcision and/or infibulation also accounts for significant incidences of PID. Unlike foot binding, practised in China till the early 1900s, genital mutilation is still practised in many parts of the world by a variety of community groups. Female genital mutilation is an extreme example of abuse resulting from a culturally driven control of female sexuality which predates most modern religions, including Christianity and Islam. The practice covers a graded series of alterations to the female genitalia, ranging from mild to most severe. 'Sunna', or circumcision, is the mildest form where only the hood of the clitoris is removed. Clitorectomy involves the removal of the entire clitoris as well as the labia minora. Infibulation, the most severe form of genital mutilation, involves the removal of the clitoris, labia minora, labia majora and parts of the vulva. After infibulation, the remaining tissue mass is sewn together with catgut or held together with thorns, leaving a tiny hole for urine and menstrual blood to pass through. Since these procedures are typically performed in non-sterile conditions and without anaesthesia, mutilation is associated with many physical complications, psychological trauma and infertility. It is believed that, worldwide, 130 million girls and women, mostly African, have been affected by the practice and that a further 2 million are at risk every year.

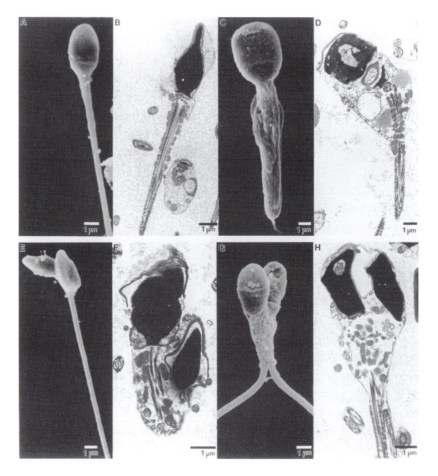

Figure 9.1 Scanning (A, C, E and G) and transmission (B, D, F and H) electron micrographs showing normal and abnormal forms of sperm from infertile semen. **A, B** Normal sperm consisting of an intact acrosome covering the anterior part of the nucleus, midpiece surrounded by the mitochondrial sheath and the principal piece of the flagellum or tail. **C, D** Large amorphous sperm characterized by vacuolations in the nucleus, separation of the acrosomal membranes and copious redundant cytoplasm. **E–H** Double-headed variants with acrosomal and flagellar abnormalities, including swelling of the midpiece mitochondria and sometimes multiple tails. Material supplied by Dr Ian Pike, Scientific Director, North Shore Fertility.

In fertile men, the sperm concentration varies between 60 and 80 million active sperm per millilitre of semen in an ejaculate volume of approximately 2.5–3.5 ml. The turning point between fertile and infertile sperm numbers is taken as 20 million active sperm per ml, but sperm density alone is insufficient

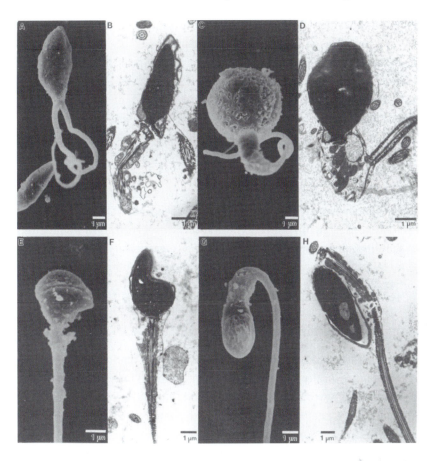

Figure 9.2 Scanning (A, C, E and G) and transmission (B, D, F and H) electron micrographs showing abnormal forms of sperm from infertile semen continued. **A, B** Pyriform sperm head, sometimes with multiple tails. **C, D** Missing acrosome (round-head-defect), excess cytoplasm and coiled tail. **E, F** Other variants with acrosomal and midpiece defects. **G, H** Faulty head–flagellum connection. Material supplied by Dr Ian Pike, Scientific Director, North Shore Fertility.

to assess the quality of a semen sample. Other parameters, such as sperm motility, morphology and DNA integrity, are especially important. Although DNA damage can be detected in fertile men, it is more pronounced in infertile men attending reproductive clinics – especially among older men whose reproductive potential is compromised. The least adequately assessed parameter of semen analysis is sperm morphology, which is, typically, examined on wet preparations or on smears of stained seminal fluid. Only morphological parameters such as head size and shape, length and appearance of flagellum, presence or absence of multiple heads or flagellae are assessed because functional faults are beyond the limits of resolution of the light microscope. The transmission and scanning electron microscopes are useful tools in evaluating the ultramorphology of sperm as they permit a detailed assessment of structural integrity of subcellular components (Figures 9.1 and 9.2).

Nowadays, a more precise assessment and method of choice employs commercial computer-assisted semen analysis systems which automatically track the position of the sperm head in successive video frames and use the stored information to calculate various parameters of sperm motion, such as velocity, progression, amplitude and frequency of head movement. These measures permit a deeper evaluation of sperm function but are expensive and routinely available only in sophisticated research centres. Once sperm have arrived on site, other qualities needed for successful fertilization involve recognition, binding, penetration through the oocyte vestments and fusion with the egg membrane (the reader is referred back to Chapter 5 Principles of reproductive ageing, p. 95).

Artificial insemination

Insemination, with or without donor semen, is one of the oldest and simplest forms of medically assisted conception. Artificial insemination (AI) as a technique has been known for centuries; it is said that in the fourteenth century Arab tribesmen impregnated enemy mares with semen of inferior stallions. In the early 1890s, Russian scientists established AI as a tool in livestock production and its application has broadened to include conservation programmes for endangered species (see The biology of conservation, p. 165). The first recorded human birth after AI with the husband's sperm was in 1790 when the Scottish physician John Hunter inseminated a woman with epididymal sperm from her husband who had an urethral defect. In recent times, partner insemination has been useful in cases of paraplegia (sperm is collected by electroejaculation), obstructed vas deferens or epididymis (sperm is aspirated from the epididymis) and forced separation of couples (prisoners on long-term sentences).

Partner insemination is also widely used for idiopathic (cause unknown) infertility. Between 15 and 30% of women become pregnant during six insemination (menstrual) treatment cycles. However, the pregnancy success rate can be improved if the sperm are first subjected to a separation procedure such as 'swim-up', which involves layering media directly upon a semen sample. After incubation, the top fraction containing the most motile (and presumably the healthiest) sperm is removed for insemination. Another popular modification of AI is intrauterine insemination. Intrauterine insemination is often successful because placing the prepared semen high up in the uterus allows sperm to bypass the cervix and its mucus that can contain antisperm antibodies.

Donor insemination (DI) is the insemination of a woman with sperm from a donor other than her husband or partner. Indications for DI may range from various types of problems with sperm (insufficient number or motility, or pathological forms), to anatomical obstructions or sexual obstacles in either the male or the female partner, or to various immunological problems (sperm antibodies, cervical mucus hostility). DI is more successful than husband insemination, with a reported 60% birth rate after six insemination cycles and is, therefore, one of the major treatments for male infertility. The technique is routinely used in Australia, Europe and the United States where, according to the US Office of Technology Assessment, women inseminated with donor sperm conceive some 30 000 infants each year. The procedure does not carry an increased risk of spontaneous abortion or congenital anomalies. It has advantages over adoption, in that the child is genetically related to the mother and the couple can experience conception, pregnancy and delivery. The disadvantage of half-siblings, related through the father, unknowingly bonding and bearing children is minimized as most AI clinics limit the number of pregnancies from each donor. It has been estimated that the chance of genetic incest occurring is one in 40 000 if sperm from one donor is used to produce six offspring in a city with a population of 3 million. All insemination centres restrict donor recruitment to men who are healthy, free from transmissible genetic disorders and sexually transmitted diseases, and have, as far as can be determined by laboratory analysis, semen with a high fertilization potential.

Fresh semen provides a higher probability of obtaining a pregnancy in any given cycle compared with frozen. However, all donor semen is frozen and quarantined in sperm banks for 6 months, after which the donor is retested for antibodies against HIV, the human immunodeficiency virus. This is essential, as antibodies may not show up for 3–6 months after infection. A semen bank, in its simplest form, is a metal container in which straws, containing semen mixed with a cryoprotective medium, is frozen in liquid nitrogen at a temperature of about -191°C.

DI is usually a response to male infertility, but there are important exceptions. For example, lesbian couples and single women – situations where physical infertility is replaced by social infertility, increasingly use DI. Historically, access to reproductive technology excluded singles and homosexual couples, who for social considerations were considered ineligible. This kind of exclusionary policy has, in the late 1990s, been successfully challenged on constitutional or discriminatory grounds. However, judges, when formulating their decisions, must also take care to familiarize themselves about the society into which the infant will be born in terms of levels of prejudice and discrimination against singles, gays and others outside the social norm. On the other hand, it may be seen as regressive and counterproductive to follow existing mores, rather than facilitating social change toward a more tolerant and open society, which would ultimately benefit all children. Research has provided good evidence that the children of gay and lesbian couples are not disadvantaged socially/economically and psychologically are similarly well adjusted, compared to those from heterosexual couples. At this stage I would remind the reader of the prevalence of child abuse and corresponding high social tolerance of cruelty experienced by children living in conformist, but dysfunctional, family units (Chapter 6).

Other important instances where DI is not used to treat male infertility are cases of known male-mediated hereditary conditions. DI may also be used in combination with other ART technologies, including sperm separation for sex preselection and for other 'designer' characteristics. The latter application raises serious concerns from the ethical, legal and biological points of view (Chapter 10).

In vitro fertilization and related technologies

The basic and, to the public, most familiar reproductive technologies are in vitro (Latin for 'within glass') fertilization (or IVF) and gamete intra-fallopian transfer (GIFT). These techniques, either alone or in conjunction with other technologies, offer additional hope to those infertile couples for whom conventional treatment has been unsuccessful. Although most appropriate as a method of achieving conception in women with absent or occluded oviducts (Fallopian tubes), IVF has also proved a useful form of treatment in many other cases of female and male infertility. In oligospermia (low sperm number), for example, the few viable sperm present are spared negotiation of the female reproductive tract and can concentrate around the oocyte in vitro. Other conditions for which IVF is useful are ovaries enclosed in adhesions, defective oocyte pick-up, male or female immunity to sperm and idiopathic infertility. The world's first IVF baby, Louise Brown, born in England in 1978, revolutionized the treatment of human infertility and opened up prospects for the plight of endangered species (see The biology of conservation, p. 165). There has been awe-inspiring technological progress since Louise Brown, including breakthroughs in quality control for embryo culture, administration of fertility drugs, successful embryo freezing and assisted fertilization for male-mediated infertility.

Because of the speed of new scientific inventions and technical improvements, the field of assisted reproduction has earned the trade a high degree of popularity and trust. IVF technology does not, however, provide all the solutions: the overall live delivery rate is low (the rates of birth do not exceed 25–30% in the best of cases), there are inherent risks, unpredictable complications and the programme is relatively costly. The extent to which women are emotionally stressed by treatment schedules and pregnancy anticipation may adversely influence the outcome of IVF, and in some men, the stress of undergoing an IVF treatment cycle may also impair the sperm quality. Counselling against heightened emotional distress is, of course, an essential component of the IVF procedure.

Put simply, the IVF procedure is a method of fertilization outside the body by adding a sample of sperm to a dish containing the collected mature ova in a synthetic nutritive medium. After an incubation period of 48–72 hours, the fertilized ova (now embryos) are transferred into the uterus through the cervix. More specifically, the IVF programme involves six consecutive manipulations: ovarian stimulation, oocyte or egg retrieval, sperm collection, in vitro fertilization, embryo culture and embryo transfer into the uterus. The aim of ovarian stimulation is to increase the number of mature oocytes available for retrieval, fertilization and embryo transfer. Freezing of extra embryos for future use further augments the pregnancy rate per stimulated cycle. Cryopreservation technology also advances legal–ethical issues of the fate of sperm, eggs and embryos who have exceeded the lifespan of their biological parents. Of particular interest in this context is the issue of posthumous conception.

The technique of ovarian hyperstimulation (superovulation) involves treatment with exogenous hormones to increase the number of oocytes matured in any given menstrual cycle. To achieve this, specific combinations of follicle stimulating hormone in sequence with other hormone analogues are used to stimulate the growth of a batch of, ideally, 8–12 ovarian follicles per cycle. Circulating ovarian steroid levels and ultrasound images of the ovaries are used to monitor the development and maturation of the pre-ovulatory follicles. Then ovulation is induced by giving an injection of luteinizing hormone (or equivalent) and the oocytes are collected by aspiration (oocyte pick-up) 36 hours later. Various laparoscopic or ultrasound-guided techniques can be used for oocyte collection, but to date the optimal technique is the transvaginal ultrasound-guided approach. This entails passing a collection needle into the ovary along a defined path visualized by ultrasound on a TV monitor. The method minimizes risk of morbidity because, unlike the older methods, it is relatively non-invasive and can be done under local anaesthesia or light intravenous sedation.

The addition of washed sperm to cultures containing the retrieved mature oocytes should result in fertilization within a few hours. Although the technique is simple, this part of the IVF procedure is the most delicate, requiring careful control of laboratory conditions if embryo viability is not to be compromised. Embryos subjectively scored as having good viability predictors, such as the ability to divide evenly, regularly and rapidly, are transferred into the uterus. Transfer is usually carried out after 48 hours when the cultured embryo is at the four-cell stage, although two-cell, eight-cell and blastocyst embryos can be transferred equally successfully. IVF also makes it possible to transfer the embryo derived from the gametes of genetic parents to a separate gestational mother. Recently, IVF technology has been extended to include menopausal and perimenopausal women who have been implanted with embryos from oocytes obtained from younger, fertile donors. Thus, embryo transfer technology has empowered medicine and, of course, veterinary science with the ability to select for sex, desirable physical characteristics, lack of deleterious genes and expanded genetic manipulations of embryos (Chapter 10).

In 1986, GIFT became a significant treatment alternative for patients with idiopathic infertility; it differs from IVF in that fertilization occurs in the oviduct. Like IVF, GIFT requires ovarian hyperstimulation and is followed by a two-step procedure: oocyte collection and subsequent transfer of oocytes and sperm into the ampulla of the oviduct. The technique has also been used in cases of infertility due to an occluded sperm-transporting system (obstructive azoospermia), when sperm aspirated from the epididymis are used. Live delivery rates following GIFT are generally higher than those for IVF, perhaps reflecting a less technological mode of reproduction in which the IVF and embryo culture steps have been omitted. ZIFT, or zygote intrafallopian transfer, involves the transfer of the fertilized conceptus before cleavage has commenced. It has been introduced as an alternative to GIFT for patients with semen abnormalities where the screening for successful fertilization is advantageous.

Superovulation by exogenous synthetic hormones, an essential part of ART, is not risk-free and can itself impair fertility. This impairment could include genetic deficiencies in the superovulated oocyte or embryo, and/or the introduction of an endocrine imbalance affecting the maternal environment. A critical stage in obtaining a clinical pregnancy is implantation where insufficient progesterone or excessive estrogenic stimulation of the reproductive tract may result in asynchrony of embryonic and uterine development.

Improper management of the implantation signal can impede the viable embryo in establishing the placenta which is required for nourishment, growth and development. Excess embryos formed by and of ART products are now routinely frozen, and the long-term effects of this have yet to be elucidated. Subtle changes in the activity of some genes have been reported following freezing, but it is not known whether these have any long-term significance (see Epigenetics, p. 163).

Ovarian hyperstimulation may also result in iatrogenic (caused by treatment or diagnostic procedures) complications, with serious health consequences for the woman. The ovarian hyperstimulation syndrome is the enlargement of the ovaries with development of multiple cysts and, in severe cases, an acute, potentially fatal generalized edema due to a fluid shift out of the intravascular space. The hyperstimulation syndrome and related concerns, such as risk of ovarian cancer and ovarian autoimmune disease, increase with each additional hormonal treatment cycle. This has heightened the demand for a milder form of ovarian stimulation in ART.

Intracytoplasmic sperm injection and cytoplasmic transfer technologies

Male infertility treatment has advanced rapidly since the early 1990s. Patients with sperm abnormalities sufficient to prevent oocyte fertilization can now father children through the techniques of sperm micromanipulation or assisted fertilization. Intracytoplasmic sperm injection (ICSI), in conjunction with IVF technology, has given hope to patients with such sperm defects as low density, poor structure, abnormal or weak motility, immotility or biochemical dysfunction at the level of binding with the oocyte's zona. In patients with azoospermia, ICSI can be performed with sperm obtained by microsurgical epididymal aspiration or by fine-needle testicular extraction. ICSI is more invasive than conventional IVF because a single functional (possibly compromised) sperm is injected directly into the cytoplasm of the oocyte.

Infants conceived as a result of sperm micromanipulation are reported to compare favourably with the IVF group of babies, but there is considerable variability since pregnancy outcome depends closely on the overall semen quality used. Patients with severely defective semen have a high risk of siring babies leading to preterm deliveries, low birthweights and early perinatal mortality when compared with the children sired with 'better-quality' sperm and those resulting from natural conceptions. Possible long-term ICSI consequences of hidden intellectual and developmental anomalies, including inherited infertility, cannot yet be established. Since certain genetic disorders predictably cause severe oligospermia and azoospermia, ICSI treatment risks the transmission, or the de novo introduction, of genetic mutations and chromosomal abnormalities in the progeny. Genetic counselling is essential to inform couples of genetic risks and likely consequences inherent in prospective ICSI technology. With proper information, some couples may prefer to explore alternatives to ICSI, including adoption or DI, or may even choose not to become parents at all.

A more recent technological breakthrough is transfer of cytoplasm from a younger donor oocyte to a recipient oocyte of an older woman who has experienced repeated IVF failure. By this 'rejuvenation' procedure the older woman is, in some instances, enabled to bear her own genetic infant. Early embryonic development, when transcription of the embryonic genome is minimal, is facilitated by the cytoplasm of the fertilized egg. Both genetic (mitochondrial DNA) and non-genetic factors appear to participate at this early stage. Two types of cytoplasm transfer procedures have been developed. In one, a small amount of cytoplasm is removed from a donor egg and injected into a mature recipient oocyte before IVF or ICSI treatment. The intention of this technique is to transfer cytoplasm but little or no mtDNA from the donor, so that the recipient egg will retain the full complement of its nuclear and mtDNA. In the second procedure, the nucleus of an immature egg from the older woman is removed and transferred to an enucleated egg obtained from a younger donor. After electrofusion and in vitro maturation, the reconstituted egg is fertilized with the partner's sperm and the embryo is transferred into the older woman's uterus. In the latter case, the oocyte has been reconstituted with the nucleus of one egg and the cytoplasm of another before fertilization. This technology is superficially similar to cloning but cytoplasmic transfer is not cloning as it involves fertilization and hence the transfer of the male genome to the conceptus.

Cytoplasmic donation widens the options (childlessness, adoption or donor oocyte programmes) available to a growing population of couples who face a high risk of failure with traditional IVF. As with ICSI, the preference provided by cytoplasmic transfer is a child genetically related to the mother. This novel method of assisted reproduction poses fresh ethical, social and legal concerns. The immediate ethical issue, of course, is to demonstrate the safety and efficacies of the procedure – a big ask since longitudinal studies take decades to bring in significant and reliable results.

Maturing human eggs in the laboratory

To create mammalian embryos using IVF techniques, embryologists need mature oocytes, which are routinely collected by ovarian superovulation.

More recently, it has been claimed that earlier stage oocytes (that is, the so-called 'resting eggs' or primordial oocytes) may be successfully grown to maturity in culture. The process is complicated and involves several steps whereby the immature primordial follicles are coached to maturity in culture media containing various growth promoters such as epidermal growth factor and hormones such as follicle stimulating hormone. The technology implies that immature human oocytes from stored frozen ovarian fragments could be utilized to create embryos. The ovarian tissue stocks can be obtained from individual patients prior to treatments such as chemotherapy. In 2007 the first baby created from an oocyte that was matured in the laboratory, frozen, thawed and then fertilized was born in Canada. Progress has also been made in related studies where scientists are hoping to preserve fertility in childhood cancer survivors by obtaining and freezing immature oocytes from girls as young as 5 years of age. Childhood cancers tend to have relatively good cure rates, of 70–90%, but the aggressive chemotherapy typically leads to sterility. It is not known whether these preserved oocytes would survive and lead to successful pregnancies in the girls when adult. By contrast, the freezing of mature eggs, followed by IVF after thawing, has resulted in the birth of a number of infants. This technology has offered some hope to patients under-going toxic drug treatments; however, it also raises serious health concerns for the babies conceived by this method.

Epigenetics, imprinting and assisted reproduction

In affluent western societies, births associated with physician-assisted reproduction now account for ~2–3% of all births, and the popularity of some technologies (such as ICSI) is rapidly increasing. Therefore, careful attention has to be focused on the longer-term effects of therapeutic interventions used to assist reproduction. While many follow up studies of ART children have suggested that ART poses minimal risk to normal development and child health, various birth registers have documented circumstantial evidence that infants conceived by means of assisted reproduction are at a greater risk of preterm delivery and low birthweight (IUGR). Other studies suggest an association between assisted reproduction and increased risk of certain birth defects such as spina bifida and cardiovascular malformations. Because the incidence of genomic imprinting defects, such as Beckwith–Wiedemann syndrome, Angelman syndrome and retinoblastoma, appear to be significantly more frequent in the ART offspring compared with the general population, the problem of a suspected connection between ART and disrupted epigenetic programming is being addressed. As described in Chapters 2 and 3, genetics focuses on how organisms retain traits by inheriting genes from their parents, while epigenetics refers to additional methods of biological inheritance that do not directly relate to the inheritance of collections of genes. Epigenetics refers to reversible, heritable changes in gene expression that regulate developmental characteristics without a change in DNA sequence. Characteristically, modulated gene expression represents a response to changed environmental dynamics, and many imprinted genes are known to play important roles in determining fetal growth. Since ART involves egg/sperm manipulations in the laboratory, an epigenetic connection for the observed increases in specific anomalies in the ART population cannot be ruled out. However, interpretation of these adverse findings is not clearcut because they may result from any combination of gamete manipulation, infertility drug treatment or an inherent defect in the infertile population.

Restrictions of confidentiality prevent, in a majority of studies, the clear association of offspring with birth disorders to specific ART approaches employed at the time of conception. Although known imprinting disorders are rare, complications of ART-generated epigenetic errors may account for a much wider spectrum of ART-related complications. Some studies have suggested that ICSI, by virtue of its invasive nature, is more likely to result in genetic and developmental abnormalities. However, it is difficult to assess whether these anomalies are a consequence of ICSI or from the underlying chromosomal defects in males with severe semen abnormalities. Further, contradictory findings may be generated from embryos with severe abnormalities not implanting, or being lost in early pregnancy, while in other studies they are observable at birth and are documented. Nature is acting as a selective evolutionary check-point in some cases. Only large long-term prospective studies, including the offspring from fertile donors, can elucidate the roles played by epigenetics and subfertility treatments in the etiology of malformations and intrauterine growth restriction.

Surrogacy

Whatever its antiquity and cultural pedigree, surrogacy, when used in conjunction with the reproductive technologies, is a relatively recent phenomenon. A surrogate is defined as a woman who agrees to bear a child on behalf of an infertile couple. Unlike adoption, an agreement is made before conception for the surrogate to become pregnant and bear a child and, in commercial cases, to be paid for her services. The most common form of technologically based surrogacy, known as genetic or partial surrogacy, occurs when the surrogate is inseminated using sperm from the partner of the infertile woman or, in situations where the partner is also infertile, by donor sperm. A couple would be likely to contract for partial surrogacy where the woman is unable or unwilling (in cases of inheritable genetic disease) to provide either the genetic (ova) or the gestational (uterus) component for childbearing. Gestatory, gestational or total surrogacy involves the surrogate being implanted with an embryo produced in vitro from donor gametes and the surrogate provides only the gestational component of reproduction. This situation is less common than genetic surrogacy because it is technically more complicated and requires extra resources such as IVF availability. An early landmark case of gestational surrogacy was that of the 'granny' surrogate, 48-year-old Pat Anthony, who gave birth to triplets in 1987 from embryos genetically belonging to her daughter and son-in-law.

A couple would be likely to contract for gestatory surrogacy where the woman has a missing or malformed uterus or has a severe medical condition (hypertension, diabetes) contraindicating pregnancy. Modern surrogacy challenges traditional assumptions about parenthood because assisted reproduction procedures make it possible to separate out the various phases of the reproductive process. It is now possible for a child to be subject to multiple parenting with two men (genetic and adoptee) fulfilling the functions of 'father' and up to three women (genetic, gestational and adoptee) fulfilling the differing functions of 'mother'. The birth of such children also holds wider kin implications for grandparents or other relatives. There is now also the distinct additional prospect that future generations of ART children will have cloned offspring in their midst, further complicating kinship relationships (Chapter 11).

Assisted reproduction, genetic diversity and the biology of conservation

In the 1970s, successful adaptation of animal research techniques revolutionized treatment of human infertility. These technologies are now being adapted to assist in the conservation of species endangered by pressing global environmental crises and vanishing bioresources. Species extinction is a natural process, but an exploding human population mixed with resource-hungry human activities are increasing extinction rates in an unprecedented manner. Immeasurable species, excepting domestic varieties, are already extinct or becoming threatened, endangered or marginalized. Biodiversity, as it measures the genetic variability of life on the planet, involves more than simply the number of species on Earth; rather it also incorporates the concept that ecological interactions among these diverse species create the existence, complexity, health and functions of ecosystems upon which all, including human, species depend for their survival. Without genetic diversity, all forms of life lose their ability to adjust to environmental change – a prerequisite for adaptive selection and the basis of evolution. Human-dominated ecosystems and related issues are the subject of Chapters 12–15; the present discussion centres on how the ARTs are being used to promote species conservation.

Inbreeding depression

Genetic diversity, or the extent of genetic variation in a population, provides all species with their evolutionary potential. The greater the variation in a population, the more likely it is that some individuals within that population will be able to withstand changing environmental conditions. Species with low genetic diversity are more prone to extinction compared with species with high genetic diversity. Genetic diversity is measured by the level of heterozygosity or the amount of allelic diversity. Heterozygosity refers to the number of individuals who are heterozygous for particular genes, while allelic diversity refers to the number of alleles present in the population. For example, humans have three blood alleles: A, B and O. Those individuals who are AB, AO, or BO are heterozygous for blood groups. When population numbers are reduced, inbreeding occurs which leads to a loss of genetic diversity, poor fertility and increased susceptibility to disease. The population's fitness may also decrease with harmful genetic traits becoming more common (Figure 9.3).

The role of ART in conservation

A well-documented problem facing animal conservationists has been the lack of success in natural breeding programmes. Typically, captivity has detrimental effects on wildlife, which can result in decreased fertility and behavioural incompatibility even if the two animals are genetically compatible. Under these circumstances, breeding programmes in conjunction with ART are the new frontiers in rebuilding the numbers of many endangered mammalian species. Artificial insemination, IVF, embryo transfer and cryo-preservation technologies allow conservation biologists, in conjunction with veterinarians, to more closely manage breeding programmes in an effort to ameliorate or avoid inbreeding depression. An example of success is the cheetah (*Acinonyx jubatus*) whose low genetic diversity and continued inbreeding has led to many problems, including a low sperm count with greater than 70% being morphologically abnormal. To date, many litters of cheetah cubs have been born through the use of the above technologies. Equally successful

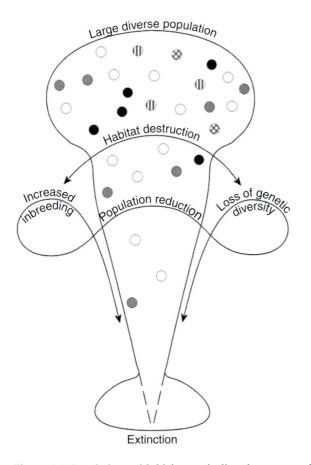

Figure 9.3 Populations with high genetic diversity are more likely to survive as greater genetic diversity provides flexibility under adverse conditions, favouring some individuals to reproduce. For example, a large diverse population with the presence of five different alleles (represented by dissimilar circles) for a particular trait experiences little selection pressure on alleles. Habitat destruction results in random reduction in population size, decreased genetic diversity (absence of hatched alleles), increased chance of inbreeding and corresponding loss of evolutionary potential risking extinction.

have been other conservation projects; such as bringing the black-footed ferret (*Mustela nigripes*), one of North America's rarest mammal species, back from the brink of extinction. Assisted reproduction also has animal welfare implications since shipping sperm, eggs and embryos from one location to another to facilitate breeding is less stressful than transporting the animals; these technologies also allow assisted breeding in wild animals without the need to keep them in captivity. Outbreeding, as facilitated by artificial insemination, for example, allows genetic contributions by those that are unable to breed naturally, or impregnation of females with males other than the dominant male. Examples of exceptional successes are the cheetah, giant panda, African and Asian elephants, black-footed ferret, gazelle and koala.

The giant panda (*Ailuropoda melanoleuca*), as the world's most widely recognized conservation icon, should be a conservation success story. However, China's panda population hangs on in only a fraction of its historic range and, with continued habitat loss and fragmentation, its future is increasingly threatened. Pandas are poor breeders in captivity, with the females being fertile for only 3 days each year. Urine tests can check when these 3 days will occur, and fertility treatments can be used to increase the rate of fertilization and increase population numbers. However, the other problem is that the males seem to have forgotten how to breed, and the females have forgotten how to rear their young. To encourage reproduction, a scheme, known as 'panda-porn', was championed by staff at the San Diego Zoo and involved showing captive pandas a video of successful panda mating strategies. Interestingly, this alternative method worked, and natural breeding was instigated in some cases. On the other side of the globe, Australian scientists are busily evaluating whether it is possible to freeze amphibian oocytes and embryos to preserve the gene base of endangered frog species and, in turn, boost population numbers of the beautiful endangered green and golden bell species. Again, the aim is to revive the genetic diversity of these depleted populations; however, with amphibians, it is necessary to learn a lot before anything practical can be carried out, as little is known about the effectiveness of ART in these species.

Preservation of animal habitats by setting aside areas free of human influence is a common and effective method of conservation; however, often the land required is not available or is not pathogen-free. An alternative approach to animal conservation has been the development of 'genome resource banks' (frozen zoos) which are repositories of cryopreserved gametes, embryos, tissues and DNA. Genome resource banks are useful in agriculture and horticulture where biomaterials from crop plants and farm animals are effectively stored to ensure future food resources. For conservation purposes, genome resource banks have the potential to preserve a wide variety of endangered species as well as to maintain the genetic diversity of others. One such initiative, called Frozen Ark, collects samples from highly endangered species, which allows for continued research and, hopefully, species renewal in future less hostile environments. In this respect, cryopreservation in conjunction with xenografting technology may offer new prospects in certain circumstances. Xenotransplantation involves grafting tissue (ovarian or testicular for reproductive purposes) from one species into another immuno-compromised species, with the subsequent purpose of harvesting mature eggs or sperm of the desired species. Host immunodeficiency ensures that the tissue graft is not rejected. Xenografting thawed ovarian tissue from the marmoset monkey, African elephant and the common wombat into mice or rats has resulted in follicular development within ovarian tissue of healthy appearance. As a consequence, it is hoped that ovarian tissue taken from dead endangered northern hairy nosed wombats could be frozen, and then xenografted to produce mature northern hairy nosed wombat eggs suitable for IVF use. The embryos would be implanted into common wombats.

For conservation and renewal of endangered species, cross-species embryo transfer is ideal as the technique allows embryos from an endangered species to be implanted in a surrogate mother of a more common species. Cross-species embryo transfers have had some success, with the birth of a zebra to a horse and an Indian desert cat born to a domestic cat. A major disadvantage of this procedure is that behaviourally and socially the two species would differ and so risk losing 'cultural' components normally acquired by learning. It may also be possible to regenerate individuals via cloning. Cloning of endangered animals, however, is fraught with physical and ethical problems since the process is species-specific and researching the peculiarities of an endangered species may not be justified due to their low numbers. Further, cloning does not increase genetic diversity – it only preserves existing gene combinations (Chapter 11).

In the final analysis, ART has helped dramatically in assisting conservation programmes, not least by increasing scientific understanding of the physiology and behaviour of a disparate group of endangered species and assisting, in practical terms, in their conservation. Knowledge about all aspects of the reproductive process, from courtship to nurturing the young, is vital to be able to assist endangered species to survive and eventually prosper in the wild. Major obstacles slowing down ART-assisted breeding programmes are the need to understand the details of the species-specific physiological essentials supporting fecundity. Breeding programmes need to be designed around the unique reproductive requirements of each species which involve, for example, monitoring the endocrinology of fertility cycles and pregnancy by analysing urine and fecal samples in the wild, as captivity data may give misleading results. Then again, ART is not the ultimate solution for the protection of endangered species because humans need to be educated on the importance of habitat preservation as well.

Principles of bioscience ethics for discussion

- The technologies driving assisted reproduction are complex and require a good grasp of human reproductive physiology; therefore, if responsible ethical judgements regarding clinical assisted reproduction are to evolve, the highest standard of biological understanding has to be conserved in the bioethical discourse. Explain, providing specifics and examples.
- In human evolution, sexual pleasure and conception are controlled by different physiological mechanisms. Discuss among yourselves the social advantages of continuous sexual receptivity and whether the assisted reproductive technologies can be considered the natural cultural consequences of our uniquely human biological heritage.
- A more recent development involves extraction and storing sperm from the body of recently deceased men with the view of inseminating the partner. Consider the bioethical implications for the cryopreserved pre-embryo whose biological father died prior to its conception. In this case do you agree or disagree that it is incumbent upon the practitioner to do what is technologically possible to alleviate loss of parenthood of the bereaved?
- In your opinion, should it be allowed to order 'desired' features of an artificially conceived child (for example, colour of eyes or mental features) and, according to this order, to select human reproductive cells, or frozen embryos?
- In the case of physician-assisted conceptions, should the resulting offspring be entitled to receive compensation in case this procedure damages his or her health? If in the affirmative, where should claims for compensation be entered and who performs the obligations of a parent towards an artificially conceived child?
- Granted that ART is expensive and has significant limitations in application, is it a valid use of conservation funds, or does it merely divert funds away from the much greater need of protecting natural habitats? Are there ethically valid reasons in being able to produce an animal in a petri dish if there is nowhere to release it?

10

The recombinant DNA technologies

... eugenics and genetics, they are clearly related.[1]

Genetic engineering and related technologies – biological perspective

Recent developments in genetic engineering have brought an unprecedented increase in our power over living things. Gene mapping, together with recombinant excising and splicing techniques, holds great promise for producing new kinds of plants, animals, drugs and for treating human genetic diseases. Transgenic plants and animals are genetically novel creatures because they carry integrated foreign genes, which are correctly expressed and inherited by subsequent generations. Modern biotechnology had its beginnings in 1973 when Herb Boyer and Stanley Cohen genetically engineered a human gene into bacteria that then produced that gene's product – in this case human insulin, which was then purified for therapeutic use. Prior to this breakthrough, individuals suffering from diabetes were treated with insulin derived from the pancreases of abattoir animals, usually pigs and cows. Needless to say, the medical and industrial possibilities were immediately recognized and venture capital was invested to create companies with the aim of genetically modifying organisms to mass-produce desired hormones, drugs, vaccines, etc. Among the many important human proteins now produced in this way are growth and fertility hormones, blood-clotting factors to treat haemophilia, and hepatitis B vaccine.

[1] The British Medical Association on Human Genetics (1998). *Choice and Responsibility*. Oxford: Oxford University Press, p. 3.

The technology used to produce transgenic organisms is known as recombinant DNA technology, or more popularly as genetic engineering and cloning. 'Recombinant DNA' means DNA made up of connected segments from mixed sources; for example, from different species or a combination of natural and synthetic DNA. Recombinant DNA technology has revolutionized experimental biology by advancing understanding of gene construction and regulation and through applications in agriculture, veterinary science, medicine, forensics and environmental pollution. In the area of environmental pollution, for example, recombinant (genetically engineered) bacteria equipped with DNA that codes for enzymes that break down constituents of oil, have been developed to help combat toxic oil spills. Biotechnology companies apply similar principles to deal with other pollutants and hazardous chemical wastes, such as sewage and dioxins. Recombinant organisms have also been developed with the goal of controlling, or eradicating, introduced feral pest species. Control of overabundant populations by immunocontraception is an important aspect of this research. Immunocontraception targets a component of the reproductive process such as ovulation, sperm maturation, fertilization or implantation, to reduce fertility by manipulating the immune system. The idea is to identify a protein essential for, say, fertilization, insert the gene(s) that encodes for that protein into a carrier organism such as a virus or species-specific parasite, and deliver the modified organism to the target species by injection, nasal spray or other means. On infection, the target species responds by producing antibodies to attack the foreign material, including the protein essential for fertilization. An important concern of this kind of research is the presence of the immunocontraceptive virus or parasite in live animal populations posing risks to non-target species and the risk of exporting the carrier beyond target areas. The term 'bioremediation' refers to the removal of unwelcome substances/species in the environment using living organisms both naturally occurring and recombinant.

At the simplest level, the major goals of recombinant DNA technology are no different from those of conventional technology. For instance, the aims of animal husbandry involve increases of fecundity, feed-use efficiency, food production and disease resistance. For centuries these characteristics have gradually been improved by slow breeding programmes designed to combine beneficent traits of individual animals. Now the animals can be radically changed in just one generation; for example, transgenic pigs expressing the human growth hormone gene grow fast and produce animals with less fat. It must be noted, however, that current biotechnology, as it relates to the environment, has the potential to have both positive and negative impacts because it usually means introducing a new organism into an existing situation. Foreign genes can have profound and unexpected effects on the overall pattern of gene expression and responsiveness to changing environmental conditions. It is imperative, therefore, that balanced risk and benefit assessments are made well before releasing any genetically modified organism to mitigate accidental environmental damage and preserve existing biodiversity.

Embryo transfer technology (Chapter 9) permits manipulation of embryos at the cellular and genetic levels. The success of this technology has empowered the veterinary and medical professions to select for sex, desirable physical characteristics, lack of deleterious genes and other genetic manipulations of embryos. Even the formerly distant prospect of mammalian cloning has become reality with the birth of Dolly – the sheep cloned from DNA taken from a live udder cell of a 6-year-old ewe (Chapter 11). Since Dolly, mice, cattle, dogs and many other animals have also been successfully cloned. This latest reproductive technology, understandably, caused an immediate preoccupation with how genetic advances will affect people's lives, often in bizarre and sensational ways. However, cloning should not obscure the more immediate positive goals of gene technology; on the other hand, science's seemingly limitless power to biotechnologically redesign our lives has raised well-grounded fears and sparked ethical concerns.

Balanced biologically informed debate has to be encouraged since innovations in genetics open up not only immediate possibilities but also for future generations, by manipulating the kind of living organisms brought into the world. On the optimistic side, manipulation of heredity in medicine and agriculture for carefully defined purposes and under appropriate supervision can both be ethically acceptable and socially desirable. Application of embryo technology for the preservation of endangered species holds broad appeal (Chapters 9 and 15). We must also acknowledge that genetic manipulation is not new – just the technology involved. Chapters 3 to 5 discuss ways that congenital risks can be heightened by parental lifestyle or sexual behaviour, and how best to protect the right of children to be born free from preventable disability. Parents have, since the earliest times, socially engineered their own children, demonstrating that human conduct and cultural manipulation are as potent as the modern gene technologies in driving human destinies.

Gene therapy

A widely discussed issue is whether deliberate intervention in the human genome is acceptable under any circumstance. Generally, gene transfer to the human genome is considered acceptable, under current therapeutic standards, only if it provides benefit to the individual and the usual safeguards for innovative therapies are observed. Since somatic cell (e.g. most of the cells of the body) gene transfer has no role in producing a new generation, it is argued that it is not ethically different from other established forms of therapy. The use of chemotherapy or radiotherapy, for example, likewise alters the cellular genome of healthy as well as cancer cells. However, the complexity of genetic manipulation, except in the most straightforward of cases, should not be underestimated. That is why much somatic cell therapy research is directed at diseases involving single gene defects which are potentially fatal (some 4000 disabilities due to single gene defects are known to affect an estimated 1–2% of the population). In cases of more complicated multigenic or polygenic gene inheritances (those arising from the interaction of a number of genes), gene therapy may just be a matter of wishful thinking. Despite the odds, scientists are attempting to identify the genes involved in polygenic illnesses because, while single gene disorders are rare, polygenic disorders are common. That polygenic disorders are common should not surprise us when we consider the 3.1 billion base pair sequences, or around 22 000 protein-coding genes, of the human genome. Progress in the identification of polygenic disorders has been made. For example, familial forms of colon or breast cancers – the most common forms of cancer in women – have been traced to certain genes called oncogenes. The relationships of known breast cancer genes such as $BRCA_1$ and $BRCA_2$ with risk factors can now be clarified, permitting evidence-based preventive action in persons at high genetic risk. Better quantification of susceptibility to disease in family units can also be made once particular disease-bearing genes have been identified.

Contradictory statements as to the heritability of complex behavioural characteristics, such as violence, criminality, intelligence, addiction or sexual orientation, abound in the scientific literature. Criminal behaviour, in particular, has at various times been attributed to the environment or to genetics, despite the fact that no single gene for criminality has ever been identified. Progress, however, is confirmed since behavioural genetics has updated the age-old 'nature versus nurture' debate to the new 'nature via nurture' perspective. Genome sequencing technology has brought recognition about ways that cultural/environmental influences can dynamically alter gene expression. Experiences that switch genes on and off have biochemical impacts: for example, in at-risk cases of heart disease, environment encompasses eating, drinking, smoking habits and exercise; in the brain, changed neurotransmitter feedback reactions triggered by some environmental impact may, in turn, increase the risk of major depression in those with a genetic predisposition to depression. Mood disorders and their predisposition are transmitted familiarly. It is reasonable, therefore, to assume that all, or almost all, polygenic disorders involve a considerable degree of interaction with the environment. The healthy solution to a particular deleterious genetic predisposition, if known, may well be to endorse a lifestyle adaptive to our genetic makeup. On the other hand, a 'corrected' general state of health does not necessarily guarantee that heart disease genes will not interact with other genes and still lead to a heart condition. Chapter 7 on wellbeing reviewed modern concepts as to why some of us become ill while others, in seemingly similar circumstances, stay well. In summary, therefore, it is important to keep the role of genetics in proper perspective and not be tempted to pursue genetic answers to every social, behavioural or medical problem. Lives are shaped by genetic background and a range of socioenvironmental factors, such as the purposeful or unconscious reinforcement from infancy of some behavioural patterns so that, eventually, they appear to be inherited. The erroneous belief that complex human behaviour is purely genetically determined would seriously undermine our sense of personal responsibility and free will, but a realistic understanding of the role played by our genes can promote responsibility and free will.

Although somatic gene therapy and germ-line modification are very similar in technique, they are quite different from an ethical perspective, as altering germ-line cells raises questions of our power to redesign human beings. Less dramatically, alteration of a defective gene in the germ cell or in the early embryo would enable future generations to benefit from the treatment, but its safety in both the short and long term cannot presently be guaranteed. In view of these transgenerational concerns, it is often stated that germ cell gene therapy should be prohibited. Caution, from the bioethical perspective, is strongly recommended when it comes to performing a manipulation which has not been properly assessed and the safety of which is not known. Were it ever possible to give reasonable assurances about the safety of a particular manipulation, it is still unclear whether society would judge its application ethically acceptable. Some argue that decisions should not be made which affect an individual prior to his or her conception. Others argue that this line of reasoning could equally be used against other procedures routinely performed for the benefit of a future child, such as ensuring that the mother has been vaccinated against rubella.

The assumption that somatic cell therapy affects only the treated individual and not the germ-line cells may also not be strictly true, especially if applied to the early embryo. The phenomenon of genomic or parental imprinting confirms that the soma, or body, influences developing germ cells during gametogenesis by selectively marking or imprinting them. At fertilization, this imprinting influences the direction of the conceptus's growth and development. The phenomenon of genomic imprinting has shown us that DNA is not passed intact through the generations because environmental influences also produce lasting inheritable changes in DNA expression. The key academic point is that soma–germ-line feedback loops exist, implying that alterations in somatic genes may be subtly echoed in germ-line gene expression.

In unscrupulous hands, technical advances in germ-line genetic modification raise the really disconcerting issue of eugenics. Eugenics, as defined in the *Concise Oxford Dictionary*, 'is the science of the production of fine (especially human) offspring' or, I may add, its driving force is to direct reproduction toward specific societal goals unrelated to health issues. In the age of genetic engineering, eugenics can also be popularly understood as the creation of 'designer' babies. Interestingly, however, eugenics is an old idea traceable to Classical Greece where Plato advocated it as a necessary aspect of the 'ideal' society: the best should mate with the best and the worst should be prevented from reproducing – reminiscent of officially sanctioned sterilization programmes of the mentally ill and homeless in Nazi Germany and Aboriginal girls in 1950s Australia. We should never forget the human capacity for excess; as demonstrated in the horrors of Hitler's racial eugenics programme.

Whether the techniques of assisted reproduction should be available to all to try to improve the health, performance abilities or the physical traits of their offspring, is controversial. It has to be faced that the demand for eugenic programmes is already a reality in advance of the technology's practicability. Parents have treated their children with growth hormone, now created in large quantities by genetic engineering, because of the belief that being tall is advantageous in both economic and social terms. Genes could be inserted that would make people taller, better looking and more intelligent according to prevailing fashions. In favour of this principle, it could be argued that if women infected with AIDS, those with a disability or with alcohol addiction have the right to bear children, surely other women can choose to have a beneficial genetic trait introduced into their eggs? Should society, through some form of regulation, impose limits on the technologies prospective parents can exploit to enhance selected features in their offspring? Biodiversity is part of the normal continuum of adaptive variation providing biological stability, and enhancing survival in the long term. To suggest that we know, in evolutionary terms, what constitutes 'improvement' or 'normality' when at times it is often difficult to define what constitutes a disease, is typical of human arrogance. Genes that appear to be deleterious may provide benefits of which we know nothing, because genes have many functions and may control entirely unrelated effects – a phenomenon known as pleiotropy. Sickle-cell anaemia, a recessive single gene disorder, is a severe abnormality of the red blood cells incompatible with an active normal lifestyle. However, a single sickle-cell anaemia gene (the heterozygous condition) provides some protection against malaria; thus, the gene has become endemic in areas where increased protection against the blood parasite *Plasmodium* is required. As a consequence, sickle-cell anaemia is common among Afro-Americans where about one in twelve is a carrier. Owing to widespread genetic ignorance back in the 1970s, blacks in the US found to be heterozygous carriers (one copy of the gene does not cause illness) were discriminated against in jobs and insurance, tragically demonstrating how voluntary screening can go badly wrong.

In summary, we may think that 'enhancement' means the elimination of genetic disease, and 'improvement' means choosing specific behavioural and intellectual traits that we want in our babies. Nevertheless, we risk misunderstanding what improvement or enhancement, in the evolutionary sense, may really mean. The social challenge, in the age of genetics, is to provide assistance to people who want to avoid passing on a severe genetic disorder, while still providing unambiguous respect and proper support for those who suffer disabling genetic conditions.

In the above context, it is comforting to know that gene technology has been in use, in various guises, for quite a while, and that its development did not take place in an ethical vacuum. Professional codes, such as the Code of Ethical Principles for Genetics Professionals and guidelines issued by hospital Institutional Ethics Committees exist, and are conscientiously enforced. Bioscience ethics aims to bring to the bioethical discussion an awareness of the biological dimension in which the technologies function. Informed consent may then balance ways in which advances in the technology can offer hope to families affected by genetic problems, whilst still recognizing inherent risks and the potential for misuse.

Many of the ethical dilemmas arising from the new genetics are very similar to those which arose in other areas of medicine; that is, do the benefits outweigh the risks. The emphasis mostly centres on the duty to act in the patient's interests, to avoid or minimize harm, respect patient confidentiality and provide up-to-date information – including being honest about medical uncertainties. Only if these criteria are respected can valid informed consent be obtained. However, the common ethical guidelines of medical practice must be modified when they are applied to genetic testing in general because genetic testing reveals important details, not only about the individual's genetic background, but also about other DNA-related people. Genetic technology can deliver information about future disease affecting ourselves, our relatives and the risk probability in future conceptions. Genetic technology differs fundamentally from treatment in other areas of medicine in which the individual's values and priorities may be the sole determinants. It is reasonable to expect that any ethical consensus reached must include an awareness of the ways in which others, including future children, may be affected by individual decisions. Extra responsibility is placed on scientists, researchers and medical professionals to ensure that the technology gained is used wisely, and that no resulting children are foreseeably disadvantaged.

As stated above, theoretically it is possible to perform gene therapy using either somatic cells or germ-line cells. Alteration of the genes in the somatic cells should affect only the individual treated, whereas altered genes in the germ cells are intended to be passed on to the next and subsequent generations. The basic principle of both types of gene therapy is to correct the fault at the source by ensuring that the cells receive the correct instructions. Theoretically, this could be achieved in a number of ways:

- if a gene is missing, it could be added
- part of an abnormal gene could be corrected to make it function correctly
- the abnormal gene could be removed and replaced with a normal one
- a normal gene could be inserted to supplement the abnormal gene which would be left in the cell

The most likely option to succeed is the insertion of a gene, either where the gene is missing or to augment an existing defective gene. Ideally, the gene should be inserted into the stem cells (these generate new cells) so when the new cells are produced, they will already have the correct gene in place. If the gene is inserted into other cells, the effect will last only as long as those cells survive and the treatment will need to be repeated at regular intervals. To date, hundreds of clinical trials, aimed at treating conditions ranging from inherited disorders such as cystic fibrosis (CF) to defects in cellular immunity, have been given the go-ahead. Private companies have raised hundreds of millions of dollars to enter the field and are now sponsoring most of the clinical trials in conjunction with academic centres of gene therapy research. For those with serious genetic disorders such as CF, gene therapy may offer the only hope of a cure. CF is a lethal autosomal recessive disorder of the epithelial glands causing major dysfunction in the pulmonary system and gastrointestinal tract. More than 400 different mutations in the CF regulator gene (the gene that produces symptoms of CF in individuals carrying two mutated alleles) have been described. Only the most frequent CF mutations are screened, but the screening only identifies approximately 70–90% of carriers in most white populations.

The major hazard of somatic gene therapy, as with all experimental treatments, is that things could go wrong. The inserted gene could be incorporated into the wrong cell, where it might not work appropriately, or it could disrupt the normal working of other genes, causing unexpected side effects. This may not be so serious if it occurs in only a single, or a few, somatic cells where death of the cells would merely render the treatment ineffective. A more serious scenario would be where the gene is integrated into tumour suppressor genes. In this case, a critical transformation in just one cell may be sufficient to activate a malignant tumour. If the gene therapy is likely to induce an occasional cancer, risk has to be evaluated in similar terms to that already undertaken for new chemotherapeutic agents, most of which are potentially carcinogenic. Recent developments directed at creating an artificial human chromosome may be a safer way of delivering genes. The point about artificial chromosomes is that the desired genes would be permanently added and, if correctly inserted, would not disturb the function of existing healthy gene sequences. Possibly the most serious scenario, not shared with other conventional treatments, is the unintentional introduction of a modified or artificial gene into the germ plasm, risking its appearance in the next generation. It is evident that, as the technologies are advancing, their therapeutic and/or preventive management places greater and greater responsibility, and accountability, on the scientific and medical communities.

In summary, the manipulation of heredity in medicine and agriculture for carefully defined purposes and under appropriate supervision can both be ethically acceptable and socially desirable. In addition, the application of recombinant DNA technology for the preservation of many endangered species may be the last option (Chapters 9 and 15). It is unlikely that gene therapy will ever become available for the majority of genetic diseases, nor benefit the majority of citizens, but we should not lose interest in prevention of inherited disorders. Prenatal genetic screening, for example, is an effective and, for many, an acceptable measure for combating genetic diseases.

Prenatal genetic screening and diagnosis

In industrialized societies, some form of prenatal genetic screening and diagnosis is now offered routinely to every pregnant woman. It involves many screening and testing techniques, some more invasive than others, which can determine whether or not the fetus is genetically 'healthy'. The more invasive diagnostic tests used are amniocentesis, performed around 16 weeks of gestation, and chorionic villus sampling (CVS) performed between 10 and 11 weeks of gestation. Chorionic villus sampling is highly accurate but carries an increased risk of spontaneous miscarriage, which needs to be balanced against the value of an earlier diagnosis. Cordocentesis and fetal tissue sampling can be used to confirm a clinical diagnosis or detect a genetic pre-disposition to a disease so that protective measures such as treatment as early as possible, preparation of the parents for the future or giving them the option of terminating the pregnancy can be canvassed.

Non-invasive prenatal screening techniques normally include screening for parental age and family history of disease or disability. It may also be by serum (blood) screening, molecular tests or ultrasound. Ultrasound scanning is rou-tinely offered to pregnant women over the age of 35 to monitor the develop-ment of the fetus, but it can also detect both major and minor defects. Maternal serum screening is becoming a more common technique as well. This relies on the small number of fetal blood cells that circulate in the mother's blood stream and which could, in theory, be isolated and tested to provide a vast amount of fetal information. However, such information can only be in the form of statistical probabilities – especially for subsequent pregnancies, as fetal cells are retained in the maternal circulation so current and previous fetal cell loads are mixed. Obtaining 'informed consent' is likely to become much more complex when it becomes possible to test with a single procedure for increasing numbers of different disorders. Where a blood sample is to be taken for screening to identify an increased risk of one or more specific disorders, it is important that parents are informed of the tests to be carried out and the implications of an unfavourable result before being asked to consent. By encouraging informed decision-making, medical ethics helps to protect the individual's self-determination and responsibility. However, in the 'genetic era', individual confidentiality cannot be easily guaranteed because genetic information is identifying and it may be possible to identify genetically related family members at any future time by identifying the individual from whom the genetic material was initially derived.

Health professionals do not necessarily discourage couples likely to be affected by severe genetic disorders from having children. Once pregnancy has been established, prenatal diagnosis may be requested for a variety of reasons. The request may imply a willingness to consider abortion, a desire to plan ahead in an informed way, or a hope for reassurance. Either termination or continu-ance involves anguish for parents who have embarked on a planned pregnancy in the hope of having a healthy child. Despite the fact that the transmission of severely disabling genetic traits contributes to a very difficult existence for the child inheriting them, society does not intervene to restrict people with genetic disorders from procreating. Nor does society put pressure on parents to ter-minate an affected pregnancy. Bringing new life into existence is one of the most important acts individuals undertake and, ideally, all intending parents should think about how to ensure the health and welfare of their future child. People who are aware of genetic problems in their families are usually more conscious than others of the need to consider the wellbeing of the future child.

Preimplantation genetic screening and diagnosis

Embryologists' search for safe and reliable methods of screening at ever earlier stages of gestation has led to the development of testing embryos for genetic disorders prior to implantation. Preimplantation genetic diagnosis (PGD) is a technique used to identify genetic defects in embryos created through IVF technology before transferring them into the uterus. Because only unaffected embryos are transferred, PGD provides an alternative to prenatal diagnostic procedures such as amniocentesis or chorionic villus sampling. The process involves testing for a range of genetic disorders in one or two cells removed from in vitro fertilized embryos at the six- to eight-cell stage. The early embryos continue to develop and only unaffected embryos are selected for transfer into the uterus. PGD allows a woman to begin a pregnancy knowing that her child will not suffer from an inherited disorder for which there is a known risk and, since determining the chromosomal makeup of embryos reduces the need to terminate a pregnancy, the service is offered to both fertile and infertile couples.

Preimplantation technology was developed in the mid 1980s in the UK for families at risk of CF but since then PGD has become a standard technique for detecting genetic disorders such as CF, Down's syndrome, Tay-Sachs disease, Duchenne's muscular dystrophy, Huntington's disease, haemophilia A, β-thalassaemia and many more. Following demand, preimplantation diagnosis technology is now widely available, with an increasing number of centres around the world having the expertise to perform the biopsy and analysis. However, it should be noted that there is no assurance that the embryo manipulation per se may not induce as yet unidentified developmental anomalies; in this context a suspected connection between Assisted Reproductive Technologies (ARTs) and disrupted epigenetic programming (Chapter 9) needs addressing. Indeed, Dutch researchers have recently found that PGD reduces pregnancies and live birth rates in older women (35–41 years) undergoing IVF. Ethical considerations and controversies also abound which revolve around the status of the preimplantation embryo and the jettisoning of positively diagnosed individuals, especially if the technology were to be applied in future to diagnosing more insignificant genetic traits.

Neonatal genetic screening and diagnosis

The main aim of neonatal screening is to identify affected newborns (neonates) in order to commence treatment at the earliest opportunity. A good example is provided by the Australian practice, effective since the early 1960s, in which all Australian newborns are screened for the inherited genetic disorder responsible for phenylketonuria (PKU). PKU is an enzyme deficiency disorder causing severe mental retardation if the infant's diet is not controlled before 6 months of age. Therefore, the benefits of routine neonatal screening for PKU are clear since the worst effects of the disorder can be avoided through early diagnosis, followed by an appropriate diet low in the amino acid phenylalanine. The advantages of early diagnosis are considered to be so great that little provision is made to provide advance information or to seek parental consent. In other parts of the world, screening for CF and hypothyroidism is also routinely provided to all newborns.

Presymptomatic screening for individuals and populations

Increasingly, genetic testing is able to identify which of those individuals with a family history of a genetic disorder will, or may, develop the condition at some time in the future. The certainty with which this prediction can be made depends upon the condition. With autosomal dominant disorders, such as Huntington's disease, the presence of the defective gene gives a clear indication that the individual will develop the condition, although age at onset and severity will vary between individuals. For other, more common, disorders which are known to have a genetic component, such as heart disease, diabetes or breast cancer, testing could indicate an increased predisposition to the disorder, but whether that individual develops the condition will depend upon a combination of genetic and environmental factors. Where it is possible to treat the condition for which an individual is at risk or where some intervention can usefully delay onset or diminish the symptoms, early diagnosis and appropriate counselling would be beneficial.

More controversial is testing for conditions for which there is no useful medical intervention. Also not so straightforward are requests for presymptomatic testing of children for adult-onset disorders because the child's future right to make informed decisions about testing, or not, would be forfeited. Young people under 16 years of age, who have sufficient maturity and cognitive understanding, can be expected to be involved in consent to treatment or testing on their own behalf.

As evidence accumulates for a genetic component of an increasing number of common disorders, the possibility of screening the susceptibility of whole populations or groups also becomes an option. However, before predisposition screening for common disorders is introduced into routine clinical practice, there has to be clear indications of benefits. Identifying the individuals at increased risk of a particular disease within a particular population is worthwhile only if there is some action which can be taken to avoid the expression of the condition or if early identification of risk would lead to improved management of the disease. People do not respond uniformly to the results of presymptomatic testing. For some, the knowledge may provide psychological benefits whatever the results – a negative test brings relief and a positive test provides release from uncertainty. Others, however, would simply prefer not to know what fate holds in store for them, even if they know that they may be at risk.

Population carrier screening for autosomal recessive disorders has been advocated as a way of permitting people more choice in reproduction. In some countries, carrier screening has progressed from prenatal screening to pre-conception screening, even of schoolchildren. Genetic screening for thalassaemia (low haemoglobin content in the red blood cells) in Cyprus and Sardinia, where the disease is endemic, is such a case. Health professionals are then involved in helping teachers in aspects of this type of prepubertal care.

The use of genetic technology for social purposes

Few potential uses of genetic information have caused as much controversy as those in the social sphere, particularly its use by insurance companies. It is often assumed that any non-medical use of genetic information is discriminatory, and thus unacceptable. However, information may be appropriately used or misused in either the social or medical spheres, so all potential uses of genetic information need to be ethically assessed and monitored. Because each person's DNA (with the exception of identical twins) is unique, the genetic markers within a small sample of blood, semen, hair, skin or other biological material can conveniently be analysed and used to match it with the donor. Genetic matching is particularly useful for some non-medical purposes, such as establishing consanguinity (kinship) and in the forensic detection of crime. For example, in 1986 DNA profiling was used for the first time in a court of law to convict a man of rape and murder. A positive DNA match was obtained from samples left at the scene of the crime and a sample obtained from the accused. At the time, the probability of this match occurring by chance was set at one in several million. Since then, claims of 'near-certain' probability from a match using this technology have been moderated. The possibility of human error, accidental or deliberate contamination of the samples and equipment malfunction has also to be taken into consideration when calculating probabilities. Whilst DNA profiling evidence alone is no longer sufficient to convict, the technology is still a powerful tool for identifying perpetrators of violent and sexual crimes, and for clearing innocent suspects.

In matters involving kinship, genetic matching has also proved very useful. Despite the fact that a person's DNA profile is unique, certain characteristics are shared between close relatives. By comparing the genetic makeup of more than one family member, it is possible to confirm or refute a claimed genetic relationship. The most common use of consanguinity technology is for paternity testing, providing the probability of an accurate match of 95.5%. The issue of paternity testing has been a hot topic in recent years, with some fathers testing paternity without the mother's consent and suing them for 'paternity fraud'. In Australia there are legal requirements for both parents to give consent, and genetic counselling to minimize the impact of an unfavourable finding. However, 'under-age' young people may be required to have a DNA paternity test against their wishes as their consent is not always seen as an essential. Genetic information is more than just clinical information – it reveals something about the individual's past and so may influence positively or negatively the child's future decision-making. The DNA paternity procedure may also be used to establish consanguinity for other purposes, such as adults seeking to identify their genetic mother or father following adoption in childhood, immigrant family reunion schemes and even babies inadvertently mixed up in maternity wards.

The Human Genome and the Human Genome Diversity Projects

The 12th February 2001 marked a major event in the history of molecular biology. Two versions of the almost complete 3.1 billion base pair sequence (or 20 000–25 000 protein-coding genes) contained in the DNA of the human genome were published simultaneously. The international Public Human Genome Consortium and the Ohio State University conducted the public version, which was published in *Nature*. Celera Genomics of Rockville, Maryland conducted the other commercial version, which was published in *Science*. Scientifically, two sequences are better than one because the opportunity for comparison and convergence is invaluable; however, it also creates tensions (see section below). The public Human Genome Project was formally established in 1988 as an international collaboration of scientists working to locate and sequence the human genome; that is, to identify all the genes contained in human cells.

Since then, progress of the Human Genome and Human Genome Diversity Projects has greatly accelerated owing to improvements in fast-paced computer-automated sequencing machines that can generate large amounts of sequence data. Once DNA fragments are sequenced, computer programs catalogue this information and compare it with databases of known sequences to determine if it represents a novel piece of chromosome sequence, or if it shares comparable sequences with other DNA fragments. The use of computer hardware and software for sequence analysis, along with many other applications such as archiving sequences in databases for storage and research, is part of a relatively new discipline called bioinformatics, which effectively integrates biology and information technology. With the assistance of such a rapid production phase, complete genome sequences and complete gene catalogues are becoming available for an increasing number of complex organisms. Thus, the completion of the whole human genome heralded a new technological era impacting on basic science and medicine and consequently on the ethical, legal and social implications of unravelling the keys to our genetic material.

To gain access to the human genome sequence depends upon which version you want to look at. The sequence from the public project is available to all those connected to the internet. The private version is less freely available since Celera does not provide its data, as is customary, to the publicly funded database GenBank, a member of the International Nucleotide Sequence Database Collaboration. GenBank makes data freely available to anyone without restrictions on use or distribution. To gain access to the entire Celera genome requires you to subscribe. In other words, they are offering to sell the information. But how do we know whether a particular sequence of human genome is representative of all humans? Most genome centres collect DNA from several different individuals. For example, scientists at Celera Genomics worked with DNA from five individuals; two males and three females self-identified as white, African American, Hispanic and Asian. It is common knowledge that, with the exception of identical twins, the genome of each person is unique, but all humans share a basic set of genes that control development and normal body functions. The Human Genome Project is an effort to produce an initial sequence as a typical 'reference' sequence of our genome. This reference sequence acts as a resource for evaluation and comparison, enabling scientists to identify human genetic similarities and to understand the range of genetic variation between individuals. The reference sequence tells us what genes are in the human genome and what some of the most common variations are, but it does not identify all variations of all genes in humans; this would necessitate sequencing every individual genome.

Now that we have a typical reference of the basic molecular blueprint of a human, scientists are beginning to see larger trends and genetic signals they were not previously aware of. Many researchers were puzzled by what seemed to be too few genes in the genome to explain the complexity of human biology and behaviour. We now know that the actual number of genes is so much lower than predicted because many genes can code for multiple proteins through a process known as alternative splicing. Specifically, genes have switches called promoters, which consist of special sequences of DNA that allow for extrinsic cultural and environmental influences to change gene expression without changing the DNA sequence. In this way, new scientific discoveries, such as RNA transcripts of single genes that can lead to the pro-duction of different proteins from the same pieces of DNA, challenge the concept of the gene alone as the dominant factor in biological development. As a result, a growing number of scientists are rethinking the orthodox view of genetic determinism and are developing novel ways of studying what a gene is and how it works. However, as explained in previous chapters, basic gene sequences are only the start as there are countless important epigenetic forces regulating gene expression, particularly in higher organisms, which play a significant role in the way the information in the genome (or genetic consti-tution) affects the phenotype (or observable properties of an individual). The Human Genome Project has, undoubtedly, increased our level of under-standing of how our bodies work, the causes of many genetic diseases and the genetic component of common anomalies. Decisively, this mammoth sequencing project has reduced the fear that we regard ourselves as nothing more than the sum of our genes and that our illnesses can be fully categorized by genetic composition, rather than by individual genes and physical symp-toms. Nature's work is far more challenging, and knowing our gene sequences will not alone provide the solution to all our ills. What is crucially important to understand is how, in holistic terms, these genes are orchestrated. A simple example may explain what is meant by orchestration. DNA hybridization technology has revealed that the DNA of humans and chimpanzees is much more similar (98.4% similar) than would be expected given the considerable morphological differences between the two species (Chapter 1). Given only 1.6% difference, evolution must also rely on other mechanisms like differential gene expression (penetrance) or transmission of variant signalling in space. The caption under Figure 11.1 (p. 194), describing the degree of epigenetic difference between monozygotic (identical) twins, is of interest in this context. Also of interest is the fact that we share 60% of our genes with chickens, 75% with dogs, 50% with fruit flies and a whopping 30% with yeast – the organism we use to make bread rise and beverages ferment. Obviously, the important genes are highly conserved from species to species.

What the Human Genome Project has established is solid evidence for the evolution of genes, providing – for those who need it – proof that we are an integral part of the great unity of life. What defines us genetically is the complexity of how our genes interact to provide the myriad functions and unique human characteristics. Ethically we cannot conduct sophisticated genetic studies on humans, but by studying the genes of 'model' organisms such as mice, yeast and fruit flies, we can form hypotheses and make predictions about how genes function in humans. For example, mutated genes that are known to give rise to disease in humans also cause disease in fruit flies and according to a report from the Howard Hughes Medical Institute,[2] approximately 61% of genes mutated in 289 human disease conditions are found in the fruit fly. Increased understanding of the causes of health and disease is leading directly to improved treatments and therapies.

Simultaneously with the rush of new scientific discoveries and insights, significant resources have been committed to examine the ethical, legal and social issues of genome research. The range of controversial issues central to the regulated manipulation of genomes and the protection of individual rights covers, broadly: privacy of genetic information; the moral, ethical and legal dilemmas posed by genetic technology; the patenting of genetic information; and educating the citizenry to make informed decisions about their personal – and beyond personal – choices and judgements. These dilemmas take on greater importance when we consider the Human Genome Diversity Project. The Human Genome Diversity Project was first proposed in 1991 by the Human Genome Organization (HUGO) to find out 'who we are as a species and how we came to be'. Its aim is to gain insight into human origins, evolution, patterns of migration and reproduction, and the global distribution of genetic disease. The last was categorized within the discipline of genetic epidemiology – the study of the distribution of disease in groups of relatives and ethnic populations and the identification of the genes responsible. By collecting DNA samples from a small number of individuals in up to 500 different indigenous population groups from around the world, a DNA database could

---

[2] Howard Hughes Medical Institute. *Blazing a Genetic Trail*, at http://www.hhmi.org/genetictrail.

be established containing information from which genetic diversity within and between population groups could be evaluated.

The diversity proposal has generated unease about a revival of eugenic practices and sparked heated ethical debate. Anxiety has been expressed about the use of indigenous populations for research purposes, largely for the benefit of wealthy industrialized societies. In this sense, genomic research goes beyond families because it involves whole population groups as research subjects even when just a few individual DNA donors contributed tissue samples for analysis. In response, the Human Genome Diversity Project has recommended that these concerns could be addressed by ensuring that all commercial gains resulting from the samples collected are used for the benefit of the local donor population. The greater medical benefits would be in the form of an increased awareness of the health needs of ethnic minority groups. With its emphasis on genetic difference between groups, there is the additional concern that the information generated could be used to attempt to justify discriminatory attitudes and behaviour, or even to develop new forms of warfare aimed at specific population groups. Specific agents would be activated only in the presence of particular sets of genetic variation, causing infertility, illness or death in the target population (Chapter 14). The question of whether and how to screen susceptible individuals and minority groups raises many ethical, legal and practical issues of who owns, and who has, the right to use such genetic information. Stem cell technologies and other advances lend commercial importance and value to the tissues and genomes of Indigenous populations with relatively homogeneous genetic makeups.

Access to the ownership of genomes

Copyright, trademarks and patents are typically grouped into an area of the law that has become known as Intellectual Property. Trade secrets are sometimes included in this area as well. Securing a patent is typically the first step in commercializing an invention or discovery. Before the invention can be marketed, however, approval from other federal and state agencies may be needed. In the USA, a new food product or drug would probably require approval from the Food and Drug Administration (FDA). When a patent for an invention or drug expires, the impact on the marketplace can be substantial, as was seen by the proliferation of marketers of the artificial sweetener aspartame (originally traded under NutraSweet) when the Monsanto company's patent expired in 1992. Since then, several other companies have marketed aspartame under their own label, or simply as a generic product. With the influx of sequence data, the rush to file patents on biotech inventions is bringing the patent system to a virtual standstill and may even create a new economic divide between the biotech-rich and the biotech-poor countries. The poorest countries are already greatly disadvantaged when it comes to developing, filing and defending patents, so it is easy to see how the present trend can further increase the impediments to creating their own intellectual property. This is happening while governments around the world are still debating whether to grant patents for specific genes such as the sequences of human genes linked to disease, or for inventions such as animals genetically modified to produce drugs in their milk.

For a patent to be granted, the focus must be on invention because a mere discovery is not patentable. Therefore, the distinction between an unpatentable discovery and a patentable invention may be, at a minimum, a new and useful application of the discovery. In general, raw products of nature are not patentable but DNA products become patentable when they have been isolated, purified or modified to produce a unique form not found in Nature. The patentability of inventions under US law, for example, is judged on four criteria. The invention must be 'useful' in a practical sense, it must be 'novel' (i.e. not known or used before the filing), it has to be 'non-obvious' (i.e. not an improvement easily made by someone trained in the relevant area), and the invention must be 'described' in sufficient detail to enable one skilled in the field to use it for the stated purpose. Applying these principles to genetic material, it becomes apparent that any change from the natural state, no matter how trivial, may be patentable. Genetic diversity, on the other hand, is the stock of genetic material resulting from the genes and gene sequences, as well as the combined effect of the expression of those genes and gene sequences within individuals, populations and communities. Genetic diversity is valuable and a resource for future economic development which has potential to improve the quality of our lives. Many scientists, however, believe that it is more appropriate to patent novel technology used to discover genes, their functions and gene therapy approaches rather than patent gene sequences themselves.

Serious concern has been articulated regarding the patenting of genetically modified organisms (GMOs). For a practical example, genetically modified rice rich in β-carotene is a product from Monsanto, who are offering it free of charge. The rice, called 'golden rice' because of the yellow colour the β-carotene gives it, is expected to provide nutritional benefits to those suffering from vitamin A deficiency-related diseases (β-carotene is converted into vitamin A by the body – an essential nutrient that boosts the immune system). By enhancing the activity of the immune system, adequate vitamin A intake can reduce the occurrence of irreversible blindness in children and reduce mortality associated with infectious diseases, such as diarrhea and childhood measles. Critics, however, are concerned that the 'golden rice' monoculture could undermine alternative low-tech and more cost-effective initiatives, such as the plan to reintroduce the many vitamin-rich food plants that were once available in these target countries. Another concern is the continued promotion of monocultures and genetic uniformity by the use of these crops, rather than by encouraging biodiversity.

Biodiversity provides a vast library of genetic material for use now and in the future and, through the application of biotechnology, this genetic information can be accessed by our economies. Australia, for example, is one of the Earth's 12 mega diverse nations, with some 85% of Australia's flowering plants, 84% of mammals, 89% of reptiles, 93% of frogs and 85% of in-shore fin fish being endemic. Such genetic diversity is a priceless genetic resource. Geneticists working for pharmaceutical and other companies have increasingly targeted communities for biomedical research material, especially in the study of genetic determinants of common diseases, and have also enjoyed some well-known successes. Particular mutations predisposing to breast, ovarian and colon cancer have been identified through studies of Ashkenazi Jews. Undoubtedly these discoveries will have important implications for cancer prevention and treatment, but the communities concerned have expressed fear that they may become the target of discrimination. Thus, there is a growing public concern that the protections existing for communities in biomedical research are inadequate. To date, the most developed protections for communities in biomedical research are found in guidelines for research involving Aboriginal communities, as demonstrated by those of the Australian National Health and Medical Research Council.

In conclusion, recombinant DNA technology offers hope to possibly millions of people and can contribute substantially in solving environmental problems. But the technology also has the potential to cause great harm. Ensuring, as far as possible, that the benefits are realized and the harms are avoided is not a responsibility solely for scientists, health professionals, bioscientists and bioethicists. These are matters for society as a whole and, without open dialogue, many of the potential benefits arising from recent advances in genetics will be lost.

Principles of bioscience ethics for discussion

- Myth no. 1: that genetic manipulation by humans is new. For centuries, coveted genetic characteristics have been gradually incorporated through slow breeding programmes designed to combine beneficent traits of individual plants and animals. What is radically new is the technology employed. Now organisms can be genetically manipulated to express products from synthetic, plant or animal genes or any combination of these. How should society formulate regulatory guidelines that balance technological progress with precaution concerning harmful unknown long-term effects?

– Myth no. 2: that multifaceted human behaviour, such as sexual orientation or addiction, is purely genetically determined. From the evolutionary perspective, what are the rewards and drawbacks of complex polygenic inheritances?

– Gene ethics probe: the publication of the human genome was a landmark in the transition of biology from 'wet' to 'dry': from essentially laboratory-based analysis to computer-driven analysis, or bioinformatics. Henceforth, scientists will be 'wet and dry', as computer-based predictions from bioinformatics laboratories lead to models that need to be tested by geneticists and molecular biologists. What laws do you consider should be put in place to regulate the use of genetic information? The human genome has been branded as a resource for everyone – like the periodic table of elements. Should this also apply to the genomes of other organisms or should biotech and pharmaceutical companies be given patent protection to provide investment incentives for continued research and development?

– Many fear that technology has created an artificial divide between Nature on the one hand and technology, politics and economics on the other. How can the individual help in the search for a constructive balance between Nature and human creative skill? What realistic goals are both sustainable and desirable?

11

Stem cells, nuclear transfer and cloning technology

Practices which are contrary to human dignity, such as reproductive cloning of human beings, shall not be permitted.[1]

Unease and apprehension about science and technology are not new in the history of science but now a new stage marked by a growing uneasiness about powerful science has been reached. Questions about the social responsibility of scientists and the applicability of their technology must be faced directly by both the lay public and the scientific community. Knowledge is dangerous in the hands of specialists who cannot always foresee detrimental implications and/or potential misapplications of their work. Although scientific understanding of a particular biotechnological or medical advancement may not be complete, responsibility to society for an understanding of the ethics surrounding its development falls specifically on those concerned with bioscience ethics and bioethics.

Probably the most publicized controversies to date have been in the area of recombinant DNA technology and its influence on biomedical and military research. Few recent science-based innovations have generated more public disapproval and misunderstanding than cloning technology. Public debate has focused on nightmare scenarios, such as large numbers of identical individuals being created for military purposes, or in the likeness of a mad dictator. In a climate of hysteria, the legitimate biological concerns and the therapeutic benefits of cloning are bound to be overlooked. However, the concerns about humans being used as subjects for cloning experiments are not totally fanciful.

---

[1] Article 11 – The Universal Declaration on the Human Genome and Human Rights (1997); elaborated by UNESCO.

Critics of reproductive cloning technology may well be justified in believing that, for some ambitious individuals, the major goal of this new technology is not alleviating the burden of disease, but to be at the forefront of the science of human reproductive cloning. The inevitable broadening of our knowledge base as concerns cell growth, differentiation and maturation may then be used to progress toward cloning humans. In a climate of scientific competition, consumer pressure and the euphoria of breaking new biological ground, caution is bound to be neglected and remedial motivation for some investigators may be to assist the infertile who have no natural way of becoming parents. Putting aside uncertain efficacy in the foreseeable future, we may well have to welcome a discrete population of cloned children. Therefore, the scientific and general community must responsibly temper the potential misapplication of this valuable technology. I'm hopeful that in this context bioscience ethics may again be a useful forum, facilitating the transition from applied science to applied bioethics.

What is a clone?

The word 'clone' itself is derived from the Greek word κλων meaning 'twig'. The earliest use of the term describes plant grafts, or the ability of plants to propagate asexually (vegetatively). We all take advantage of these natural forms of vegetative propagation when we take cuttings of favoured plants and, by simply sticking them into the ground, look forward to their becoming autonomous plants. Asexual reproduction is based on the mitotic division of the nucleus and so produces offspring that are nearly genetically identical to the parent. It is a rapid, effective means of making new individuals, widely practised in Nature. A serious drawback of asexual reproduction is its very equivalence that leads to the production of a genetically identical (or near identical, see below, p. 194) progeny or clone. Although a clone may be well adapted to its existing environment, it is at risk should conditions change. This is the reason why organisms that produce genetically different offspring (diversity fostered by sexual reproduction) are more successful when the environment alters unpredictably in time and space. In the latter circumstance, at least some of the genetically diverse offspring may be adapted to the new environmental conditions. Since the 1970s, the word 'clone' has also come to designate a viable mammalian offspring generated from a single parent; that is, an artificially generated identical genetic copy of an existing life form.

In the animal world, spontaneous splitting of the early mammalian embryo results in monozygotic twins, or a clone pair. In humans, for example, the

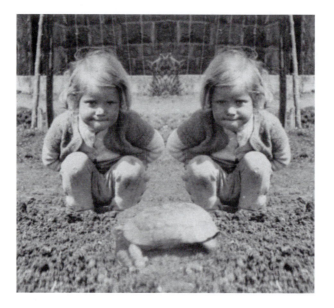

Figure 11.1 Monozygotic pairs are considered perfect clones of each other because they share all their genes. However, despite the importance of genetic factors in common, it is interesting to note that for monozygotic twins the concordance of genetic disease (that is, the proportion who are both affected) seldom exceeds 40%. Variations in the timing and pattern of growth and differentiation might, in part, explain the unexpected differences in disease expression.

separation of one embryo into two masses at the 64-cell stage or beyond and the subsequent development of each mass into a fetus, produces identical or monozygotic twins. Despite the fact that such twins have the same genetic constitution, possess identical blood groups and closely resemble each other, they are not perfectly identical. Subtle genetic–epigenetic variations, such as a more favourable uterine position or genetic mutation in one twin, are significant in differentially affecting the pattern of growth and development of each twin (see caption under Figure 11.1). In this context, it is significant that the first cloned domestic cat had a different fur colouring from its gene donor. Cat fur colouring involves several genes situated on the X-chromosome and, since females have two X-chromosomes, some of these genes were randomly inactivated during X-dosage compensation early in female embryonic development, which works to equalize the expression of X-chromosomes in both sexes (Chapter 2). Subtle differences in clones may be considered as evolution on a small scale, but this is of practical importance only in situations where the generational turn-around is short. The chance arrival of an antibiotic-resistant mutant bacterium in a population of bacterial clones, for example, would provide a selective advantage provided that this type of antibiotic forms part of the bacterium's environment.

Cloning technology in conjunction with recombinant DNA technology has long been applied in research involving microorganisms and some invertebrates; but when the technology was successfully applied in a mammal, the political situation abruptly changed. The basics of recombinant DNA technology were described in Chapter 10. By 'recombinant DNA', it is meant DNA made up of connected segments from mixed sources – possibly from two different species, or a combination of natural and synthetic DNA. An example of combining DNA from different species is the insertion of a gene from a human into the DNA of a yeast which, with luck, may manipulate the yeast cells into 'factories' producing the protein product of the human gene (Chapter 10). A typical goal of recombinant DNA research is to obtain many copies of the transgenic cell containing the gene of interest. Detection of the desired cell and its cloning is routinely accomplished by various techniques available to the molecular biologist. For example, one form of cloning technology is being used as a treatment for cancer and involves the production of monoclonal antibodies employed in immunotherapy for tumours. White blood cells are removed from the patient and exposed to cancer cells in the hope that they will produce the correct antibodies to destroy the cancer. Only about one in 100 000 cells will react, producing the required antibodies; these cells are then cultured (cloned), isolated and injected back into the patient to seek out and destroy the tumour. Another use of these cells is to produce identical monoclonal antibodies which, when isolated and injected, can detect specific types of cancers. Diagnostic kits using the latter technology for colon cancer are available. Drugs directed against the tumour can also be attached to the specific monoclonal antibodies as a form of cancer treatment.

It was not until cloning technology was combined with stem cell research and Dolly – the cloned sheep – was created that the implications reached into our collective consciousness; as demonstrated by Bill Clinton's (the then President of the United States) immediate response to request an ethics report. The prompt formation of the Shapiro Committee clearly demonstrated that, in the mind of the government, cloning technology needed immediate attention. The ethical implications of Dolly's existence affected the whole of society, requiring broad discourse among peoples of widely differing opinions and expertise.

There are two main types of cloning – reproductive cloning and embryonic stem cell or therapeutic cloning.

Reproductive cloning: basic principles

Cloning in the reproductive context describes the process by which an animal cell, or group of cells, is used to derive a new but identical organism. The defining feature is that the cloned individual is genetically identical to the ancestral organism from which it was derived. Cloning from animal cells is very different from asexual propagation because differentiated animal cells are greatly restricted in their developmental capacity. With the exception of sperm, eggs and early embryos (technically named blastocysts), each adult cell is committed to perform a specialized function. To perform its specialized function, only a defined set of genes (those necessary to perform the allotted task) are actively expressed, with the remainder of the cell's genome being switched off. Therefore, to reprogramme a differentiated cell to the undifferentiated state, laboratory intervention is necessary. The biological breakthrough came in 1997 when a Scottish team headed by Ian Wilmut at the Roslin Institute, announced the birth of Dolly, the sheep cloned from a 6-year old differentiated cell. She was the product of fusion of an unfertilized egg, stripped of its nuclear DNA, with the donor cell obtained from the mammary gland of her sole parent. The process of inserting the nucleus of a diploid somatic cell into an oocyte stripped of its nucleus is known as somatic cell nuclear transfer. The reason for using an unfertilized egg host cell with its nucleus removed is that it is stocked full of signal proteins and other products essential for early development. The developmental process is initiated by the donor nucleus, and growth and cell division follows.

Contrary to popular belief, Dolly did not have precisely the same genetic makeup as her parent but rather was only a near genetic copy. In the first instance, she possessed genes from mitochondrial DNA which were donated by the enucleated egg cell (0.05% to 0.1% of genes are carried unchanged in the cytoplasm, contrasting with the nuclear component of random genetic combinations from two parents). In other ways too, Dolly's identity differed from her parent by the inheritance of any somatic mutations which may have been acquired during the ancestral cell's life. Such mutations may not have prevented the specialized somatic cell from functioning perfectly well in its original site, but could provide potentially fatal flaws to the proper functioning of other organs in the new embryo. When considering Dolly's uniqueness, we should remember the phenomenon of epigenetic inheritance and genomic imprinting. Epigenetic programming defines the developmental process that fine-tunes growth and differentiation according to environmental determinants (Chapter 3). Subtle effects throughout the various in vitro manipulations and prenatal development in the surrogate's unique uterine environment would have influenced variable genetic expressions. For example, altered hormonal influences during the clone's development in utero may change regulatory settings of the clone's own, still flexible, hormonal feedback systems. Since somatic cells do not live indefinitely, another unknown variable is whether the clone's lifespan would be foreshortened by being pre-programmed to die at the age at which the original cell would have been discarded. There is evidence in support of the early death hypothesis. Japanese researchers have found that cloned mice sickened and died of pneumonia and liver disease earlier than their normal counterparts, and researchers from the United States identified imprinting disruptions in cloned cattle that suffered from developmental abnormalities at birth. Dolly, critically ill, was finally put to death in 2003 at the age of only $6\frac{1}{2}$ years, even though many sheep live more than 10 years. In middle age she suffered from a progressive lung disease found in older sheep as well as premature arthritis. Although unconfirmed, these maladies may be a consequence of her origin. Thus, any or all of the above variables may have challenged the clone genetically.

Embryonic stem cell (aka therapeutic or biomedical) cloning

When looking at the ethical and regulatory aspects of human reproductive cloning, the western nations were quick to support a ban on human cloning but were prepared to use human embryos for therapeutic stem cell research. The goal of stem cell cloning is to create an embryo in the same manner as for reproductive cloning but to derive embryonic stem cells for research and potential therapeutic purposes instead of producing a child. Since better hygiene and the discovery of antibiotics and vaccines have significantly decreased the problem of infectious diseases, degenerative ailments have become the chief health problem in industrialized nations. The major degenerative diseases, in decreasing frequency, are heart disease, cancer, stroke, chronic lung and liver disease, diabetes and Alzheimer's disease.

Stem cell lines, once established, can be multiplied indefinitely and used to create cultures of particular cell types for introduction to the human body where needed. Consequently, a constant supply of new embryos or blastocysts is not required for many of the anticipated treatments. An implant of cultured stock stem cell lines is said to be allogeneic because the implanted cells and the recipient patient differ genetically. For allogeneic purposes, stem cells are derived from early human blastocysts, as these are not yet committed to specialization, or from embryonic germ cells as these are protected from commitment because they are destined to become the next generation of eggs and sperm.

The embryos come from IVF clinics and are either incapable of further development or are surplus to requirements. In both circumstances they are used only after informed consent has been obtained. Thousands of embryos preserved in liquid nitrogen exist in laboratories with, according to a 2003 study, some 400 000 in the United States alone.

Diseases or injuries affecting the central nervous system (CNS) are particularly receptive to allogeneic stem cell therapies because, due to the blood–brain barrier, the introduced cells are less likely to be rejected. Consequently, a major effort in allogeneic stem cell research is aimed at finding effective treatments for neurological diseases and injuries such as Parkinson's disease, Alzheimer's disease, stroke, spinal cord injury and brain cancer. The treatment protocol for Parkinson's disease, for example, may be to design a catheter which can accurately implant a bolus of healthy stem cells into a particular part of the brain. These cells are then expected to develop into functional dopamine-producing neurons (death of the cells that produce dopamine is the underlying cause of Parkinson's).

For the treatment of diseases not within the CNS, such as diabetes or heart disease, autologous cloning is required to avoid immune rejection by the patient. Autologous cloning is where the implanted cells are derived from the recipient patient. To obtain a 'personalized' autologous stem cell line, the first step is to create a blastocyst from one of the patient's own body cells and a DNA-stripped unfertilized donor oocyte or egg cell. Donor oocytes are typically obtained from aborted fetuses or spare oocytes donated by couples undergoing IVF treatment. The process of inserting the patient's genetic material into a host egg cell is known as 'reprogramming' because this fusion (nuclear transfer) technology allows the differentiated to dedifferentiate and the oocyte nucleus combination to develop, in vitro, into a blastocyst. The cultured stem cells are then directed down different developmental pathways to become heart, liver, bone marrow or other cells, according to need. For example, in the event of a heart attack, which occurs when blood flow to a section of heart muscle becomes blocked, the damaged heart muscle begins to die. If a blood supply is not restored, the weakened heart can lead to further difficulties, including death. In this scenario, the hope is that compatible stem cells would be used to repair and restore function. Before reaching their final stages of differentiation, the 'about-to-be' stem cells would be injected into the patient's ailing organ. Guided by the body's own regulatory signals, the cells would differentiate into tissues supplementing or replacing the old damaged muscle cells, restoring healthy tissue function. Figure 11.2 diagrammatically illustrates the principle behind growing tissues and organs for transplants.

Growing body parts to order

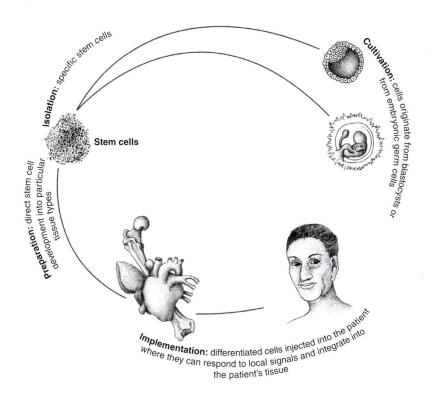

Figure 11.2 Growing spare body parts to order. See text for explanation.

By using the therapeutic cloning technology described above, it is also possible to insert new or modified genes into the stem cells and then deliver the genetically manipulated cells into body tissues. An obvious example is therapeutic cloning of pancreatic insulin-producing stem cells for patients with diabetes. The great advantage of this type of cloning is that the use of genetically engineered stem cells generated from the patient's own genetic information avoids allogeneic host-versus-graft reactions. Cultured insulin-producing pancreatic cells would also in future solve the current shortage of insulin-producing cells from donor islets, and reduce the personal and societal burden of morbidity from diabetic complications. In this way, researchers hope to use genetically modified stem cells to repair human disorders that are currently incurable.

Adult stem cell alternatives

In future it may also be possible to use adult- or somatic-derived stem cells from sources such as bone marrow from adult individuals or from umbilical cord blood rather than from embryos or fetuses. Small numbers of adult stem cells exist to maintain and repair tissue cells and it seems possible to transform them into specific cell types in the laboratory. For example, adult-derived stem cells, including haematopoietic stem cells (from bone marrow), have given rise to a variety of tissues such as connective, blood, bone, cartilage, striated muscle, nervous, lung and liver. Of foremost importance, however, is the need to successfully control and streamline the transformation of the stem cells into their specific cell types in experimental animals, before adult-derived stem cell technology becomes valuable in curing human ailments. The immediate advantage of adult stem cells is that they do not derive from an embryo, thus circumventing objections based on protection of potential human life. The disadvantages of using adult-derived stem cells are twofold. Firstly, unlike embryonic stem cells, which can be grown in large quantities, they do not readily multiply in culture and, secondly, they are less proficient at turning into certain specific cell types; that is, they are multipotent (produce many but not all cell types) compared to the pluripotent (capable of generating all cell types) embryonic cells.

Reproductive cloning: ethical considerations

Cloning technology has provided many valuable insights into cellular function, developmental physiology and ageing processes. Likewise, practical applications now include better animal models for human diseases, leading to new or improved therapies. Many technical problems remain, since the art of directing embryonic stem cells down specific pathways is still in its infancy and the reprogramming step in autologous cloning is inefficient, requiring a very large number of egg cells. However, under intense medical and commercial pressure these major technical difficulties are likely to be solved in the very near future. Greater rates of success with autologous therapeutic cloning, of course, will create separate complications because the resulting blastocysts, being genetically identical to the patient, can be directed to form particular stem cells, or can be surrogated to produce a child clone of the patient. There is a world of difference between the objectives of therapeutic and reproductive cloning, but the difficulty is that the technologies overlap and can be utilized to serve either purpose. Given the rewards in alleviating disease and suffering from the development of both allogeneic and autologous stem cell therapy, we must decide which aspects of cloning technology are ethically acceptable.

The ethical status of stem cells is a matter of controversy because the label 'embryo' or 'fetus' is associated with the technology. In fact, the early pre-implantation blastocyst is not yet an embryo and is more properly called a pre-embryo. For this reason, ethics commissions in several nations, including Australia, the United Kingdom, the United States and Europe, have approved research on the human pre-embryo up to 14 days because the conceptus is not differentiated. In this sense, the pre-embryo cells are no different from those in standard tissue cultures. On the other hand, it is true that a human pre-embryo could, given the right conditions, develop into a human being. The protagonists against cloning maintain that by virtue of the pre-embryo's special status, it is wrong to carry out destructive experiments on them.

Up to now the discussion in this chapter has centred almost exclusively on the technological aspects of cloning. The following focuses on those who may be the most vulnerable group – the children resulting from this technology. What are the rights and needs of these cloned offspring, both as children and as adults? Who would like to speculate on how the cloned offspring may respond to the realization that an arbitrary decision was made that he/she would live a life in genetic likeness of a pre-existing person? It might be argued that identical twins have the same genes and do not seem to suffer from identity problems. Twins are, nevertheless, a unique mixture of their biological parents, and their future life, unto their old age, is relatively unknown; that is, not displayed in advance. Further, those who maintain that embryo cloning is akin to mimicking the natural occurrence of twins – artificial twinning in fact – should reflect on the confusing relationship, twin or offspring? In the biological context, there is no confusion – the newcomer is a twin or sibling but never the offspring. The term genetically-identical-different-aged or GIDA twins is used to describe this relationship. Given this insight, we could further speculate on what psychological and physical stresses the younger twin may be subjected to by its older GIDA twin. In such a relationship, do the comforting terms of belonging such as 'my son' or 'my daughter' and 'my mum' or 'my dad' have real meaning? What about a clone's right to family identity, feelings and self-image? Could the clone legitimately claim that society has acted against its best interests and voice strong objections to having been created by means of risky, experimental procedures, especially if injured or maimed?

Proponents of cloning may argue that in future the question of genetic uniqueness may be bypassed by combining reproductive and therapeutic cloning technologies. It may be possible to insert a few chosen genes from another donor in order to create a genetically 'unique' clone. Could this type of reproduction still be called cloning, and would it not amount to frivolous experimentation on unconsenting subjects? How would the younger GIDA twin cope with the tension between seemingly conflicting rights and obligation? Some deny that parents can ever wrong their children by deliberately bringing them into being, even with avoidable genetic impairments. Does this not amount to virtually unlimited autonomy of parents in their reproductive decision-making? Such parents may even decide not to reveal to the child its origins, to reduce any psychological ill effects arising from being a clone, or perhaps out of fear of the social stigma.

Western societies in particular are increasingly calling parents to account for decisions and behaviours that adversely affect their children, whether it be drug abuse (Chapter 4) or dysfunctional parenting (Chapter 6). On the surface it seems that we have come a long way from the days when children were considered the property of their parents. Compassionate societies demand that children's needs, desires and fears have to be considered seriously. Certainly, the secular community is promoting social change as seen in the UN Convention on the Rights of the Child, which extends the full range of human rights – civil, political, economic, social and cultural – to children. It is a sign of a mature society when the best interests of the most vulnerable are at the centre of legal judgements – a process unprecedented in human history.

Other serious concerns can be categorized as integral to the family unit. For example, will the birth of the baby clone resolve parental vulnerability associated with infertility or old age or, if posthumously conceived, grieving for the dead? The desire by older or infertile individuals to be cloned can lead to speculation about the psychological motivations. Do they desire immortality? Are they attempting to re-fill an empty nest? Is this an exaggerated narcissistic investment in staying young? Is it the selfish imposition of their needs on a sibling masquerading as a child or children? Would the younger be pressured to accept the standards of the older, rectify its mistakes, omissions or sins, and, if so, what about its right to lead a free previously untold life? Or may the motivation be more practical, such as a source of self-compatible transplants? What is reasonably certain is that most individuals looking forward to cloning themselves are expecting the birth of a healthy baby, but what about the medical risks? Since Dolly, scientists have succeeded in cloning several species of mammals: goats, pigs, sheep, cows, rodents and a mule. However, the high failure rates (>90%) comprising miscarriage, stillbirth, disability and morphological deformity suggest that the technology is inapplicable for human reproductive cloning. To give the reader some idea, from 277 reconstructed embryos, only 29 were implanted in ewes and only one – Dolly – developed successfully. Cloning primates may even be a greater challenge, as demonstrated in one centre where an unknown number of attempts resulted in the cloning of a human male embryo using the nucleus of an epidermal cell from the leg transferred into the cytoplasm of an enucleated cow's oocyte. This embryo was allowed to grow to nearly 400 cells before being incinerated in accordance with legal requirements.

The argument that autonomous individuals have the right to do what they will with their genes does not always make good sense – not least because infertile couples are too vulnerable to make an objective decision. Couples desperate to reproduce do not pay attention to risk assessments, bioethical considerations and the like because all they hear is that there's hope. Such an attitude is understandable because the desire to have genetic offspring – 'having a child of one's own' – is one of the strongest biological drives. Should desperate, infertile couples be given access to cloning technology permitting them to perpetuate the desolation of infertility?

Principles of bioscience ethics for discussion

- The twenty-first century has already been identified as the biotechnology century. Modern biotechnology has the potential to solve many of the world's problems, including food, health and the environment. However, as with all-powerful new technologies there are risks, both real and perceived, along with the benefits. It is, therefore, crucial that the community better understand what's really going on in high-tech laboratories and what scientists are trying to achieve. Given that it is irresponsible not to be knowledgeable about the science of cloning when formulating ethical and regulatory guidelines, how should we organize ourselves communally and influence each other individually?
- Using animals, researchers have demonstrated that genetically modified neural stem cells can track and destroy cancerous brain cells. The transplanted stem cells were seen to migrate significant distances through healthy tissues to reach the cancer cells, an unexpectedly good result. What are the ethical requirements regarding follow-up research and at what stage should the technique be tested on humans?
- As a society we have never been in favour of regulating reproduction. Should we now regulate the reproduction of those wanting to be cloned? Which should be given greater weight, infertile couples' right of reproductive freedom and access to any available technology, or the duty of care argument cautioning against cloning humans?

12

Human-dominated ecosystems: re-evaluating environmental priorities

If psychosis is the attempt to live a lie, the epidemic psychosis of our time is the lie of believing we have no ethical obligation to our planetary home.[1]

The lack of union between short-term pursuit of profit and long-term sustainability of our planet is the most fundamental threat to our existence. Ignorance, driven by the peculiarly human quest to conquer natural ecosystems, is at the source of contemporary environmental predicaments. This chapter is dedicated to an explanation of fundamental biological principles governing environmental integrity; that is, the relationship of the biosphere within its habitat.

Population growth and economic activity – are we overstraining our limits?

The biggest problems facing humankind – problems which link the environment, health and social issues – are those of population growth and levels of resource consumption. Presently, there are over six billion people living on this planet. It took approximately four million years for the world's human population to grow from just over zero to one billion in 1850; two billion in 1930; then, as antibiotics, vaccines and technology increased life expectancy, three billion in 1960; four billion in 1975; five billion in 1987; six

[1] Roszak, T. (1993). *The Voice of the Earth: An Exploration of Ecopsychology*. New York: Touchstone Simon & Schuster, p. 14.

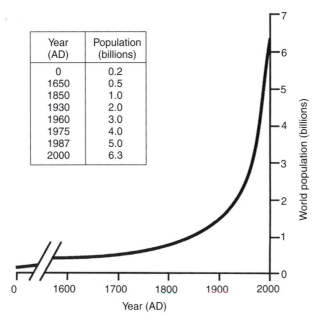

Year (AD)	Population (billions)
0	0.2
1650	0.5
1850	1.0
1930	2.0
1960	3.0
1975	4.0
1987	5.0
2000	6.3

Figure 12.1 Exponential growth of the world's human population. (Reproduced from Pollard, I. (1994). *A Guide to Reproduction, Social Issues and Human Concerns.* Cambridge: Cambridge University Press, p. 226, with permission.)

billion in 1999, with the projected estimate to reach seven billion in 2013 (Figure 12.1). If this is not a sufficiently strong wake-up call, then the impact of such a growth rate can be better appreciated by considering the time taken for the population to double in size. Growth rates of around 2% per annum (a doubling time of 35 years) are particularly relevant, since large parts of the world have a population growth rate close to this. If we similarly look at economic activity, at a 3% per annum rate of growth, the world economy would double in approximately 23 years, triple in approximately 37 years, quadruple in approximately 47 years, and increase fivefold in approximately 54 years, clearly an unsustainable state of affairs. Population growth and economic activity, however, have not been uniform; a typical resident of the industrialized quarter of the world uses approximately 15 times as much paper, 12 times as much fuel and 10 times as much steel as a resident of an overcrowded, developing country. Not surprisingly, the environment has not escaped unscathed from the rapid growth of both population and economic activity, and the results of unsustainable growth are increasingly apparent everywhere. Yet, since the 1960s when concern peaked, as expressed by Paul Ehrlich's book The Population Bomb, the world has behaved as if the issues of human-carrying capacity and the need for population control are taboo subjects. Human-carrying capacity is the maximum population that can be supported at a given living standard by the interaction of any given human–ecological system.

On the other hand, due to rising age at marriage and increasing availability and use of safe, effective contraceptive methods, global population growth has slowed. According to the latest estimates from the US Census Bureau, the actual annual increase in world population peaked at about 88 million in the late 1980s and declined steadily thereafter to a low 75 million per annum in 2002, at which it stabilized before rising to 77 million per annum in 2007. Specifically, the world's population rose 64% between 1950 and 1975, then 47% in the last quarter of the twentieth century. The United Nations' prediction is a rise of 30% between 2000 and 2025, then 14% between 2025 and 2050. Currently, population growth rate remains high in the Middle East, South Asia, South East Asia, Latin America and sub-Saharan Africa. Negative population growth rate is especially noticeable in central and eastern Europe (due to low fertility rates) and southern Africa (due to high HIV-related deaths). It is predicted that Japan and some countries in western Europe will encounter negative growth due to sub-replacement fertility rates in the near future.

We know that demography is influenced by issues of economics, culture (including social and environmental values), politics and migration. We also know that Earth's overall capacity to support people is determined by natural constraints. Now that previous United Nations' projections have to be revised downwards, it can be assumed that developing nations, as they modernize, will behave reproductively like industrialized nations. Given a global fertility rate of around 1.85 children per woman in 2050, for instance, then the global population would peak at about 8.5 billion people and subsequently start declining. Programmes which directly help to meet demands for family planning have been most effective in alleviating poverty, reducing suffering and promoting economic and social development. Programmes which emphasize and support women's reproductive rights have been especially effective. Human beings are empowered when they are more able to make effective decisions about children, such as when and how many children to have. At the same time they gain dignity and energy to reduce the insatiable drive for expansion and exploitative destruction of the world's biodiversity and its remaining wilderness. On a more optimistic note, people are better fed, better educated, healthier and live longer compared with 25 years ago, so effective reconciliation may still be under our control.

The extant environmental problems facing all nations – developed and developing – are similarly matched in their destructiveness and require urgent attention. The predominant biological problems for the industrialized countries concern air and water pollution, contaminated food and lack of open space. These all contribute to an increased incidence of stress-induced lifestyle diseases, such as cardiovascular disease, diabetes, cancer and depression. Stress-induced conditions are also called diseases of adaptation; that is, diseases of an exogenous and non-infectious etiology (Chapter 7). Interestingly, diseases of adaptation are also sometimes called 'diseases of affluence'. The predominant biological problems for the overcrowded developing countries are lack of arable land, social instability, civil war, famine and infectious disease, all contributing to an increased incidence of desperation and despondency.

Extinction and conservation of biodiversity

While it is true that technological developments have provided overall improvements in human welfare in many parts of the world, it is also true that our local, regional and global environments are becoming increasingly stressed. Whether highly urbanized or industrialized, every country makes heavy demands on their ecosystems. Both city and country life are dependent on massive power consumption, much of which is drawn from non-renewable and polluting sources. Much of our wealth, the wealth that has directly and indirectly supported our urban growth, has come from resources buried under the ground. Most of the world's habitable land is under heavy competitive pressure for housing, farming, mining, industry, forestry, transport or recreation, a fact illustrated by the cost of land of any kind for any purpose within or nearby major cities. Pollutants are flushed by natural rainfall into the rivers and hence into the oceans. River systems and the oceans need special attention because of the difficulties inherent in determining underwater impacts. Introduced aquatic species, agriculture and dammed rivers cause extinctions in places where humans are fairly scarce. A decreasing supply of pristine estuaries and wetlands presents us with an acute conflict between their technological use and their natural biological function as nursery and breeding grounds.

With the human appropriation of natural habitats and the ongoing decline in air and water quality, countless plant and animal species are becoming extinct every day. A particularly spectacular but not unique correspondent's report (BBC, 1996 and www.abc.net.au/news/stories/2004/01/20/1028651.htm) from Bihar State, India, can serve as one example. The report described how disorientated and starving elephants were now raiding homes looking for food because of loss of their land by human encroachment. The animals naturally caused an upheaval, especially after finding stocks of rice wine, which they consumed together with whatever else they could find. A dangerous war

ensued between enraged human and beast, effectively destroying the traditional mutual respect between the two; what we are really witnessing is the
last desperate act of a unique and vanishing ancient species.

At the other end of the world, melting Arctic Ocean ice is pushing polar
bears to suicidal swims and cannibalism, while an unprecedented number of
lone walrus calves, far from shore, drown or starve because their mothers
follow the rapidly retreating ice edge north. Pacific walrus, *Odobenus rosmarus
divergens*, have to forage for food by going further and diving deeper towards
the sea floor and, not surprisingly, the young are unable to keep up or forage
for themselves. Shallow continental shelf areas are the traditional feeding
grounds for many marine mammal species and it is precisely these grounds
where the first effects of global warming are felt. The unrestrained ecological
destruction of coral reefs in South East Asia and other parts of the world is
another example of humans losing control. When the demand for fresh fish is
so lucrative, dealers encourage fishermen to catch as many fish as quickly as
they can, with devastating environmental consequences. According to some
studies, overfishing and coastal development have already caused greater
devastation since the 1970s than at any time in the past 220 000 years; it is not
just the fish that are depleted but the whole reef complex with its associated
invertebrate communities as well. Much of the destruction seems irreversible
due to the disappearance of corals in favour of algae, and seaweed consequent
to the disappearance of seaweed-eating herbivores such as large fish, turtle and
dugong. Seaweed competes with coral for reef space and, if seaweed over-
abundance is not kept in check, corals are unable to recolonize depleted areas.
Current trade in reef fish is unsustainable and is the marine equivalent of the
'clear felling' of forests. Must we really stand aside and see a sustainable source
of food disappear forever in the space of a few years?

As commodities become increasingly scarce they, of course, also rise in
value. For example, one of the world's rarest plants – an African cycad, *Ence-
phalartos woodii,* now the star of Cape Town's Kirshtenbosch Botanic Garden,
has a microchip implanted in its stem to protect it from smugglers and thieves.
Rare animals in the wild are also being tagged in this way so that conservation
authorities can use satellite tracking systems to keep tabs on them. The high
value of disappearing plants and animals makes it inevitable, however, that
smugglers will eventually find ways around the system. Many of the lions,
tigers and bears that still delight circus audiences across the world are illegally
obtained according to TRAFFIC, the arm of the World Wide Fund for Nature
which monitors trade in wild animals. TRAFFIC Europe says that circuses
are flouting the international treaty set up to protect rare species. What we are
so effectively destroying is the unique Quaternary diversity – the species

(ourselves included) which developed over the last two million years of geological time, from the Pleistocene to the present. The Quaternary is characterized by the appearance of an astonishing diversity of flora and fauna – but for how much longer will our fellow travellers exist if we persist in systematically destroying their future?

The worldwide disappearance of many amphibian species must be taken more seriously because it suggests that the impacts of global warming and pollution have reached even remote waterways and rainforests. Amphibians are extremely vulnerable to water pollution because of their dependence on water for breeding, and the powerful synergy between pathogen transmission and rising temperature creates favourable conditions for the spread of disease. For example, a particularly virulent chytrid fungus disease that affects amphibians has been implicated in the worldwide decline and extinction of many frog species. Chytridiomycosis is an infectious disease caused by the chytrid fungus *Batrachochytrium dendrobatidis* which damages the frog's skin, and, since frogs use their skin in respiration, the infection is capable of causing sporadic deaths in some populations and 100% mortality in others. Global warming tends to accelerate the life cycle of parasites, which is having a significant impact on host survival. Frogs are important indicator species of general environmental health – like the miner's canary – thus their disappearance represents more than just an aesthetic loss of a wonderfully diverse group of creatures. These animals are crucial components of the ecology, and their absence from ecosystems can seriously disrupt the functioning of the rest of the community. Adult amphibians are hunters of various animals, including mosquitoes and flies, while amphibian larvae serve as a food supply for aquatic insects, fish, mammals and birds. Although habitat degradation, water pollution and the chytrid fungus are the most powerful causes of amphibian disappearance, depletion of the ozone shield in the stratosphere and concomitant increases in ultraviolet radiation can also disrupt amphibian embryology. This highlights the complexity of the forces leading to the extinction of species. It does not need ecological training to see that the greatest threat to biodiversity is the activity of just one species, our own. Dead-end extinctions are irreversible, and over the past two centuries we have accelerated the rate of extinction of species far beyond the natural replacement rate. Our planet has been traumatized by five major extinctions in its four-billion-year history of life and most have been associated with climate change. Now we are entering the 'sixth mass extinction event' of our own making which, additionally, represents the greatest mass extinction of species since the extinction of the dinosaurs 65 million years ago. If we do not proactively begin to protect our unique biodiversity, our future will be the poorer or even in doubt (Figure 12.2).

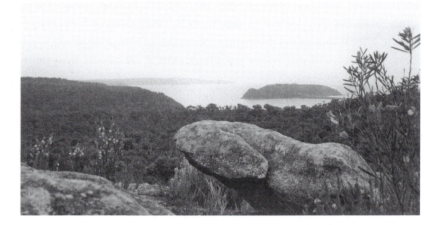

Figure 12.2 Unique natural landscapes need protection from siege by humans and their pollutants. Kuringai Chase National Park, Sydney, Australia.

In brief, the impact of human activity on our natural, finite resources is so great that there is now good evidence to suggest that we are already living on 'environmental credit' to sustain a lifestyle that is beyond the long-term capacity of the Earth. Unhappily, we still do not seem to be able to escape the population-driven trap of the need to produce increasing amounts of food to feed the hungry; in many parts of the world, an increased food supply is rapidly transformed into more people, and therefore more hunger. So the expanding human population is relentlessly demanding an increasing share of the resources of the biosphere. As each life support system is systematically depleted, humans will fight for the remnants and in the process destroy what remains with explosives. The waters of the Nile, Tigris, Jordan and Euphrates have nourished civilizations for more than 10 000 years but in recent times Iraq, Egypt, Israel and Syria have all threatened to go to war over these rivers' precious waters. It is also likely that future disputes will involve underground water reserves which stretch, like rivers, across national borders. Colonel Gaddafi of Libya spent a fortune on his 'Great Manmade River' project which collects ancient water held in rocks beneath the remote Sahara. By piping this precious water to coastal farms, he is drying out Egyptian oases; once aquifers are emptied, they may remain empty forever. Yet the culture of waste endemic to the use of water in many, especially western nations, has not been given the critical emphasis it is due. If you have paid for it then, it seems, there are no ethical obligations to respect this precious resource. During drought conditions, many parts of Australia are under water restrictions, and most will be for the foreseeable future. But there is also a need to distinguish between temporary restrictions, which are a drought response, and permanent water conservation measures that put a prohibition on wasteful uses of water.

Genetic diversity and environmental adaptability

Species are disappearing rapidly as a result of being over-harvested and over-polluted, but more importantly through the destruction of habitat, especially wetlands and tropical rainforests. With the loss of species diversity, we are also witnessing a loss of genetic diversity within species at a rate far exceeding anything known from palaeontological records. Human-driven change to our biosphere is unique in two major aspects. Firstly, it is caused by a single species, which was until recently a subsidiary member of the natural biosphere; and secondly, it is characterized by a growing proportion of artificial ecosystems which have substantially lower species diversity and lower genetic variation compared to that of the natural systems.

Scientists have estimated that the tropical rainforests, covering about 7% of the world's land surface, may contain over 90% of Earth's living species. This richness in natural ecosystems contrasts greatly with human-dominated eco-systems, which consist of a few cultivated, pampered agricultural plants and domestic animals, each with relatively low genetic diversity. Inbred cultivated species may be evolutionarily successful over the short term, while humans keep their environment stable, but they may not be a long-term proposition when requiring natural adaptability in times of climatic uncertainty and environmental change. Scientists have repeatedly warned us against replacing global biodiversity with human monotony, especially at a time when we are pushing Nature's limits. Inbreeding is the biological phenomenon of individuals sharing common ancestors, resulting in a more uniform population. Inbreeding is known to cause overall decreased population fitness, as demonstrated by an increased susceptibility to disease and the presence of a range of physical anomalies. The biological reason for discouraging breeding between close relatives is the greatly increased chance of homozygosity of recessive genes coding for deleterious characters. Please refer back to Chapter 9, Inbreeding depression, p. 166, particularly the legend under Figure 9.3. Cunning plans to keep geneticists busy searching for new pest-resistant genes in inbred crop plants, for example, are not a sensible biological or business proposition, since the future of species diversity is dependent upon genetic diversity within species. Instead of reducing genetic diversity, we should do all in our power to maintain it to facilitate adaptation and survival of species in a changing world.

Human diversity, despite our 3.1 billion base pair DNA alphabet, must also be maintained, as we are not exempt from the laws of genetics. Neonatal mortality, for instance, is correlated with the degree of cousin marriages, as is the incidence of major congenital malformations and other deleterious health effects. Major postnatal morbidity in the progeny of first cousins is elevated some fourfold, together with prenatal mortality in excess of sixfold when compared to non-consanguineous offspring. Because conservation scientists are acutely aware of the importance of biodiversity at the DNA level, they have created gene resource banks around the world which hold collections of the genetic resources of crop plants for long-term conservation and for use by plant breeders and scientists (Chapter 9). In the wild, however, the current high rate of extinction cannot in justice be allowed to continue.

We are responsible not only for the global loss of both species and their genetic diversity, but are also taking up what little native habitat space remains. Currently, 40% of total photosynthetic activity on land is claimed for human consumption. With increasing human numbers, consumption could soon appropriate all of the products of photosynthesis, leaving nothing for the non-human species and the ecosystems that support us. Many of us witnessing such a losing strategy feel outraged, and want to encourage a general acceptance of the sentiment expressed by the US Environmental Protection Agency: 'The value of natural ecosystems is not limited to their immediate utility to humans. They have an intrinsic, moral value that must be measured in its own terms and protected for its own sake.'[2]

Human-driven climate change

Globally, human power to alter the environment has become awe-inspiring in its immediacy. Before we know whether a newly invented product can warp the biosphere, it is marketed and put to use around the world. The chlorofluorocarbons (CFCs) used as propellants and refrigerating agents were an instructive example of such dangerous, and yet utterly casual, commercialization. Following their release in the 1930s, CFCs were heavily distributed worldwide and are now actively destroying the ozone shield that protects life from lethal ultraviolet radiation. Some terrestrial plants have responded to increasing ultraviolet stress by reducing photosynthetic productivity which, indirectly, reduces growth and retards carbon assimilation from the carbon dioxide (CO_2) weighed-down atmosphere. Thus far, no one can really predict

---

[2] US Environmental Protection Agency Science Advisory Board. (1990). *Reducing Risk: Setting Priorities and Strategies for Environmental Protection.* Washington DC, p. 9.

the extent of the influences that increased ultraviolet radiation will have on the plankton of the southern oceans, nor whether existing photosynthetic balances will be disturbed. With deforestation, the oceans are now the major carbon sink removing industry-driven CO_2 from the atmosphere and it is very likely that human-driven disturbances will adversely impact on the role of the oceans as a carbon sink.

Currently, climate change is conceivably the largest environmental and health challenge which requires an international response. Global warming refers to the effect on the climate of human activities, in particular the burning of fossil fuels (coal, oil and gas) and large-scale deforestation which causes an accumulation of greenhouse gases, of which the most important is CO_2. Carbon dioxide in the atmosphere traps heat and plays an important role in keeping the temperature of the Earth within a habitable range; however, increases in CO_2 emissions from human-made greenhouse gases are leading to rapid alterations of the climate. Powerful greenhouse gases other than CO_2 include methane (CH_4), nitrous oxide (N_2O) and CFCs, but since the atmospheric concentration of CO_2 is much greater, it plays a greater role in greenhouse warming and climate change than these other compounds. Methane's contribution is, however, predicted to rise following permafrost thaws encroaching wetlands and lakes hitherto iced over in northern Canada and Siberia. The methane (natural gas) is a legacy of decomposed primordial vegetation and long-dead animals where it remained until rising temperature initiated the 'ebullition' phenomenon or bubbling methane gas into the atmosphere. Between 1974 and 2000, a period that coincides with global warming, the spread of thaw lakes caused methane emissions in Siberia to rise by 58%. Volume for volume, methane is 21 times more effective in trapping solar heat than is CO_2. Fortunately, methane has a relatively short chemical lifetime in the atmosphere (approximately 12 years) compared with CO_2 which stays much longer (50–100 years). There are also many other air pollutants in the atmosphere but they persist for short periods, of hours or days, while the greenhouse gases persist in the atmosphere for periods of decades to hundreds of years.

The basic underlying principle is that greenhouse gases absorb the radiation emitted by the Earth's surface and act as a blanket by keeping the heat from radiating out; it is this process which increases the average temperature in the Earth's air and oceans – a process projected to continue. Global mean temperature has already risen by almost 1°C, with much of the warming occurring during the last few decades of the twentieth century. Furthermore, by the year 2100 the mean global temperature is predicted to increase from 1.4 to 5.8°C, there will be an elevation in mean sea level of 9–88 cm, and increases in heatwave frequency of 25–31%. A 2°C increase in global temperature would severely damage tropical wilderness areas like Australia's Great Barrier Reef and Kakadu's wetlands, and melting polar and alpine ice would decrease snow cover and increase sea levels worldwide, effectively wiping out many remaining habitats. Warming air and ocean temperatures also have an effect on rainfall, placing some regions under drought conditions for extended periods, while others experience more powerful storms such as hurricanes and typhoons. Should climate change continue at today's rates, it will threaten everyone's way of life at the most basic level: access to water, food and use of land for yielding crops, especially in already arid areas such as Africa. Accelerating melting of polar and alpine ice would raise sea levels, further causing flooding and erosion, and resulting in possibly hundreds of millions of people displaced from their coastal city homes or, more seriously, their countries. Nations such as India, Bangladesh, parts of Africa, Netherlands and the Pacific Nations would lose land or be completely inundated, even though they do not play a big role in contributing to global warming. Over the past decade, sea levels have been rising at twice the rate of previous years and in 2002 a large Antarctic ice shelf collapsed dramatically, forcing many scientists to modify upwards their projections of the deleterious effects of climate change. Some researchers believe that global warming is accelerating and may be approaching a tipping point – a point at which climate change acquires a momentum that makes it irreversible. Despite the strong evidence for global warming, however, some political strategists and other 'doubters' still do not support constructive efforts to ameliorate the severity of climate change. This is mostly for economic or industrial reasons rather than not accepting the science. In addition to the geophysical changes, we need to be aware of the interactions between rising temperature and global health effects such as the emergence of new pathogens, the wider distributions of existing disease-carrying pests, spores and pollens, and the production of photochemical air pollutants which will affect all – advantaged and disadvantaged. Ironically, Africa, with the world's lowest emission of greenhouse gases, could suffer the greatest health impact.

That the Earth's climatic system has occasionally jumped from one mode of operation to another is well established. Regrettably, researchers have yet to discover the causes of these abrupt climatic shifts, and until they do the situation leaves us in limbo with regard to accurate climatic predictions. It is possible that large-scale reorganizations of the ocean's circulation following atmospheric triggers may be involved in climatic control. If so, the current build-up of greenhouse gases may well set in motion a reorganization of deep water ocean dynamics and change the weather patterns that depend on it.

Recently, great interest has been expressed in the El Niño Southern Oscillation phenomenon (El Niño meaning 'the Child' of change, as opposed to La Niña, 'the Child' of constancy) and whether its currently increasing frequency is linked to global warming and human increases in atmospheric CO_2. One model postulates such a relationship in which trapped heat in the CO_2-rich atmosphere increases the temperature of the oceans, triggering cycles of drought and rain. While putative mechanisms of action may be debatable, accurate measurements are not. There is no doubt that the Oceania region, from the tropical rainforests of Indonesia to the interior deserts of Australia, is strongly influenced by the ocean and El Niño phenomenon. Nor is there any doubt that the small island nations and coastal regions of the Pacific are very vulnerable to increasing coastal flooding and erosion. Warming sea temperatures in recent years have damaged many of the region's spectacular coral reefs, disrupting one of the world's most diverse ecosystems.

El Nino and its supposedly 7-year cycle aside, a scientific consensus on global warming now exists. As far back as 1995, the United Nations' main advisory panel endorsed a scientific report concluding that the balance of evidence suggests that there is a discernible human influence on the global climate. As a result, the United Nations Framework Convention on Climate Change (UNFCCC), which is an international environmental convention designed to address environmental and social issues concerned with climate change, imposed obligations to limit greenhouse gas emissions. The UNFCCC was the first legal device to address climate change, and from it formed the Kyoto Protocol. The Kyoto Protocol has been approved by many nations, and its objective is to limit greenhouse emissions in a cost-effective way. Each party under the Kyoto Protocol has a set target for CO_2 reduction over a set time period. Consequences exist for those who do not follow the protocol and who have agreed to its terms. However, the current targets are weak and must be redesigned to reach the cut of 70% by 2050 to avoid a major climatic upheaval. CO_2 emission is considered a pollutant, and those under the Kyoto Protocol have a legal right to pollute within limitations, whereas those not confined to the Protocol continue to pollute indiscriminately.

It is hard to control a matter as large as climate change and laws will only help if the majority accept them. Therefore, we must all do what we feel is fair for our shared biosphere and apply significant pressure in favour of greenhouse gas reductions. Imagine what wealth the markets for low carbon energy products will generate if every nation changed to low-emission energy systems! Imagine the follow-on global economic opportunities that will encourage further development in low-emission systems! And this is already happening where, for example, some 60 million Europeans now get their residential electricity from advanced-design wind farms, 40 million Chinese get their hot water from roof top solar water heaters, and Iceland heats close to 90% of its homes with geothermal energy. Therefore, the bioscience-bioethical focus now has to be about profitability in an environmentally friendly manner. The good thing is that in a new environmentally conscious ambience, the businesses and governments perceived to be green will be favoured, obligating other players in the same market economy to follow suit and also become greener global citizens.

Stress and adaptation

The discovery of the ozone hole over the Antarctic forced us to acknowledge the ecological gambles in which we are engaged. Yet, there remains some dispute as to the 'reliability' of the scientific data, as if it might make political sense not to act until we are absolutely certain that our survival is at stake. It looks suspiciously as if we, as a species, lack some essential instinctive survival mechanism when responding to an extreme emergency concerning our very existence. Biological experiments have unequivocally demonstrated that the hormonal response of an individual to a particular stress must be well timed and mediated by the most appropriate response selected from a multiplicity of possible pathways within the central nervous system. A well-directed stress response has survival value and increases fitness. An ineffectual stress response without a proper resolution creates a situation of chronic stress which, in the long term, leads to immune compromise, illness, social dislocation and aggression (Chapter 7). The crucial point may be the large-scale, long-term nature of the present global emergency and the fact that we have evolved only to comprehend those emergencies which are at the scale of immediate, short-term danger to the individual or small tribal clan. Since natural selection may not favour global, intergenerational thinking, miscalculated responses to our environmental crises may deprive the biosphere of much of its present diversity and beauty, and also carry the risk of our own extinction. Should our worst fears be realized, however, we can be partially consoled in the knowledge that the planet will endure and will generate new, and hopefully more benign, forms of life in the eons to come.

Stresses are cumulative, with multiple stresses being synergistic rather than additive; the body does not, however, distinguish between stress categories or etiology (that is, whether originating from mental, physical, infectious or chemical quarters). For all living organisms, the chances of escape from unacceptable levels of stress are becoming vanishingly small; we are all unwilling environmental victims. The world of synthetic chemicals can serve as an instructive example. Toxic members of the dioxin family have been detected virtually everywhere; in our air, water, soil, sediment and food. Although some dioxin is naturally released by volcanoes and forest fires, the chemical we are being exposed to is, for the most part, an inadvertent byproduct of the industrial way of life.

Dioxin is a contaminant created during the manufacture of certain chemicals such as pesticides and wood preservatives, and industrial processes such as paper and nappy bleaching, the incineration of wastes containing plastics, and the burning of fossil fuels. The dioxin family contains 74 persistent problematic chemicals that accumulate in body fat deposits. The prolonged Agent Orange controversy, for example, centres on this general group of chemicals. Agent Orange, a synthetic herbicide, was dropped by the US military over Vietnam between 1962 and 1971 in an effort to strip away the rainforest canopy under which the Communist forces were hiding. Agent Orange is readily contaminated with dioxins during its manufacture, but it took years of debate surrounding reported illnesses before a panel from the US National Academy of Sciences actually undertook a review of the scientific evidence. In their 1993 report, the group found sufficient evidence to link exposure to dioxin-contaminated herbicides to three cancers: soft-tissue carcinoma, non-Hodgkin's lymphoma and Hodgkin's disease. Since then, the carcinogenic status of dioxin has been confirmed, as has its deleterious association with a wider range of additional effects on the body. These include skin disorders, liver problems, impaired immune response, endocrine and reproductive dysfunction, and functional effects on the developing nervous system and other adverse developmental effects. Human-made synthetic hormone disruptors, including transgenerational consequences, are discussed in Chapter 13.

Living within Nature's constraints

The fundamental truth that the systems of people, the economy and nature are interdependent, and that life-sustaining systems are closed and not open ended, is now widely accepted. Yet economists have acted as if we live in an open system which has an infinite capacity to provide life's most fundamental requirements and to absorb its waste byproducts. Yet, most data-based studies in sustainable development provide evidence and a clear warning that Nature's limits are being exceeded. But what about the environmental consequences of human needs and human greed? The destructive power of human interaction with the infinitely complex global ecosystem is influencing the planet's future. Scientific data from disciplines such as ecology, anthropology, demography, economics, nutrition and political science have long identified that population growth, poverty and unsustainable degradation of local and global resources fuel a vicious cycle. Yet in politics, as in private life, there are widely differing opinions about what constitutes an ideal economy. Some point to rapid population growth as the cause of poverty and environmental degradation; others would argue that poverty is the cause rather than the consequence of inadequate economic activity. It remains a mystery why economists have seriously failed to respond in an integrated manner to the interconnected problems of poverty, population growth and environmental destruction (Chapter 13).

Given that humankind is now the ecologically dominant species in the global ecosystem, and given that we can manipulate natural processes with an intelligence unsurpassed by any other living organism, it is high time that we take seriously the preservation of the vital ecosystem services built into these natural systems. Let us, as sentient beings, choose to use our power responsibly. Given the intellectual capacity of our species, all we need is a critical mass of human beings working for change. We have the advantage of cultural evolution, and cultural change can transform society blindingly fast. For example, 4000 years ago the environmental impact of *Homo sapiens* was hardly detectable but, particularly during the last two centuries, cultural evolution has brought us to our present predicament. By comparison, genetic evolution takes hundreds of thousands of times longer than human-directed cultural change (Chapter 1). It would be ironic if we cannot use our exceptional brain, which has brought about revolutions in technology and medicine, to also balance population growth and resource consumption with the new benefits we have gained. Scientifically, we know how to control our numbers; new methods of contraception are increasingly being developed which give many effective choices for population control. What is missing is the will to use these technologies responsibly to reinstate a fair and just balance in the biosphere.

Clearly, the fundamental issue is whether we will learn to use Earth's natural resources in a sustainable manner and maintain an acceptable quality environment, or whether we will overwhelm the capacity of the natural systems with our human demands. As social creatures, we each have a very low fitness unless we cooperate with our fellows, and as animals we cannot survive independent of the rest of the biosphere. There is a lot to be optimistic about because we value true learning and have an unrequited quest for knowledge and understanding. We are also capable of deep feeling and should be asking for much more from the ongoing conservation debates than mere personal survival. We should be asking for a rich and varied life shared with the other species of our planet. Most of us now wish to see ourselves as a part of

Nature. This new sense of the interdependence of all living systems and their further dependence on physical cycles is a significant intellectual advance as it undercuts the dualistic view of human and natural systems being distinct from one another (Chapter 15). To live up to our responsibility of being in partnership with the planet is the ultimate human challenge and, if successful, will be our highest achievement. The next section is designed to provide the reader with scientific information, insights and mechanisms considered necessary bioscience background in order for us to move forward bioethically.

Understanding living cycles and anticipating environmental policies rather than relying on remedial measures

Take care of the Planet and it will take care of you and your children.[3]

It is clear, even to the most unobservant, that *Homo sapiens*' manipulation of the environment is enormous and ranges from the obvious, like the damming of great rivers, to subtle effects such as those of DDT on the reproduction of wildlife (Chapter 13). It is also clear that we are choosing to change the Earth more rapidly than we are able to comprehend the consequences of our actions. Equipped with a different perspective, we can, however, accelerate our efforts to understand the Earth's ecosystems and the ways these interact with the various global changes of human making. Educating ourselves is crucial, since the human dimension of global change is such that our involvement is now essential if any biodiversity is to be maintained in the wild. Since the survival of the biosphere needs our assistance, we cannot escape our responsibility of nurturing the planet back to health, and we need to do this from a basis of scientific knowledge and ethical decency. Most importantly, we need to integrate our scientific analyses with previously neglected ethical dimensions if we are to pass on a healthier planet for subsequent generations to enjoy. To do this effectively, we need cross-cultural agreement in formulating new rights and obligations, rights of access to environmental information, consultation in environmental decision-making, and equality of opportunity in securing the kind of environmental policies we want throughout the world. These issues concern us all because our 'right' to environmental quality involves the quality of life on Earth. An Environmental Code of Conduct (akin to the Human Rights Code), which reflects and transcends the best of historical, cultural and societal

---

[3] Anonymous author.

mores, may prove effective in bringing about attitudinal change as they relate to environmental concerns.

Access to reliable information is crucial if we are to exercise our democratic rights and participate effectively in environmental decision-making. Environmental concerns are multi-layered, ranging from major global issues such as depletion of the Earth's natural resources, the destruction of the ozone layer and the greenhouse effect, through regional concerns such as water and soil pollution, biodiversity and acid rain, to local effects such as individual quality of life and the aesthetic beauty of the local landscape. With such a diverse range of possible environmental concerns, misinformation and conflict are inevitable. For example, what is best for the environment may not be the most profitable for business in the short term. Business is beginning to realize, however, that if it is going to thrive in the long term, both economic growth and global environmental exploitation need to be sustainable.

Choosing the optimum way forward is complex, but good work has long been done by various environmental pressure groups, such as Greenpeace, in moving environmental concerns up the political agenda. As a consequence, information about the environmental impacts of products is being made available to consumers through ecolabelling schemes, and the environmental impacts of companies are being publicized through compulsory environmental assessments and eco-auditing. Measures such as these not only improve environmental quality but also strengthen the environmental power of the individual. A major complicating factor is that the public's perception of environmental priorities is generally governed by the extent and/or bias of media coverage. This deficiency can easily be rectified if, before making policy decisions, businesses and legislators make sure that any action made is to the benefit (or at least not to the detriment) of the environment, as judged by the best scientific advice and taking into account global, regional and local concerns. And, in fact, many businesses are already profiting from the triple bottom line accounting system where the social and environmental impacts are factored in, as well as profit. Despite this practice being still in its infancy, the triple bottom line has positioned business on a more stable footing – not just in the long term but also short-term benefits, such as goodwill, are evident. More on multiple-entry bookkeeping practices can be accessed from Chapter 15.

Fundamental symbiosis: the biogeochemical or nutrient cycle

There is an increasing appreciation within mainstream ecology about the central role that symbionts play in ecological processes. The term 'symbiosis' simply means 'living together', without any implied value judgements. In the biological literature, however, the term is also used to describe a particular category of relationship where all parties benefit from the interaction. In this case, the relationship is called either symbiosis or mutualism, and the idiom is used in its biological sense here. Populations of organisms interact with one another in complex and often surprising ways. It is common for two (or more) organisms to evolve together for mutual benefit; for example, many plants have mutualistic relationships with their pollinators. Usually the interactions are not highly species-specific. Symbioses underpinning biogeochemical or nutrient cycles involve specific relationships with microorganisms and are essential in the production of energy and nutrients. In other words, nutrient cycles, in cycling chemical elements through the biotic and geological components of all ecosystems, are well-balanced, fundamental ecological processes. The synthesizing component of the cycle involves nutrients being taken up from the soil by plant roots, translocated within the plant and eventually, via the process of photosynthesis, food being distributed throughout the food web. The recycling component of the cycle returns to the soil the nutrients contained within the dead biomass so that the whole process can be repeated.

There are three main pathways by which nutrients enter the ecosystem. These are rainfall and dust deposition, weathering of parent rocks and nitrogen fixation. Nitrogen enters the ecosystem by a process known as 'fixation', whereby inorganic nitrogen from the atmosphere is converted, or fixed, to a form usable by all living organisms for the synthesis of amino acids, proteins and other nitrogen-containing compounds. The organisms responsible for nitrogen fixation are either symbiotic bacteria living in association with a plant, such as those living in the root nodules of leguminous plants, or inside lichens, or free-living forms such as blue–green algae. Other nutrients, such as phosphorus and potassium, enter the biogeochemical cycle by the weathering of rocks and soil material. Likewise, there are three main pathways whereby nutrients leave the ecosystem. These are leaching from the soil by rainfall, being carried away into streams and rivers in surface run-off containing topsoil, and dispersal by wind. Typically, loss in natural ecosystems, if left undisturbed, is minimal. Local vertebrate and invertebrate animals such as fish and insects respectively, as well as fungi and bacteria, utilize the organic matter washed away and in turn make nutrients available to the roots of streamside vegetation.

Tropical rainforests are the most productive biome on Earth, but their biodiversity is based on a very tight cycling of mineral nutrients, most of which are tied up in the vegetation (Figure 12.3). These wet tropical forests may have up to 500 different species of trees per square kilometre. Most of the species

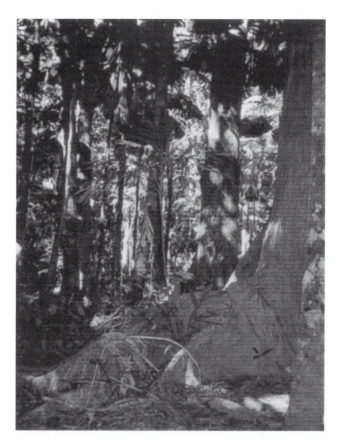

Figure 12.3 Old-growth tropical rainforests are the most productive biome on Earth. The luxurious vegetation is interconnected by an extensive, shallow root system and anchored by the buttress complex of mature trees. Because many endemic rainforest species can survive only in the ecological communities in which they evolved, conservation biologists are most concerned about the preservation of complete communities. Daintree National Park, Queensland, Australia.

are rare, and nearly all of them rely on animals to transport their pollen and disperse their fruits. In rainforests, large biomasses of dead leaves, flowers, fruits and branches, referred to as litter fall, are continuously shed from the forest canopy. Litterfall is significant because nutrients in litter accumulated on the forest floor are returned to the soil after it is decomposed by small soil-living organisms and fungi. These nutrients are then available for re-uptake by plant roots, alone or in combination with a fungus that has formed a mutualistic relationship with a particular plant. These symbiotic fungi, called mycorrhiza, are more efficient at gathering nutrients from the soil (particularly phosphorus) than are the plant's roots, and so promote the plant's nutrition. Again we are witnessing, as with the symbiotic relationship between nitrogen-fixing bacteria and host plants, another type of relationship which benefits both organisms – the plant gains because it is supplied with nutrients, while the fungus gains because the plant, via photosynthesis, supplies it with energy. At any particular time a tree contains only a small fraction of the nutrients it absorbs over its lifetime; but because of natural cycling and the reuse of nutrients, luxuriant rainforests can grow on soils that an agriculturist would regard as infertile unless supplied with large amounts of fertilizers. Australia's verdant Cooloola and Frazer Island rainforests, for example, are evolving on sand dunes, a soil type usually considered very non-productive.

On land, the roots of most plant species are associated with symbiotic mycorrhizal fungi, but in those terrestrial environments where vascular plants do not flourish (in many alpine–arctic habitats and some deserts, for instance) the dominant primary producers are the lichens. Lichens are symbiotic associations of a fungus and unicellular algae or cyanobacteria, where the combination effectively functions as a plant. In this union the fungus draws nutrition from the photosynthetic bacterium or alga, while providing structure and shelter. In marine environments, the symbiosis between corals and the algae contained within them (zooanthellae) is the architectural foundation for all shallow water coral reef communities, communities which are renowned for both their high productivity and their biodiversity.

It may be useful to point out that scientists have estimated that the overall photosynthetic contribution by algae amounts to some 50–60% of all photosynthesis on Earth, with the kingdom Plantae accounting for most of the rest.

Losing the food race

The impact of human activities on some symbioses is well known. For example, local extinction of many lichens by sulphur dioxide or other pollutants has long been used in pollution monitoring, and the abundance and distribution of many mycorrhizal fungi in central Europe has severely declined as a result of the combination of pollution and ecosystem disturbance. In the tropics and subtropics, the coral reefs are facing multiple human insults, including eutrophication, increased sedimentation and a progressive rise in temperature. It is widely believed that deteriorating conditions are contributing to the breakdown of many algal/coral symbioses, as observed in the mass expulsion of the algae and the concomitant bleaching of the corals. Extreme bleaching in many parts of the Great Barrier Reef in Australia has caused large-scale coral mortality, and a shift in the community from one dominated by corals to one dominated by micro-algae is becoming increasingly evident.

Nutrient cycles are also strongly affected by other environmentally disturbing human activities, in particular logging, clearing in forests, and burning
habitats. To what extent biogeochemical cycles are affected depends on the
intensity of the disturbance, with selective logging being considered a low-
to-moderate disturbance. The most obvious and immediate effect of selective
logging is the removal of nutrients from the ecosystem in the log harvest.
Additional, long-term nutrient loss occurs due to topsoil erosion, which can be
considerable if logging is uncontrolled and intensive. Clear felling and burning
of forests represents a more intense disturbance, and is commonly carried out
over large areas of the tropics to allow for agricultural development. With
clearing and burning, both the living and dead biomass nutrient pools are
effectively ravished; and nutrient recycling is reduced, or even halted, if the
disturbance has resulted in excessive destruction of plants, mycorrhiza and
microbial populations. Despite these losses, however, many reports show that
soil fertility is usually maintained for at least several years after clearing and
burning. Further, if forest regrowth is allowed to occur (i.e. agriculture ceases
and fires are excluded), a succession back to tall forest can take place, demonstrating that in many cases Nature's nutrient cycling can be re-established.
However, the restoration process takes a long time, and 'restoration' does not
necessarily mean complete reversion back to the originally destroyed ecosystem. Old-growth forests, for instance, take thousands of years to develop, and
past plant and animal species or symbiotic relationships may have become
extinct or disrupted in the interim. If a particular disturbance persists, or is
repeated at short intervals, nutrient cycling cannot re-establish, and in these
situations nutrients continue to be lost from the ecosystem by volatilization
and leaching. Eventually, the land declines into a state of severe degradation.

When bacterial nitrogen fixation can no longer support the needs of plant
growth, then the only remedy is larger and larger quantities of fertilizers,
which are now usually produced by industrial activity. Visible symptoms of
continuing degradation of the world's soil reserves, and an accelerating need
to feed an ever-expanding human population, is forcing many scientists to
believe that technology alone cannot solve our food crises and, in order to
escape from the trap called 'winning the food race', an alternative environmental approach is required. Winning the food race requires a scientific,
coordinated approach to increase agricultural production, to improve food
distribution, to manage resources sustainably and to provide family planning.
To achieve food security, we must address Nature's needs while simultaneously providing essential education and health care, eradicating poverty,
stabilizing the population and restoring the Earth's natural systems; a significant but not impossible harnessing of human adaptive intelligences.

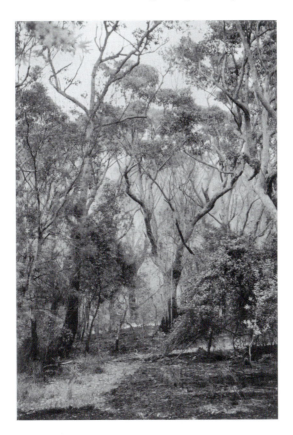

Figure 12.4 Clearing and burning represents an intense disturbance. The result of a deliberately lit bush fire in Murramarang National Park, south coast of New South Wales, Australia.

By contrast, each year during the dry Australian summer months, vast areas of remote bushland are needlessly destroyed by people who get pleasure from deliberately starting bush fires (Figure 12.4). The destruction wreaked on otherwise healthy bush by these people cannot be evaluated in terms of the suffering of burning animals, frequently including endangered species, which cannot escape to safety.

Deep design: the synthesis of Nature and culture

The single most important drawback for future management and conservation programmes is the dearth of basic biological information, particularly about the ecology of relationships, including those of symbiotic microorganisms. At every level, the biology of the ecosystem is shaped by long-term intimate associations with larger organisms such as animals and plants, and microorganisms. Valuing natural biodiversity in purely economic or monetary terms is an insult to the Biosphere. Furthermore, how can anyone make a value judgement by valuing present damage done to the environment which also belongs to future generations? To redress this dilemma, an increasing number of green activists are advocating a process called 'deep design'. Deep design is the simple idea of assigning a realistic value to environmental systems, and reflects the synthesis of nature and human culture. In the deep design value system, wider issues such as sustainability, aesthetics and bioethics are considered within a holistic framework. This approach starkly contrasts with simplistic and materialistically driven short-term approaches, which could well be described as 'shallow design'. Deep design principles, or some modification of them, may be successful in tapping the human potential to adaptively change behaviour. As social animals, we should construct a modern evolutionary ethics which will make it inevitable for us to respect the continuing existence of other species as an integral part of our own existence. Biodiversity has a value in its own right, as well as being an integral part of our cultural inheritance.

Major changes in the way we use synthetic chemicals and other products in our industrial processes can be facilitated by following Nature's example. Guided by natural systems where chemicals, nutrients and organic matter are continuously recycled, waste from one industrial process should feed another industrial venture. In a well-designed system, worn-out parts could be returned to the makers, where components would be disassembled and the materials recycled and used again in parts for new appliances. This concept is already having a profound impact on some industries, including sections of the automobile industry where products are designed for disassembly and re-use. Several automobile makers are working jointly to design cars that can be easily taken apart at the end of their life and reprocessed for recycling into new automobile parts. By simulating natural cycles, industry can close the loop of waste and recycle materials over and over again, thus eliminating the demand for new raw materials and reducing the contaminated waste disposed into the environment. The essence of such closed loop recycling can be called 'intelligent design'.

A brief summary of the Australian experience may demonstrate how detachment between Nature and culture can easily become a catastrophe. It is an embarrassment to see how the Europeans, when they settled this continent just over 200 years ago, did not respect Australia's deep design. If they had, the large-scale destructive impact of the alien plants and animals which they brought with them could have been prevented. In the absence of natural checks and balances, the behaviour of introduced plants, animals and pathogens has been devastating. Feral cats, dogs, pigs and horses are incompatible with the native fauna, yet are now well established over most of the Australian continent such that their complete eradication is now almost impossible. 'Biological pollution' describes those forms of environmental degradation that are not caused by the usual offending industrial and agricultural activities. Belated attempts at biological control, such as the release of the calicivirus aimed at controlling rabbits, are expensive and often unsuccessful in the long term. Clearing of native vegetation for agriculture and the introduction of sheep, cattle and other cloven-hoofed animals from the northern hemisphere have had devastating, and permanent, environmental effects.

The hoofed mammals of Eurasia evolved on rocky mountain landscapes, whilst the Australian fauna evolved on landscapes consisting largely of alluvial plains covered with soft sandy soils. It is no accident that all Australian indigenous mammals have soft-padded feet, well adapted to their fragile environment. They are also adapted in other physiological respects; the marsupial fauna has evolved adaptations suitable for an environment that is mostly arid and has very high climatic variability. Their amazingly efficient reproduction may involve the presence of three sequential stages of offspring associated with their mother at the same time. An almost-weaned young kangaroo (a 'joey') may still go back to the pouch for an occasional suckle when a newly arrived sibling is attached to another nipple while, in the uterus, another early embryo is waiting in embryonic diapause (a physiological block to further development) for its turn to enter the pouch. When both older and younger joeys are feeding in the same pouch, the mother is producing two different types of milk, one richer in proteins secreted from the nipple where the younger joey is feeding, and one richer in lipids secreted from the nipple used by the older joey.

Presently, millions of sheep and cattle are stocked even in the arid interior regions, and feral horses (brumbies), goats, pigs and donkeys run wild. Australia has the international record for the greatest number of extinctions in the shortest period of history, and South Australia heads the national list of states in this regard. Early settlers in Australia saw the wilderness as a deadly enemy to be tamed, conquered and changed without pity or sympathy; today we are only a little more enlightened. The inheritance bequeathed to us has been the loss or reduction of a richly unique indigenous fauna and flora. We are left to grieve for this aesthetic, scientific and spiritual loss; none deeper than that felt by Australia's original inhabitants, who were custodians of this land for over

40 000 years. The theme of how disconnection between Nature and culture precipitates environmental deterioration is continued in the next chapter, which addresses transgenerational ethics.

Principles of bioscience ethics for discussion

- Nature's most successful evolutionary strategy is based on symbiotic associations (cooperative relationships for mutual benefit) which favour ecocommunities outstanding for their high productivity and biodiversity. Such a strategy permits, for example, the development of luxuriant rainforests on soils that an agriculturist would regard as infertile unless supplied with large amounts of fertilizers. Discuss what it takes, in your opinion, to favour human-generated symbioses over human-generated conflict.
- Conservation biology is a relatively new discipline that draws together information from a number of biological subdisciplines to determine how best to manage ecosystems for the benefit for all species, including *Homo sapiens*. Why is valuing natural biodiversity in purely economic or monetary terms an insult to the Biosphere?
- Logic tells us that death control has to be balanced by birth control, but how can we best balance the tension between population control and conservation maintenance? Could it be politically correct, in certain circumstances, to ask the question, 'should we use medical science to prolong human life when this means large-scale environmental extermination?' Justify your viewpoint.

13

Human-dominated ecosystems: reclaiming the future for following generations

Only after the last tree has been cut down
Only after the last river has been poisoned
Only after the last fish has been caught
Only then will you find that money cannot be eaten

Cree[1] (Indian prophecy)

Self-destructive behaviour and overexploitation of the environment

Our motives for having children are many. They include the evolutionary drive to immortalize our genes, to realize our own procreational potential, to follow the dictates of tradition, or even to exploit them as a source of unpaid labour or security in old age. The previous chapter analysed the positive correlation between fertility, economic activity and environmental deterioration. This chapter develops the theme further, though from different perspectives. In particular, it examines ways that societies lock themselves into a self-sustaining destructive mode of behaviour characterized by high fertility, overexploitation of the local environment and low regard for the rights of future generations.

The tragedy of the commons

Although 'the tragedy of the commons' was originally used in a philosophical context, it was eagerly taken up by population ecologists

---

[1] The Cree people are indigenous hunters of north-eastern Canada.

inquiring into the practicalities of ecology, social justice and the natural limits to human reproductive rights. Prominent among those was Garrett Hardin, whose steady contributions since the 1950s were a crucial driving force in the debate's advancement – both from the biological and bioethical points of view. If we are to protect the quality of life of our children, then we must question the corresponding right to breed freely. A quote from Hardin's early manuscripts provides an insight into this important debate: '. . . how shall we deal with the family, the religion, the race, or the class (or indeed any distinguishable and cohesive group) that adopts overbreeding as a policy to secure its own aggrandizement? To couple the concept of freedom to breed with the belief that everyone born has an equal right to the commons is to lock the world into a tragic course of action' (*Science* (1968) **162**, 1243). Acceptance of the unrestricted right to breed regardless of circumstance implies child ownership, an attitude no longer acceptable in the ethically mature society.

Within rural economies, a destructive cycle can readily be generated if parents do not take full responsibility for rearing their children, but distribute some of the costs to their relatives or to the community. Rural communities have traditionally owned communal assets, such as village ponds, threshing grounds, grazing fields and local forests. Control of these local 'commons' enabled households, especially in semi-arid regions, to pool their risks and resources while invoking behavioural standards which ensured protection of these community facilities or assets against overexploitation. In an increasingly competitive environment, however, the processes of economic development, urbanization and increased mobility erode traditional lifestyles and methods of protective control. In communities where access to shared resources is continued but within a deteriorating environment, the value of children also becomes degraded because parents then pass some of the costs of their children onto the community. The parents may produce many children in the hope of receiving more than their fair share of the 'commons'. Typical examples can be seen in parts of West Africa where as many as one-third of the local children are living not with their parents but with kin. In these communities, nephews and nieces have the same rights of accommodation and support as do the biological offspring. The inevitable overprocreation leads to yet greater crowding, greater pressure on environmental resources, and consequent overexploitation of the commons.

Child exploitation is practised in many developing countries, including parts of India where children as young as 6 years of age are required, without educational or recreational breaks, to tend domestic animals and crops, care for younger siblings, fetch water, collect firewood, dung and fodder, or weave carpets for sale. By the time these children reach the ages 10–15, their daily unpaid working hours are often one and a half times those of the community's adult males. As resources are depleted, more labourers are needed to gather scarce fuel, water, etc., so more children are produced, and the local environment deteriorates still further – providing households with the incentive to enlarge the family yet again! The 'tragedy of the commons' happens when each household is locked into a system where fertility and environmental degradation reinforce each other in an escalating spiral. No one gains and millions of children waste their potential in a community where they are insufficiently valued; parenthood comes cheap in a cultural setting where producing a child is not a privilege accompanied by a lifelong commitment, but viewed as a right without constraints.

Education has proven to be the most effective tool in reversing destructive fertility cycles. Therefore, the world community has an obligation to identify policies that will change the options available to men and women so that couples will find it economically preferable to limit the number of offspring they produce. Fertility is lower in countries where citizens enjoy more civil and political freedoms, and where a number of social policies, such as the provision of health and family planning services, compulsory education and other couple-empowering measures, are deployed. Improving social coordination and directly increasing the economic security of the poor is essential, as is a targeted literacy and employment drive for women. The aim would be for children to be perceived as sufficiently costly or valuable to dislodge the mercenary hold of the cycle of disproportionately high human fertility. An increased middle class usually results in greater democracy and greater environmental awareness.

The tragedy of the commons is repeated in industrialized and industrializing countries through the effects of pollution. In this situation, it is not a question of taking something out of, but of putting something into the commons. Sewage, chemical, radioactive and heat wastes are deposited into the water, dangerous fumes and particles into the air, and toxic, non-degradable substances into the soil. The thinking behind the polluting enterprise's behaviour is strikingly similar to the rationale driving competitive procreation: discharge of waste into the commons saves the cost of purification and passes the responsibility onto others. In societies where money means power, such reckless behaviour pays because it is politically tolerated. Every day we witness examples of governments caving in to powerful pressure groups campaigning to ignore environmental protection regulations on land, ocean and reef commons which, as a result, are disappearing through unsustainable

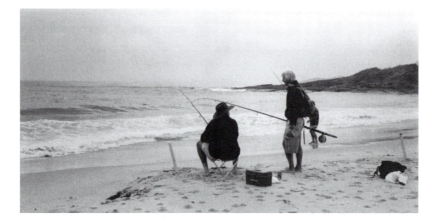

Figure 13.1 We must protect our right to roam the commons. Gannet Beach, south coast of New South Wales, Australia.

economic activities. The present focus on climate change is based on the recognition that the atmosphere, oceans, forests, biodiversity and Antarctica are global commons; yet an assortment of polluting industrialized nations are unwilling to recognize their unmistakeable responsibilities to the rest of the world. The question then arises as to what degree should a polluting nation take responsibility for climate change? We must urgently preserve what is left of our birthright; the right to roam the commons, go fishing and commune with species other than our own (Figure 13.1).

By discovering more about the world we can make it more difficult for the politicians because institutionalized control over landscape is also a convenient means of controlling human beings. If nothing is done, we will have to negotiate accelerating population pressures, unimaginable pollution, stress-induced violence, and social and personal despair. Such a situation will further increase the expanding underclass of unwanted, undervalued, unemployed homeless children roaming city streets. Vulnerable kids with such poor prospects are tempted to seek a solution for their alienation in substance abuse, antisocial behaviour or suicide. Is that the future we want the next generation to inherit? Of course not; so we must set our collective minds to the hard problems, about the individual's primary obligation being social, and about the need of scientific savvy being part of the educational backdrop to social decision-making. Therefore, in the spirit of bioscience ethics, the rest of this chapter attempts to display scientific developments from which bioethical lessons may be drawn.

Chemical exposure, sex determination and sexual behaviour

The endocrine system: an overview

The body's endocrine system is an internal chemical messenger system which regulates all physiological functions through a complex system of neuroendocrine feedback loops. Hormones are produced by a variety of glands in different parts of the body and are released into the blood stream. Hormones then bind to special receptors in organs or tissues and cause these to respond in genetically modulated ways. Since hormones are extremely powerful, having effects at levels of parts per trillion, our bodies strictly control their blood concentrations. One of the most familiar hormones is adrenaline, which is released in response to danger and prepares the body for swift action – the 'fight or flight' reaction. Others include the glucocorticoids, especially cortisol, which enables the body to withstand non-transient stresses (Chapter 7). Also well understood are the sex hormones. The female hormones progesterone and estrogen control the menstrual cycle, pregnancy and childbirth. The male counterpart, testosterone, is responsible for sperm production and also controls masculine libido and behaviour. These same sex hormones perform fundamental functions during prenatal sex determination and postnatal sexual behaviour (Chapter 2).

Chemical insults to any part of the body's physiological control systems by synthetic chemical pollutants (xenohormones) that mimic specific hormonal activities may initiate a series of adverse neuroendocrine ripple-on effects. As detailed in Chapter 3, children are particularly at risk to chemical insults because they face greater exposure per kilogram of body weight and are physiologically more susceptible to reactive chemical pollutants in their environment. Toxicological exposure may begin during gametogenesis and continue to adversely affect the fertilization process or embryonic and fetal development during critical periods of gestation. Even after birth, children's bodies remain vulnerable, with underdeveloped protective detoxification mechanisms. Because adverse effects on intellectual ability, social behaviours, fertility and a genetic predisposition for certain diseases may take decades to be identified, precautionary measures must be taken to minimize exposing children to xenohormones and other pollutants carrying long-term epigenetic consequences.

The polychlorinated biphenyls (PCBs) and the organochlorine insecticides exhibit considerable estrogenic activity, and their effects on sexual differentiation, fertility, early pregnancy loss and immune function have been well documented. The effects of environmental exposure to contaminants in humans are difficult to assess accurately against a continuum of confounding genetic and epigenetic factors. Exposure to the estrogenic pesticide DDT (dichloro-diphenyl-trichloroethane) and a number of closely related chlorinated hydrocarbons is a well-known risk factor in both human and other animal species. Equally, DDE (dichloro-diphenyl-ethane), the major metabolite of DDT, is recognized as an anti-androgen by virtue of its power to block testosterone function. Since testosterone is the major parent compound from which estradiol and dihydrotestosterone are synthesized, prenatal exposure to anti-androgenic xenohormones may disturb steroid hormone production, leading to potential disturbances in fetal growth and differentiation (Figure 2.1, p. 29 illustrates normal sexual differentiation). In summary then, the pathophysiological mechanisms of synthetic chemical hormone disruptors may be via: a) prevention of hormone production; b) acceleration of hormone metabolism and excretion; or c) inhibition of hormone metabolism and excretion. Anomalous hormone levels can lead to abnormal development since too little hormone can be as harmful as too much. Steroid hormone disruptors are just one polluting agent disturbing the complicated, integrated system of animal control systems. Other synthetic hormone mimics target different neuroendocrine systems – in particular, the adrenal and thyroid glands, involved in stress management and metabolic rate, respectively. In turn, abnormal stress management depletes immune competency.

Epigenetic transgenerational actions of synthetic endocrine disruptors

Of the many possible environmental concerns, the long-term legacy of common pollutants that affect reproductive health and resultant wellbeing of subsequent generations is examined here in detail. Persistent contaminants are now spread throughout the planet, and their adverse effects on humans and wildlife are increasingly well recognized. For example, that exposure to periods of high air pollution is associated with sperm DNA fragmentation is seriously significant. Numerous compounds linked to several different chemical classes with demonstrated adverse reproductive effect include the polychlorinated biphenyls or PCBs (industrial chemicals used as heat transfer and hydraulic fluids, flame retardants and dielectric fluids for capacitors and transformers), the organochlorine insecticides methoxychlor, kepone and DDT, as well as a number of closely related chlorinated hydrocarbons (chlordane, dieldrin, endin, heptachlor) used in aerial crop spraying. Other homely examples are:

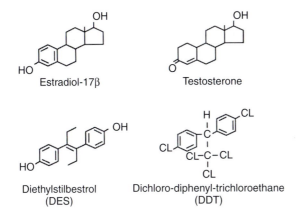

Figure 13.2 A comparison of the chemical structures of the natural steroids estradiol-17β and testosterone with the synthetic estrogen DES and the insecticide DDT. Despite its non-steroidal structure, DDT is an effective estrogen mimic.

-   The organochlorine contaminants dioxin and furan, an accidental byproduct of the chlorine industry, especially the manufacture, disposal and combustion of the chlorinated plastic PVC.
-   The alkylphenols, a breakdown product of industrial detergents.
-   The phthalates, chemical plasticizers extensively used in making soft PVC products for food packaging, plastic toys and numerous other products.
-   Butylated hydroxyanisole, a food antioxidant.
-   Bisphenol A, a key ingredient of the plastic polycarbonate coatings inside some tin cans, some reusable milk bottles and in dental fillings

As briefly described above, many laboratory-made chemicals mimic the action of naturally occurring estrogens. Unlike the synthetic estrogens such as diethylstilbestrol (DES), chemicals akin to DDT were not intended as drugs or hormone mimics (Figure 13.2) but were invented to kill insects and to give manufacturers new materials such as plastics. Inadvertently, the industrial chemists created products that could jeopardize fetal development and adult fertility, a characteristic not recognized until adverse reproductive effects showed up in wildlife. Most discussion of hormone-disrupting chemicals focuses on estrogenic compounds like the polychlorinated biphenyls, the organochlorine insecticides and dioxin, so the concerned reader may get the false impression that xenoestrogens pose the only threat. This is not so, but since the first hormone-disrupting chemicals that scientists discovered in the 1960s were the estrogen mimics, they have been studied and written about in greatest depth. Since then, researchers have identified numerous other endocrine-disrupting synthetic chemicals which are also ubiquitous in the environment. Some mimic estrogen, but others interfere with other parts of the endocrine system, including testosterone, thyroid and adrenal metabolism.

Important properties contributing to the biological potency of xenohormones include their extreme chemical stability, allowing them to resist natural detoxifying processes; their high volatility, enabling them to be endlessly recycled around the planet; and their lipid solubility, ensuring their accumulation in animal body fats. Unlike natural hormones, which the body is able to detoxify and excrete as harmless compounds, these synthetic hormones resist physiological breakdown. Their accumulation in body fat gives humans and animals low level but long-term exposure. The belief that exposure to xenohormones is benign unless exposure is relatively high is misleading because mixtures of biologically active compounds have synergistic actions. Prenatal and/or postnatal exposure to a mix of persistent organochlorine pollutants is an excellent predictor of impaired immune function in children. Children who have been exposed to PCB-related compounds through their mother's contaminated diet display reduced antibody responses following common childhood vaccinations, suffer increased frequency of childhood infections and risk immune-related diseases such as asthma.

The greatest danger from persistent toxic materials in the environment (which also applies to radioactive chemicals) is that they accumulate exponentially up the food chain. Chapter 12 discussed how every food chain or food web is made up of producers (green plants), consumers of various types, and finally decomposers, all of which are important in one way or another in maintaining the dynamic equilibrium and evolutionary progress of the ecosystem. Through this natural process of biomagnification, the concentration of any single pollutant can be millions of times greater in the body of a top predator (carnivores like the eagle, tiger or human) compared with the surrounding environment. Biomagnification of PCBs in fish, for example, can reach an accumulation factor exceeding 250 000 times.

The first public warning about the dangers of persistent pesticides was sounded in 1962 with the publication of Rachel Carson's seminal work *Silent Spring*. 'Silent Spring' referred to a world without birdsong, and her book propelled hormone disruptors to the top of the list of most urgent environmental concerns. In 1996, a second popular book, *Our Stolen Future* (Colborn *et al.*), raised general awareness further by providing a comprehensive, updated guide for the concerned general reader. Since *Silent Spring*, thousands of scientific papers have been published on the subject. In the twenty-first century, circumstantial evidence strongly indicates that persistent contaminant hand-me-downs are amongst the most destructive legacies of our time. Only time will reveal how this will affect future evolutionary trends. Inappropriate chronic hormonal exposure is unprecedented in our evolutionary experience, and no one knows how delicately balanced physiological systems will respond to this new chronic stress.

Wildlife and laboratory findings

Health problems in wildlife have been repeatedly linked to accidental spills or deliberate release of contaminants in their habitats. Many reports involve defective sexual organ anatomy, impaired fertility, the loss of young, or the sudden disappearance of entire animal populations. DDT has been particularly devastating to birds of prey (ospreys, condors, bald eagles) because it alters calcium metabolism, resulting in the production of thin eggshells which cannot support the incubating bird's weight and so break before hatching. Behavioural abnormalities, which are less immediately apparent, have also been documented. A puzzling 1970s report from the Channel Islands in southern California noted female herring gulls nesting together instead of with males. With modern scientific insight, such out of the ordinary behaviour is not difficult to understand. Exposing young chicks to excess estrogen affects brain as well as reproductive tract development, resulting in permanently suppressed adult male sexual behaviour and fertility. The female gulls were nesting together because of a shortage of competent males, which were dis-interested in mating or incapable of courtship. Sadly, despite the female pairs' desperate efforts to raise chicks, their eggs would have been sterile.

Other studies have found that air pollution in urban areas appears to be linked to a significant decrease in the male:female sex ratio at birth. Mice were exposed to either filtered air or unfiltered air for the first 4 months of their lives. Both groups were then mated with female mice that were not exposed to pollution. Males not exposed produced an expected male:female sex ratio of 1.34:1 compared with a ratio of 0.86:1 in those exposed to pollution. It has also been reported that exposure to contaminants transmitted via either air or aquatic routes produces elevated rates of heritable DNA mutation which, interestingly, were due primarily to an increase in mutations inherited through the paternal germ-line. Spermatogenesis in the experimental groups was also negatively affected.

Numerous other examples of reproductive dysfunction (physiological, ana-tomical and behavioural) experienced by fish, amphibian, reptile, bird and mammalian species have been documented. Transgenerational effects are also common; the adults breed successfully but their offspring do not survive or are in turn sterile. Because wildlife is being exposed to hundreds of chemicals simultaneously, it is usually impossible to pin any specific abnormality to any particular chemical or group of chemicals. As explained in Chapter 7, the body's protective stress response does not distinguish between differing categories of stress, which are cumulative, with multiple stresses being synergistic rather than additive. Another serious problem is that, despite noteworthy advances, toxicologists are falling further and further behind in their ability to analyse and identify the contaminants and contaminant mixtures increasingly encountered in the environment. This is not due to a lack of available analytical methods, which are better than ever, but to a lack of resource investment and the sheer magnitude of the problem.

Human findings and the precautionary principle

Ominously, the damage seen in wildlife and replicated in laboratory animal experiments has foreshadowed symptoms that appear to be increasing in the human population. While a much-quoted epidemiological study reported a greater than halving in average sperm count per unit volume in normal men since the 1940s, others have been more conservative. For example, among men with sperm counts within the normal range (above 20 million sperm per millilitre), the average sperm count over the period between 1989 and 2002 had fallen from around 87 million per ml to 62 million per ml. Although still well within the normal range, this decrease in sperm count does represent a considerable drop over just a 14-year period, especially when the average age-related level of blood testosterone is said to decline faster than can be attributed to the ageing process alone. The next goal needs to be an investigation of sperm quality; measured motility or increasing DNA damage to determine whether this has also declined over recent years. It is also notable that over a similar time-frame, male reproductive anomalies such as cryptorchidism (maldescended testes), hypospadias (structural abnormalities of the genitalia) and testicular cancers have increased significantly.

Multiple potential causes for falling sperm counts have been proposed, including environmental mutagens, chemical toxins, obesity, and lifestyle factors such as smoking, drinking and drug use. However, falling sperm counts and increasing incidence of male reproductive abnormalities have coincided with the introduction into the environment of xenoestrogens. In the early 1990s, psychologists reported that the greater the concentration of PCBs, DDT, dieldrin, chlordane and lindane in the mother's umbilical cord blood (a measure of her level of contamination easily collected at birthing), the more poorly her infant scored on various measures assessing neurological development. These assessments included short-term memory, which is a useful indicator in predicting the child's future IQ. Postnatally, the chemical contaminants present in the mother's blood are also present in the fat of her breast milk. Contamination of breast milk has been particularly severe among indigenous Inuit people living on Broughton Island in the high Arctic off Greenland, because these communities still eat the traditional wild food, particularly succulent seal blubber, but which is now loaded with an additional synthetic chemical legacy. Inuit babies take in seven times more PCBs than a typical infant living in southern Canada or the United States. The PCBs and other chemicals that contaminate the infants have almost all arrived by wind and water currents and have been passed up the food web to humans. Broughton Island people have the highest levels of PCBs found in any human populations except those directly contaminated in industrial accidents.

The plasticizer bisphenol A, a key ingredient in polycarbonate plastics used in the production of water bottles, resin coating in food containers and white dental sealants, is another example of a widely dispersed xenoestrogen. Regardless of its known ability to alter the expression of numerous genes with varying effects among specific tissues, bisphenol A is also used as an additive in other types of plastic products such as children's toys and baby bottles. Animal and epidemiological studies suggest that exposure – even at very low doses – of this xenoestrogen can be linked to a large number of health problems, including prostate and breast cancer, obesity, attention-deficit hyperactivity disorder, brain damage, altered immune system, lowered sperm counts and early puberty.

When contemplating our place in the evolutionary lineage, we tend to focus excessively on the characteristics that make us unique, instead of reflecting on those we share not only with other close relatives such as chimpanzees, but with all life forms. Humans and other animals share a common environment as well as a common evolutionary legacy. Transgenerational effects, such as changes in behaviour and diminished fertility, will show up faster in wildlife because most animals mature and reproduce more quickly than we do so, inevitably, the lag time before human damage becomes evident is longer.

Many current regulations designed to protect human and wildlife health are based on risk assessments, which attempt to determine 'safe' doses of individual chemicals; that is, doses which will not cause 'unacceptable' levels of clearly identifiable health effects such as cancer. This approach tries to identify how much pollution people have to be exposed to before too many of them become sick. The same approach is used when pollutants are released by industrial processes into the environment. Again, the assumption is made that there is a 'safe' level of pollution that the environment can cope with. Such

safe limits do not take into account the synergistic effect of multiple pollutants, and since the safe level is usually calculated in terms of adult males, it
assumes that fetuses and children have the same safe level as their adult
counterparts. Clearly such a permissive approach based on an arbitrary identifiable health target cannot protect all those for whom it is intended. For
example, it was impossible to predict the damage caused to the ozone layer by
CFCs, nor could scientists have predicted that many industrial chemicals, safe
at the doses individuals were exposed to, would turn out to be hormone disruptors causing permanent damage to fetuses and children. It is clear that
regulators and industry will have to accept that there is no environmentally
safe level for many chemicals, and that often the traditional risk assessment
approach does not even begin to address potential problems such as that of
hormone pollution. New strategies are needed which are based on the precautionary principle, which calls for preventative action against, in the present
case, chemicals where there is any evidence of harm.

The precautionary principle is a rule about handling uncertainty in the
assessment and management of risk. This rule recommends that, when
deciding about actions, a cautious (or precautionary) approach should be taken
in the face of uncertainty, particularly when dealing with human health and
the environment. The idea behind the principle is that appropriate action
should be taken to avoid the risk of serious and irreversible damage to human
and environmental health, but it does not mean that no action should take
place if there is identifiable risk. The principle ensures that in circumstances
where our best predictions turn out to be wrong, it is better to have erred on
the side of safety; that is, forgoing potential benefits of a particular technology
is better than experiencing harmful consequences from failing to predict
the risks. The precautionary principle emerged in the 1970s, and is currently
invoked in numerous international laws, treaties and protocols in, for example,
environmental management, control of toxic chemicals, food standards, fish-
eries management, species introductions and wildlife trade. The overarching
aim is to support ecologically sustainable development in managing natural
resources, and to conserve biodiversity while continuing to develop the
economy. The principle can, however, be equally called upon to assess risk–
benefit equations posed by technological applications. It can be seen that the
precautionary principle is a most useful tool to flag ignorance and uncertainty
about certain eventualities, and to hold policy until overall scientific understanding of the problem has been gained. It is probable that, more than any
other environmental problem, environmental uncertainty applies to loss of
biodiversity and associated climatic change. The general principle of caution
would then also prevent the release of chemicals into the environment,

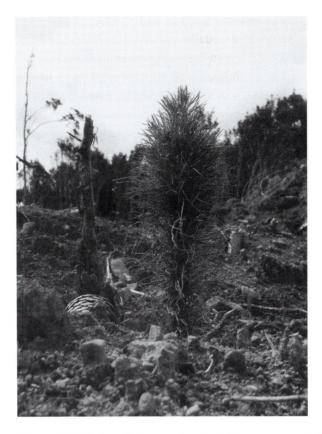

Figure 13.3 Biodiversity is strongly affected by environmentally disturbing human activities, in particular logging, clearing of forests and burning. If we do not break the destructive cycle of overexploiting the Global commons and begin to maintain sustainable environmental integrity, countless species will be doomed to extinction. (Please see the back cover for the colour version.)

particularly those which persist and build up in animal and human bodies and which can, therefore, be passed on to the next generation.

Much of the essential thrust of the environmental movement is to preserve the Earth's resources for coming generations. Temporal issues of inter-generational fairness, justice and equity have evolved out of past catastrophes associated with nuclear energy, toxic waste, depletion of the ozone layer, habitat destruction, overfishing, the clearing of rainforests and global warming (Chapter 12). Science and technology yield advances in knowledge, but this knowledge must be exercised with cautious responsibility. We should remind ourselves that hormone disruptors are the same chemicals which have given us, in the past 30 years, increased crop productivity and an increase in the general level of health by bringing hygiene and comfort to everyone's home. But, if we do not break the destructive cycle of overexploitation of the Global commons, any ability we still have to maintain environmental integrity will be forever lost (Figure 13.3). By providing all couples with the power to decide how many children they wish to have and when they wish to have them, family planning services will promote the democratic principle that individuals be free to make choices for themselves. In addition, programmes which empower women by providing education and target child health issues will also increase women's confidence that the children which they do have, will survive.

Political and religious leaders who fail to consider the Earth's limited resources and who advocate policies that result in unsustainable population growth, may in future be judged to have been negligent in their duty of care. The failure to persuade the world that unsustainable population and economic growth is robbing our children of their future is the ultimate in selfishness.

Principles of bioscience ethics for discussion

- If a desirable social aim is for children to be sufficiently valued as individuals, then directly increasing the economic security of the poor is non-negotiable. How can the self-destructive behaviour where environmental degradation boosts further an already disproportionately high fertility rate be best stabilized?
- We can develop our knowledge base through either trial and error or a more systematic approach using science, which provides us with appropriate targets for change. Often to our detriment we have been quick to believe that a new advance was the easy answer to a particular problem. For example, the pesticide DDT was going to kill off mosquitoes, making malaria a disease of the past, but DDT has contributed to all manner of health problems, from reduced immunity to infertility to extinction. Discuss ways that the precautionary principle acknowledges that modern science raises unique ethical questions that demand a cautious (or precautionary) approach in their application. How can the precautionary principle best be applied?

14

Human-dominated ecosystems: warfare = fitness enhancement or losing strategy?

He was ... beginning to wonder if discord were not a more powerful principle than harmony. Communal violence everywhere was an intimate crime. When it burst out one was not murdered by strangers. It was your neighbours, the people with whom you had shared the high and low points of life, the people whose children your own children had been playing with just yesterday. These were the people in whom the fire of hatred would suddenly light up, who would hammer on your door in the middle of the night with burning torches in their hands.[1]

On the face of things, institutionalized violence, in particular the deployment of scientific expertise in advancing technologies of destruction, is certainly a losing evolutionary strategy. On the other hand, fundamental differences do exist among scientists' ethical values relating to territorial defence and 'justified' environmental destruction. Nevertheless, without a doubt, many are of the opinion that a mature society can no longer tolerate the hideousness of warfare on the following grounds. Firstly, since modern large-scale conflict can no longer lead to the monopolizing of coveted scarce resources (unlike the situation in our tribal past), the activity is self-destructive and has no biological survival value. Old notions of national security are outmoded, and military spending must be diverted towards sustainable development and the alleviation of disaffecting poverty. Secondly, dysfunctional, non-adaptive human behaviour – not the power of science and technology – is the key factor threatening human survival. It needs to be re-emphasized that the greatest

---

[1] Rushdie, S. (2005). *Shalimar the Clown*. London: Vintage Books, p. 390.

challenge for humanity is to balance developmental needs and environmental preservation, and that the principal problems facing us – problems which link the environment, health and social issues – are those of population growth, poverty on a large scale and inappropriate economic activity. We have to curb senseless environmental destruction and intuitively re-recognize our need to expand respect for the nested systems that serve life on Earth (Chapter 15).

The aggressive way we are multiplying, consuming natural resources, using energy and producing waste, is irredeemably destroying our planetary home. *Homo sapiens'* relentless demands are putting at risk the natural balance of our global commons. Wholesale species extermination is not the means by which selection of the fittest is made; rather cooperative symbiosis – biophilia if you like – may yet secure our last chance for survival. An early hallmark of human evolution was the capacity to reason, to reflect on actions and to engage in sophisticated discourse. So why not now harness our uniquely flexible intelligence to advance, develop and engage our brains in diverse and new fitness-enhancing tasks? Instead, we are consistently following the primitive brain's limited repertoire where there is little connection between rational thought and the primordial expression of collective reptilian impulses. As described in Chapter 1, the misuse of instinctive primal group behaviour engages the brain's limbic system to inflame further the basic objectives nested in the unthinking portions of our primitive brains. The lower our engagement with intellectual activity, the stronger is our collective conformity where, typically, disputes are loaded with semiconscious emotional compulsions. When alienation, resentment and anger reaches a critical number, the mob instinct is set free, the momentum of which may expediently be manipulated by 'leaders' who wish to focus this great force on identifiable groups of people or nations of convenience. For instance, the 1940s saw Nazis slaughter an estimated 4.1–6.0 million Jews and another estimated 5–6 million non-Jews comprising the Romani of western Europe, homosexuals, prisoners of war – especially Russians, among other sought-after targeted groups. None of us need to be reminded that state-run destructive goals are only achievable by immeasurable cooperation from the people. During times of stress, would it not be better to 'work' for constructive instead of destructive social goals? Instead of waging war, would it not be better to participate in cooperative goals such as greening the environment, improving self-knowledge or strengthening our emotional intelligence?

A fresh, alternative fitness-enhancing survival model could be to expand beyond bioethics' existing framework governing the traditional strictly delineated guidelines of human and animal bioethics, and include responsibility for sustaining the life support structures existing within ecological systems. In essence, transcend the restrictive anthropocentric in favour for the unrestrictive biocentric. By acknowledging that humankind is not at the centre of our shared universe, but stands there as an integral part of Nature's biodiversity, consisting of other animals, plants and microorganisms, we will already have expanded the framework governing bioethics and, serendipitously, increased our chances for survival. Acceptance of ecological rights should facilitate maturation and guide us toward questions of responsible development and ecosystem stewardship. Environmental stewardship was once a key characteristic of all belief systems, but the rapid changes in society brought about by science and technology have unfavourably impacted on human relationships and practices. In turn, fundamental lifestyle change has affected, often in unpredictable ways, the continued maintenance of a healthy human society in harmony with the environment. Present-day ecological imperialism needs to give way to a modern understanding of life support structures and the evolution of a more appropriate and flexible set of humane priorities.

Within the above context it seems most appropriate to quote Darryl Macer, 'A mature society is one which has developed some of the social and behavioural tools to balance bioethical principles, and apply them to new situations raised by technology' (from *Bioethics is Love of Life*, p. 84). Certainly there is an urgent need to develop a heightened ethical discretion in our personal and social use of technology, but to do this effectively we need first to inform ourselves and acquire a good working knowledge of biological systems. Now is the time, when we are choosing to redesign life-sustaining ecosystems biotechnologically, to adapt by also redesigning human ingenuity and ethical attitudes. Consequently, the two strands of this text – bioscience ethics (information extending our understanding of biological systems) and bioethics (adaptive living by applying this understanding) should jolt our consciousness toward a more mature ethical debate within science-based endeavours. For that reason, this chapter is devoted to how we may further develop the environmental debate by asking the question whether the evolution of human aggression, as experienced in institutionalized warfare, can still be regarded as a fitness-enhancing behaviour, or can it be classified as a losing strategy.

The institution of war

The scientific basis of human aggression, including war, has been extensively studied by academics from many disciplines. To recapitulate briefly; when one individual intentionally harms another, we describe this behaviour as aggression. Aggression during wartime is a form of collective, institutionalized violence because it is driven by a diversity of carefully planned strategies that maintain the structure of war. To understand individual aggression we have to understand the basis of aggressiveness in specific individuals, while to understand war we must also come to terms with repugnant aspects of group behaviour. It is surely curious that the repulsiveness of military conflict is not legislatively forbidden, as is infanticide, child abuse, torture, murder, rape and other forms of barbaric aggressive behaviour. It seems that the most important difference between individual aggression and war is the presence in the latter of pervasive cultural factors influencing the acceptability and aggrandizement of war. The ugly consequences of the self-reinforcing mass ecstasy generated through our primitive herd instincts are not seen as an unthinkable abomination because every culture, now and in the past, has been guilty of this sanitized form of bloodletting. Institutionalized warfare provides the excuse and absolves the herd gene from performing acts of violence that no sane person would entertain acting out alone. All cultures have popularized it in fiction, art, film and now on the Internet, and warriors have always been glorified in secular and religious propaganda. In essence, therefore, militarization is much more than preparing for and taking part in armed operations by trained personnel; rather it is a psychologically well-orchestrated process promoting senseless aggression, hostility and violence which then becomes institutionalized throughout the entire society.

The nature of warfare has changed over the past 200 years. Wars of the nineteenth century involved professional and mercenary armies that had little or no effect on the general population. The twentieth- and twenty-first-century wars are characterized by unparalleled ethnopolitical violence fought on a mechanized scale that impacts on civilians who are the primary victims of military aggression. This development was most evident during World War II, and since then most technologically enhanced wars are being fought by militia, with the objective of infringing civic rights through the targeting of economic and public health resources. This strategy has the greatest effect on the more vulnerable groups of women, children and the elderly. In 2002, all 37 wars in progress were civil wars which in total involved 2.29 billion people. Carnage rates before and after the 2003 invasion of Iraq alone are quoted as: 100 000 civilian deaths, one million children orphaned and 12 million people made homeless. The horrendous psychological effects on children living in war zones are discussed in a separate section.

Proof of the profitability of war, which sustains the military mind-set, is everywhere. The 1990s have seen more than 20% of the world's qualified scientists and engineers engaged in military research, while annual global military expenditure had exceeded world spending on health by 28%.

Regionally, the economies of many countries have long been operating on a war footing. Bosnia–Herzegovina, Croatia and Serbia are good examples of war economies, where 85% of all the region's earnings in 1994–5 were directed towards its war effort, at an estimated cost in excess of US$20 billion. The 2005 United States' defence spending amounted to more than double that of the combined 24 participating European Member States, with US military expenditure as a percentage of GDP being 4.06% compared to Europe's 1.81%. To place the United States' military expenditure into perspective; its 2008 operating costs of the war in Iraq ran at a whopping $12.5 billion a month, rising to $16 billion if Afghanistan is included. In contrast, $16 billion dollars is the annual budget of the United Nations, or four times that of the World Health Organization, or 2 years' funding for the campaign to eradicate illiteracy worldwide.

Military extravagance is not difficult to understand when we think of the ongoing costs of military personnel, equipment procurement, operations maintenance and research intended to 'improve' technological applications; or, in more homely terms, the cost of rifles, ammunition, hand grenades, land mines, automatic and semiautomatic guns, jeeps, trucks, other military supplies and basic necessities such as food, footwear and clothing. Yet, defying all logic, the global community still accepts as tolerable the tragic consequences on the populations, economies and the territorial structures of the communities in conflict. Rather than condemning this unique form of human behaviour, it seems that wars are rewarded in various culturally approved ways. Australians celebrate 25th April with a public holiday to commemorate ANZAC Day – the anniversary of the Australian and New Zealand Army Corps landing which ended in defeat, at Gallipoli (Turkey) in 1915. Other nations generally choose to commemorate their victories. Either way, a majority of people around the world would probably give much to be able to celebrate the end of all wars, and the end of mortgaging future wealth to pay for present violence.

Much has been written about the concept that warriors are caught up in a web of altruism; that is, warfare, despite it being an aggressive act, also entails cooperation and alliance, which has provided, in our tribal past, Darwinian fitness. For example, the 'balance-of-power' hypothesis holds that the primary function of human groups is to compete with other human groups, and that the optimal size of human groups is determined by the need to maintain balanced power. Gluing together this balance of power is balanced reciprocity or reciprocal altruism - or, may I suggest, the balance of cost and benefits where world military expenditure as a percentage of GDP is roughly 2% of gross world product.

The tragedy of conflict

The reptilian brain in mammals plays a crucial role in selecting its leaders.[2]

It seems that we are increasingly engaging in ecologically based conflict, conveniently categorized as 'the ecology of violence'. The ecology of violence can be viewed as the inevitable consequence of enforced poverty, land and resource mismanagement, greed, population pressures and overexploitation of natural resources. In this respect, the ecology of violence is reminiscent of the tragedy of the commons (Chapter 13), where ecological marginalization is the primary cause of conflict, which can then easily escalate into warfare, further self-perpetuating the cycle of environmental and human degradation. Figure 14.1 summarizes the self-sustaining characteristics of the ecology of violence.

Once war is established, the economy becomes predatory by consuming scarce resources to further the conflict, trapping its inhabitants in an increasing cycle of war-related debt and further poverty. The most common consequences of institutional warfare are reduced national income, destruction of former productive territories, and fleeing refugees adding to the existing large numbers of displaced persons. Within towns and settlements, industry, hospitals, administrative offices and their documentation are damaged or destroyed, along with spiritual, cultural, historical and national monuments, such as churches, museums, libraries and important protected natural areas. Indirect damage caused by the interruption of communication and traffic routes, and the need to care for refugees, displaced persons, war invalids and orphaned children, takes on transgenerational significance.

One unifying characteristic of all war operations is the low regard given to human and environmental rights, especially of future generations. War violates fundamental human decency when action is taken against non-military targets and when the civilian population is subjected to atrocities such as rape, assassinations, massacres, torture and ethnic cleansing. All of the above have been perpetrated under the banner of justice and righteousness. Most of the above can also be seen on our television screens, where we regularly view images of nations being slaughtered, increasingly on a scale of unbelievable magnitude. At the same time we invariably see well-fed soldiers alongside starving refugees, mostly women and children. Altruistic rhetoric or not, isn't

---

[2] MacLean, P. (1990). *The Triune Brain in Evolution: Role in Paleocerebral Functions.* New York: Plenum Press, p. 247.

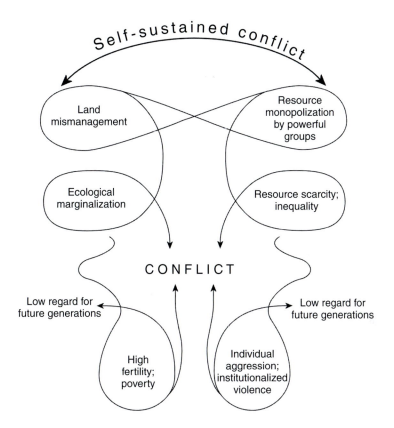

Figure 14.1 Civil unrest is typically a consequence of severe overcrowding, poverty, insufficient resources or inequality of resource distribution. The need for reform may generate dominance conflict among unstable hierarchies, monopolizing scarce resources which, in turn, promulgates a self-sustaining spiral of socioecological unrest across generations.

it time for the tribal human animal, equipped with its unique capacity for social intelligence, to evolve up to a minimal standard of behaviour and resolve its disputes by means of peace mediation and peace-keeping skills? Instead of seeing institutionalized warfare as a winnable endeavour, we must regard it as an evolutionary failure. To quote France's ex-president Jacques Chirac, 'War is always a sign of failure, and is always the worst solution'.

For the unfortunates trapped in war-torn zones, conflict can become a way of life. Millions of children grow up not knowing what peace is. In recent decades, sharp increases in the number of environmental refugees fleeing landlessness and poverty in their homelands should be seen as a global warning. In its 2006 publication, the United Nations High Commissioner for

Refugees (UNHCR) estimated that the global population of registered refugees was nudging close to 10 million, with a further 23.7 million internally displaced persons in more than 50 countries. The statistics on internally displaced persons includes only those who are displaced by conflict and persecution – millions more are being uprooted within their own countries by natural disasters or marginalized to make way for national projects by the ruling hierarchy (Fig. 14.1). It has also been estimated that half of these internally displaced persons are children.

Many factors have been responsible for the growing number of displaced persons. In Africa, Europe and Asia, long-simmering ethnic conflicts have turned violent, with accompanying civilian casualties and population migration. A particular event can quickly trigger massive migrations, such as the flight of an estimated 2 million Hutu Rwandans fleeing into neighbouring Zaire and Tanzania in 1994. Many feared retaliation at the hands of the victorious, mainly Tutsi, Rwandan Patriotic Front for the Hutu-led genocide of the Tutsis. However, emigration is a viable option only if there is somewhere to emigrate to. Uncontrollable mass human migrations pose severe biological problems (not least in terms of the fertility and psychological dislocation of the émigrés) and are a serious destabilizing influence in already overpopulated host countries. Fears about the loss of land or social influence may create ethnically based conflicts between new and old settlers, often resulting in campaigns of terror against the émigrés.

Environmental scientists have been claiming for decades that mismanagement of the environment and the problems that this generates increase a community's vulnerability to conflict. Three principal factors causing increased tension over resources can be clearly identified. These are the degradation and depletion of a key resource, population growth increasing the demand for the key resource, and injustice in its distribution, where one sector of society takes a disproportionate share, leaving insufficient for the others. Unfortunately, the will for reform frequently degenerates into a power struggle among unstable hierarchies professing differing ideologies. The ensuing violence is easily spread to neighbouring countries and increases overall aggression in the vicinity, with the regional environment being doubly the loser (Fig. 14.1). Lack of land, deforestation and population growth lay behind the 1994 Zapatista rebellion in Chiapas, Mexico, and water scarcity has contributed to ongoing violence in Gaza (Israel). The connection between environmental security and peace will become even more apparent in the future. Climate change, desertification and increasing scarcity of fresh water, in particular, are likely to cause violent competition for what remains, increasing the existing magnitude of environmental destruction. Desertification is not just the natural expansion of existing deserts but the degradation of fought-over land in arid, semi-arid and dry sub-humid areas. Another crucial issue facing us all is acceptance of the fact that there is nothing that conventional military notions of threat and defence can do to give security for the environment. At times of military conflict, the institution of war places a very low priority on environmental protection; this is exemplified by the environmental terrorism perpetrated by the retreating Iraqi army which ignited Kuwait's oilfields in the aftermath of the Gulf War of 1991. Or the continuing legacy of chemical contamination of people living near former US military installations in Vietnam more than 40 years after the Americans discharged their dioxin-laden herbicide Agent Orange into the once pristine environment. Or the accelerating rise in leukaemia and other debilitating illnesses among children and NATO troops living/stationed in regions contaminated with depleted uranium as inherited from depleted uranium armour-piercing weapons employed to penetrate buildings, bunkers, tank armour and other militarily targeted solid objects. Exposure to depleted uranium (a low alpha radiation emitter) waste is a known causal factor in cancer, birth defects and other key dysfunctions, and is believed to be a contributing factor in the ongoing 'Gulf-war syndrome'. The Pentagon used depleted uranium in large amounts in Iraq in 1991, in Bosnia in 1995 and in Kosovo in 1999.

War ravages industries, including chemical industries which, in turn, cause immediate and ongoing pollution problems by contaminating soil and water resources. Local environmental contamination then spreads to neighbouring and downstream countries, which depend on these basic resources. The environmental consequences also have profound effects on wildlife. These effects are related to the disturbance and intimidation of animals, especially mammals and birds, and the contamination and destruction of their habitats. This, in turn, can lead to severe consequences, such as the extinction of some animal populations (especially the most threatened) or reduction of populations of vulnerable species and the permanent loss of fragile and unique ecosystems. The stress of intimidation and suffering of the animals trapped by war chaos affects their overall long-term resilience, including their reproductive capability. Reproductive dysfunction then adversely affects fertility, mating behaviour and the raising of young.

Within more stable nations not in effect engaged in warfare, social deprivation generates deep tensions which may also lead to violence and a desire to destabilize the existing hierarchy. Some of the ethnic riots in the USA and Britain are, in the depth of emotion generated, civil wars kept in check by virtue of their small size and these countries' relative economic stability. Thus, there is also the related problem of pursuing a culture of aggression at times of national peace, when civilians can easily arm themselves with automatic military-style weapons. Because the manufacture of weapons is so lucrative, both developed and developing nations worldwide are equally guilty in not insisting on adequate nationwide registration of firearms and stringent limitations to firearm ownership. The United States leads the industrial world in gun-related murders, suicides and accidental deaths. In 1996, for example, handguns were used to murder 9390 people in the US compared with 2 people in New Zealand, 15 in Japan, 30 in Great Britain, 106 in Canada, and 213 in Germany. It is estimated that for every gun death three others are injured, often in the long term, when the survivors are left with serious injuries, permanent disabilities and trauma that can impede a normal way of life. The following is a fitting quote from the UN Programme of Action on Small Arms: 'Global gun violence is a multidimensional problem requiring action at all levels – international, regional, national, local, in the home and in the mind. Effective solutions must be comprehensive and based in law and policy, enforcement and information, awareness and culture. The UN and its Member States have a critical role to play in all of these.'[3]

Biological warfare

When mass human migrations are uncontrolled, the spread of disease, particularly sexually transmitted disease, is an ever-present threat. The opportunistic spread of the human immunodeficiency virus (HIV) and AIDS, for instance, is significant at times of war, when poverty and ignorance forces women, who do not necessarily consider themselves as prostitutes, to sell unprotected sex on a massive scale. Rape, which has occurred throughout history in all cultures, is also at its highest level during wars. As a consequence, the incidence of disease is higher at times of war, although this is usually localized. Conditions inducing chronic ill health are also elevated at times of war due to stress and the dearth of medical staff, who are monopolized by the war machine. Until recently, however, no one gave serious consideration to human-engineered pandemics, in which nearly 100% of the targeted populace could suffer a horrific death.

To those studying modern warfare strategies it is increasingly apparent that the world needs to be better prepared to deal with disease epidemics resulting from terrorist attacks using biological weapons. Unfortunately, the threat of biological warfare did not decrease with the signing of the 1972 worldwide treaty on Biological and Toxic Weapons which, in theory, prohibits their

---

[3] http://www.iansa.org/campaigns_events/gun-control-2006.htm; p. 8.

development and deployment. On the contrary, the danger of institutionalized terrorism has become more real to the ordinary citizen since the Gulf War and the September 11th (2001) terrorist attacks on US soil. It is well documented that military powers, including the United States and the former Soviet Union, have undertaken basic research programmes on biological weapons, with the alleged stockpiling of many agents of germ warfare. In addition, several smaller nations have access to microorganisms and toxins that could be used as biological weapons. In recent decades there have also been isolated attempts to use biological weapons as agents of terror.

The potential for the development of biological agents as weapons has been due to recent scientific advances in basic and applied microbiology. The close parallel development of science and its application to war should not come as a surprise, since humans have always used the latest available technology for destructive as well as for constructive purposes. Biological warfare is not new because cadavers, animal carcasses and contagious matter have been used as weapons to contaminate enemy water sources, such as wells and reservoirs, since time immemorial. Infected rams and donkeys were deliberately driven into enemy territory by the Hittites during the Anatolian wars when fighting the Arzawans between 1320 and 1318 BCE. The animals were carriers of *Francisella tularensis* – the causative agent of tularaemia – a fatal disease even today if not treated with antibiotics. The ensuing tularaemia epidemic is known as the Hittite plague, with the contaminated territories stretching from Cyprus to Iraq and from Israel to Syria. Cuneiform tablets from Sumer (modern Syria) dating back to 1170 BCE document that the ancients were well informed about the processes of contagion and its application in biological weapons. History also reveals that biological weapons have not only been used between warring nations but have been deployed against specific ethnic minorities within one nation as, for example, the use of smallpox (caused by the variola virus) as a biological weapon against the First Nation people of America in the eighteenth century. In this instance, blankets from smallpox victims were given to the Indigenous people. The resulting epidemic killed as many as 50% of the members of the affected tribal group.

The deliberate use of microorganisms and biological toxins, such as neurotoxins produced by marine dinoflagellates or some cyanobacteria, are effective, low cost, easy-to-use weapons of mass destruction. These agents also require a minimum of scientific knowledge for their production and deployment. Because the same biological agents are used for legitimate medical purposes, as in the development of antibiotics and vaccines, the procedures of production and handling are generally available. Any interested civilian can find recipes for making biological weapons in the scientific literature or, for that matter, on the Internet. Moreover, unlike nuclear weapons or missile placements, specialized equipment is not required for the delivery of these lethal pathogens.

Most fatalities and injuries from conventional bombing occur immediately; however, the effects of a biological attack can be delayed and depend on the incubation period of the virus or bacterium involved. In addition, modern concentrated forms of biological agents are invisible, odourless and tasteless, making it difficult to know when, or if, a terrorist attack has taken place or is under way. Biological warfare is becoming the most feared form of global terrorism because any one of hundreds of cultured agents can stealthily be introduced and quickly claim millions of casualties. Civilians who are not generally immunized or do not possess protective equipment are especially vulnerable. A millionth of a gram of anthrax, for example, constitutes a lethal dose, while a kilogram of it has the potential of killing hundreds of thousands of people in a metropolitan area. Ever more sophisticated genetically engineered forms of viruses are being manufactured by scientists. For example, at a now defunct USSR virology centre, it is claimed that researchers were experimenting with chimeras made from genes of two different species of virus. A particular chimera mentioned was a genetically engineered form of smallpox virus which contained material from the Venezuelan equine encephalitis – a brain virus that causes near-coma but need not be fatal. The surreptitious release of a biological agent can easily be facilitated via crop dusters, trucks equipped with spray tanks, timing devices in subways and airports, or released through the air conditioning systems in buildings and other crowded places.

Future generations of biological weapons may become so powerful as to push them up to the top of the list of all weapons, including nuclear, in terms of potential lethality. This scenario may result from the misapplication of sophisticated technologies made possible through the knowledge gained from the Human Genome and the Human Genome Diversity Projects (Chapter 10). In theory at least, the successful manufacture of population-specific genetic weaponry for use in the deployment in what is loosely termed 'ethnic cleansing' may become a horrifying reality. The possibility arises because the above mentioned projects are not just gene mapping endeavours but, in addition, reveal genetic differences between groups of people living within one population.

An aim of the Human Genome Diversity Project is to identify sets of genetic markers that distinguish specific population subgroups. An identified difference could be diverted, from an ethically neutral identification of genetic difference to the targeting of specific genetic variance found in ethnic subgroups living in conflict-ridden territories and war zones. Although the intent of the genome projects is for ultimate benefit, as in medical applications and gene therapy, the same technology can be misused in the development of genetically modified lethal microbes, which selectively infect people belonging to one specific human population. The attraction from the aggressor's point of view is that genetic-specific biological weapons make them more controllable because the aggressors themselves are, in theory at least, protected from catching the disease. Scientists working for good must now be more aware than ever before that their considerable and valuable contributions may be misapplied or misused.

Since there is now a real possibility that wars of the future may not be fought on traditional battlefields, new contingency plans have to be made. Biological weapons are not respectful of traditional boundaries or geography, so the challenge and expense involved in providing protective measures is enormous. The first goal has to be to counteract the terrorists' goal of creating unprecedented fear and chaos, so that remedial action can be swift. Since valuable resources will have to be expended to withstand this new form of aggression, it will be the wealthy nations who will make these contingency plans. These privileged nations, if they do not already, will soon have in place capabilities and response measures. For example, physicians will have to become familiar with the organisms that are most often used, and have access to antidotes and effective drugs to treat the diseases these organisms cause. Additional personnel will have to be trained to recognize the early symptoms of disease caused by biological warfare agents. Stress debriefing teams will have to be trained to help cope with the psychological/emotional aspects of treating exposed survivors and their families. Development will have to be directed towards the refinement of biodetectors, and medical units with expertise in prophylactics, hazard mitigation and decontamination will have to be established. Vaccine and antibiotic research will have to be accelerated in the event of terrorist use of new genetically engineered organisms intended for biological warfare. The technology to manipulate the genes of harmless bacteria so that they produce potent toxins, such as ricin, has already been in existence for some time. Simple things like protective clothing and masks with improved air filtration systems will have to be mass manufactured. Personnel will have to be trained in specific biological weaponry intelligence collection, analysis and pre-emptive response to terrorist attack.

It is sobering to reflect that the US government is taking the threat of biological warfare so seriously that in 1996 it passed a 'Defence Against Weapons of Mass Destruction' act. Under the provisions of this legislation, major cities are designated as centres for specialist biological weapons training within the fire, police, rescue and hospital emergency services. Let us hope that this new expertise will never have to be used in a serious terrorist or war situation.

Computer technology, cyber-electronics and virtual warfare

Another area of astonishing technological progress is the potential application of computer-dependent and related electronic technologies in virtual warfare. Through computer games, our children are very familiar with autonomous weapons equipped with their robo-warriors engaged in their gun-toting teleo-operations. These may familiarize and prepare our children for future catastrophes – or, perhaps, toughen them up for a military career! In any event, the use of robotics in civilian systems is negligent, compared with their increasing use in the military sphere where serious money is being spent on furthering the research and development of sophisticated teleo-operator systems. Teleo-operations at remote work locations carry special advantages for dangerous peacetime jobs when the precise nature of the task cannot be predicted. But it is a different mission when it involves military operations with robot drivers circling around the globe in their gunning vehicles, fighter planes or invisible submarines.

Weapons of mass destruction are, unfortunately, often technologically indistinguishable from tools that save lives. A remotely operated vehicle can enter a building to save or kill those trapped within; whether the robot wields a scalpel or a gun is a matter of human intention, not mechanical ability. The technology already exists, so the question is whether there can be adequate controls placed on the proliferation of sophisticated military cyber-technologies suitable for the deployment of chemical and biological weapons. In its 2006 report, the International Commission on Weapons of Mass Destruction[4] – an independent body instigated by the Swedish government – released recommendations for action restricting the production, deployment and use of the types of weapons that come under the generic title of 'weapons of mass destruction'. 'Weapons of mass destruction' covers nuclear, biological and chemical weapons and their delivery systems such as missiles or bombers. This is a positive step towards peace but, interestingly, explosives, small arms, and napalm do not qualify as weapons of mass destruction. Still, progress towards global peace is being made in some quarters, as demonstrated by the European nations who have changed the fundamental nature of their armies from one intended to protect territorial integrity to one of peacekeeping. European peacekeeping forces are actively dispatched wherever required and, for the

[4] www.wmdcommission.org/sida.asp?id=1

first time, preference is given to recruits who are willing to serve as peace-keepers rather than traditional fighters, further promoting a healthier preventative, rather than conflict-orientated, state of mind. The economic integration of European countries has been distinctly triumphal in the establishment of peace in the area, especially when we consider Europe's long turbulent history.

Although the underlying cause of conflict is usually resource-related, wars are often fought on ethnic/religious grounds. This is because the individual conscience is more assured when the protagonists believe that they are fighting for a 'cause' based on religious/moral principles. Possibly it could be made more explicit that religion can be exploited in this way, which might then generate a positive feedback for transformation and a willingness to bring about real reductions in all kinds of violence, including sectarian. Given our technological powers, to move the world by force is neither adaptive nor worthy of human intellect. Our relentless killer instinct and ecological imperialism is massively non-adaptive, so to survive we must learn to stop. Religious leaders have, therefore, grave responsibilities in this respect because, in the final analysis, religion has to be worked through the practice of bioethics, meaning 'life ethics'.

The legacy of war on future generations

More and more of the world is being sucked into a space in which children are slaughtered, raped, and maimed; a space in which children are exploited as soldiers; a space in which children are starved and exposed to extreme brutality. Such unregulated terror and violence speak of deliberate victimization. There are few further depths to which humanity can sink.[5]

When discussing the environmental hazards of war, we must also take into consideration their long-term consequences and, in particular, their effects on future generations of children. Environmental issues are a matter of relations between generations: radioactive waste, once produced, is there and cannot be easily destroyed; the gases known as the chlorofluorocarbons (CFCs) already released into the atmosphere now will damage the ozone layer in 30–80 years. Although the use of the polychlorinated biphenyls (PCBs) ceased in western countries in the late 1970s, they were subsequently manufactured and used in South East Asia, and central and eastern Europe in a wide variety of

---

[5] UN Report on the Impact of Armed Conflict on Children, 1996. www.unicef.org/graca/

commercial applications like electrical transformers, condensers and in vehicular hydraulic fluids. To make matters worse, some of these locally manufactured PCBs contain higher levels of persistent, highly toxic byproducts such as chlorinated dioxins and furans than those PCBs formerly synthesized in western Europe or the United States. During warfare, huge quantities of persistent organic pollutants are released into the environment. Within war-torn zones, as experienced in the political entities of the former republic of Yugoslavia (Croatia, Bosnia and Herzegovina), local and 'Allied Force' operations resulted in the release of considerable quantities of PCBs and other chemical pollutants into the environment. Widespread release of PCBs originating from shelled and burnt electrical transformers and condensers, and from abandoned and severely damaged military vehicles, placed the Balkan Peninsula citizenry, particularly vulnerable children, in long-term chemical jeopardy. On top of everything else, during uncontrolled PCB combustion, ever more toxic polyhalogenated dibenzofurans and dibenzodioxins are formed.

As well as PCBs and byproducts of their incomplete combustion, other war-generated pollutants such as heavy metals, depleted uranium, fuel oils, petroleum products and a large variety of toxic chemicals are recklessly spread into the environment. These toxic mixtures leach into the soil and ultimately find their way into water sources. Thus, widespread environmental contamination with pollutants of all sorts surrounding any conflict zone is inevitable. Pollutants enter international waters via ground, surface and marine water transport, so the contamination of potable water resources, rivers, fish, cattle, dairy products and crops in neighbouring nations also becomes an environmental tragedy. Many synthetic manmade chemicals, including the PCBs and the organochlorine insecticides, are serious hormone disruptors. As already noted (Chapter 13), xenohormones that mimic specific reproductive hormonal activities are a hazard to normal sexual development, fertility and pregnancy, and so are instrumental in setting up a transgenerational legacy of war-related environmental pollution. This toxic legacy is passed on to the next generation preconceptionally, prenatally and in early infancy via contaminated breast milk and post-weaning contaminated foods. An extensive epidemiological study analysing human milk samples collected during 1998/99 from the general population in Zagreb (Croatia) revealed that all samples were heavily contaminated with hazardous levels of PCBs.

The above situations underscore the urgent need to improve human and environmental protection measures which minimize exposure, through the food chain, of persistent bioaccumulative toxins in war-zone and neighbouring countries. However, post-war reconstruction of industry and remediation of contaminated soil and water requires a mammoth effort through provision of large amounts of international aid, which are then not available for competing projects such as relief of poverty in other areas.

Child soldiers

War-zone children are not only victims of violence but are also adversely affected as active participants. In 2003 there were more than 30 armed conflicts occurring in over 25 countries, and half of these involved child soldiers under the age of 15. These children, in direct infringement of the UN Charter for the Rights of the Child, were brainwashed by violent recruiters into serving renegade political gangs in exchange for food, shelter and security of sorts. Human Rights Watch further documented that there are over 300 000 children at any given time participating in hostilities while 'serving' in rebel groups and government forces around the world. These child soldiers perform a range of tasks in addition to armed combat participation. These tasks include laying mines and explosives, scouting, spying, acting as decoys, couriers or guards, cooking, as well as sexual slavery. The abundance of child soldiers is a direct reflection of the deterioration of societies where disintegration of schools, homes and families leave armed groups as the child's greatest chance for survival.

A child's reaction to the traumas of war varies with age and level of development. Typically, children under the age of 6 lack well-developed cognitive, social and emotional qualities, which makes them especially vulnerable. Their inability to comprehend the political and social issues responsible for their situation leads to confusion, feelings of guilt and difficulty in developing ethical competence as adults. Older children have the ability to think abstractly, leading to heightened awareness of morality and ethics, and this may influence their understanding of and response to war. In the best scenario, the experience of irrational cruelty induces in children a healthy scepticism for adult values; at worst, cruelties are perpetuated down the line. Whatever the case, disregard for human needs and incursions into the lives of family units causes emotional pain and confusion in children and adults alike, and hinders normal brain development, including a natural progression in the capacity for intellectual and emotional thought. Abnormal brain function consequent to the terror of war may initiate post-traumatic stress disorders (PTSDs) where sufferers lose their connection with reality. PTSD refers to severe and continuous emotional reactions to an intense psychological traumatic event. Symptoms include nightmares, emotional dissociations, insomnia, memory loss, depression and anxiety. The word *trauma* is derived from the Greek word for *wound* and includes harm to the body, mind and spirit. PTSD is especially evident in children from war-zone regions. War-zone traumatic stress responses in some children tend to show as hardened intrapsychic defences that have evolved to cope with the extraordinary conditions of living amongst social and political upheaval. It is not uncommon for the children of war zones to appear emotionally anaesthetized, which may play out as adults unable to connect with their surroundings. PTSD and related syndromes can also cause the onset of risk-taking behaviours, including drug and alcohol abuse, adding to pre-existing personal afflictions (Chapter 6).

Uganda, Rwanda, Palestine, Israel, Sri Lanka, Iraq, Afghanistan and many more countries have suffered generations of political, civil and military unrest. Children born and raised in these societies often grow up without knowing what it can be like to live in an environment free of war and accompanying sociocultural prejudices. For the new generations of children growing up in displaced communities, continuous distress, ingrained poverty, chronic malnutrition, little or no access to basic health care facilities, the breakdown of family units, exploitation and sexual abuse seem to be the way of being. Attempts to estimate these costs of war are futile because how can one begin to calculate the indirect consequences of wars on the human and natural environments?

A new approach to problem-solving by pre-empting population and poverty crises is essential if we are to overcome the futility of waging wars and suffering the consequent environmental degradation. It is sobering to reflect that biological evolution over more than three billion years has resulted in the millions of species of organisms living today and the many millions more that lived in the past but are now extinct. We are part of this union of life and our characteristic contribution could be creative intelligence, but creative intelligence also postulates choice, moral reflection and ethical rules. Our exceptional creativity – also the basis of freedom – gave us technology and art, but technological inventiveness as a species can result in progress or ruthless destruction. Will we continue to heedlessly destroy the fruits of evolution unable to adapt and handle change because we are too closely bound to our primitive fighting heritage? Survival obliges us to silence our overzealous support for military ideals and protect essential ecosystems for the maintenance of life on Earth. Humans are not only shaped by genes but also by ideas or 'memes' (Chapter 1) and it is significant that, in all cultures, symbolic art is used to satisfy deep psychological needs. To strengthen and provide courage to combatants of all ethnic affiliations, warrior masks were traditionally worn to invoke terror in the enemy (Fig. 14.2). We have now come to a time in our evolution when, as a matter of survival, we have to remove those malevolent

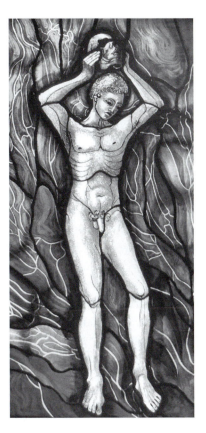

Figure 14.2 Stained glass window of a transformed combatant stripping off his warrior mask. Edged and painted glass worked in traditional techniques on thin-sheet stained glass held together by soldered lead strips (created in the 1980s by the author Irina Pollard).

expressions of hostility and take on a more mature, intellectually creative look at the world.

Since traditional notions of national security are outmoded, military spending should be diverted away from the acquisition of weaponry and towards environmentally sustainable development. Given that environmental stress is a major cause of civil unrest, it follows that, in the interests of peace, governments must invest in such things as sustainable fishing, forestry, soil and water conservation, and land reform. Finally we have to face the fact that our evolutionary heritage, which provided us when threatened with two different survival strategies – to fight and obtain high social rank in spite of upheaval or to flee to pastures new – are, in the modern context, both losing strategies. An intelligent approach may be to orchestrate a global referendum which declares war illegal and consequently releases untold wealth for reconstruction and egalitarian reformation.

Principles of bioscience ethics for discussion

- Cyber-ethics probe: given our increasing scientific knowledge, the future should be a positive time to shape up our mores and enjoy a healthy, invigorating presence. Yet the astonishing progress in electronics, which possibly has the greatest potential to humanize our collective history, has been hijacked to serve in the arena of virtual warfare. What shared aspects of identity and individuality are important in identifying constructive ways of conflict resolution?
- Neither ethnicity nor cultural identity is sufficiently reinforced by genetics to warrant the classification of 'race'. Consequently, other differences must exist among individual groups of humans to prevent them approaching one another in mutual understanding and sympathy. Why can so many global problems be identified as targeted racism, and in the absence of 'biological race' why has this scientific insight been marginalized by an equivalent weapon dubbed 'sociological race'?
- Human rights and human security are not mutually exclusive but mutually dependent; please comment. The decades since the signing of 'The Universal Declaration of Human Rights' have been characterized by war, waged primarily by the very states that were instrumental in making The Declaration in 1948. What in your opinion is the use of The Declaration to those who cannot read it?

15

Human-dominated ecosystems: reworking bioethical frontiers

I would suggest that our real role as stewards on the Earth is more like that of the proud trades union functionary, the shop steward. We are not managers or masters of the Earth, we are just shop stewards, workers chosen because of our intelligence, as representatives for the others, the rest of life on our planet. Our union represents the bacteria, the fungi, the slime moulds and invertebrates, as well as the nouveau riche fish, birds, reptiles and mammals and the landed establishment of noble trees and their lesser plants. Indeed, all living are members of our union and they are angry at the diabolical liberties taken with their planet and their lives by people. People should be living in union with the other members, not exploiting them and their habitats. When I see the misery we inflict upon them and upon ourselves, I have to speak out as a shop steward. I have to warn my fellow humans that they must learn to live with the Earth in partnership, otherwise the rest of creation will, as part of Gaia, unconsciously move the Earth itself to a new state, one where humans may no longer be welcome.[1]

The unprecedented and awesome power of science and technology, combined with the sheer number of people living on the planet, has transformed the scale of human impact from local and regional to global. It was pointed out in Chapter 12 that lag times, before the effects of human-driven change emerge, can often be long. We design new technologies and deploy them on an unprecedented scale around the world long before we can begin to fathom

---

[1] Lovelock, J. (1995). The greening of science. In T. Wakeford and M. Walters (eds.) *Science for the Earth: Can Science Make the World a Better Place?* Chichester: John Wiley & Sons, p. 62.

their possible impact on the global system or ourselves. The time has certainly come, at the beginning of a new millennium, to ask the ethical questions that have been overlooked in the headlong technological euphoria of the twentieth century. Is it right to change the composition of the Earth's atmosphere? Is it right to alter the chemical environment and genetic potential of every unborn child? It is critical that humans, as a global community, give serious consideration to these questions and begin a multi-faceted discussion that reaches far beyond the usual participants – the chemical companies, government regulators, farmers, economists, scientists and environmental groups. This important initiative must engage everyone – teachers, parents, physicians, philosophers, artists, historians, spiritual leaders and scientists. We all have to reflect on the richness and diversity of human experience and wisdom, and pool our resources. We have to find better, safer and cleverer ways to meet basic human needs, which includes all our fellow travellers on Earth. We must learn to responsibly represent ourselves in symbiotic union with the rest of life on our planet.

Global responsibility – a transboundary détente to developmental needs and environmental preservation

Climate change is a significant new additional stress on global systems, both natural and human. Climate change will affect all countries as the oceans are warming, ice is melting, the North Atlantic current is weakening, soils and forests are releasing methane and carbon, and tropical diseases are spreading (Chapter 12). In addition, considerable advances in energy technology will be needed to stabilize atmospheric carbon dioxide concentrations at acceptable levels. Amazingly, only now, when the scientific evidence is indisputable, have arguments about global warming shifted from questions such as, 'Is it happening and if so should we err on the side of caution or just forge ahead regardless?' to 'Has the point of no return been reached, will the inevitable change be slow or will it catastrophically flip to a new state and if so how will we cope?' Because the cost and technological challenge of coping with these changes is so great, the developing world in general is more vulnerable than are the developed countries. The expansion of the tropical and subtropical areas that favour malaria-transmitting mosquitoes would lead to an estimated additional 10–15% increase in cases of malaria each year. Dengue, yellow fever and viral encephalitis would in all probability also increase. It may be possible that some of these effects and a litany of others, such as increased coastal flooding due to sea-level rise, loss of mountain glaciers, shifting agricultural areas and land losses on low-lying coasts, could be mitigated with the right technology. Savings would come from greater efficiencies and, in the long run, lower expenditure. For example, the energy-efficient domestic lightbulb, solar water heaters, etc., are already quickly paying back the initially higher costs of purchase and installation. Clearly, clean (possibly initially subsidized under certain circumstances) energy will have to be utilized on domestic, national and international fronts without delay if we are to ameliorate the worst predictions of climate change.

The power of the collective – endorsing multiple-entry bookkeeping

Over the past few decades, public attitudes towards environmental issues have undergone marked change. Since the end of World War II, social analysts have described value shifts associated with environmental matters as being the most profound of all changes in values. However, real progress can only be made when a critical mass of people have fundamentally changed their way of thinking. Once it has been generally accepted that a healthy environment is essential, not only for our physical but also our emotional and psychological wellbeing, environmental conservation will become an established part of our ethical conscience. It will become natural to foster sustainable development and make it a cornerstone of domestic and foreign policy. However, an essential shift in values and conduct can only follow if the collective mind-set challenges the status quo.

Since the destruction of land is an infringement of the rights of both present and future generations, we would be well advised to exert ourselves in peaceful political protest against any specific environmental abuse. We must relearn to respect wild things as having intrinsic value in themselves, irrespective of the value placed upon them in monetary terms. Peoples from all nations ought to be united with an ethics inclusive of both humans and Nature. In Chapter 12 I referred to the 'triple bottom line' accounting system where the power of ethics within some businesses has already resulted in progressive attitudinal change, particularly the acceptance that profit is not the only reward to be pursued. For example, in 1998 the trans-national company Mitsubishi Electric Corporation, under the managing directorship of Tachi Kiuchi, included three new categories in the company's accounts: pollution intensity, resource productivity and quality of life. A decade on, the concept of the triple bottom line has taken off, indeed many of the world's top companies have responded to stakeholder pressure and other institutional forces for value change and publish triple bottom line reports. In sustainable communities, the real wealth of the market revolves around sufficient material goods, sustainable ecological systems and optimal quality of life based on the abundance of personal and community-orientated services. Issues of happiness and spirituality become more important inner measures of quality of life, moving away from the quantity of things; thus, in an ideal world, the economics of the commons ranges from the integrity of the environment to the social fabric of our communities.

The triple bottom line accounting system also embraces 'industrial symbioses' where products, byproducts and waste materials are exchanged and recycled according to Nature's principles. In addition to reducing the ecological footprint, industrial symbioses carry broad financial benefits. New multiple-entry bookkeeping practices, such as the quadruple bottom line, are also driving a beneficial social conscience. The quadruple bottom line embraces a further component, that of governance, where the key element is leadership which focuses on the ethical responsibilities of employees through good managerial practices. Communities are increasingly repelled by the lack of ethics in boardroom disclosures, and the quadruple bottom line accounting system is having a beneficial impact as witnessed by the recent fall of certain corporate giants. Associated with heightened consumer expectations, businesses, if they are to succeed, must seriously begin to take into account cultural value shifts and focus on establishing ethics within their organizations. For example, in communities valuing sustainability, businesses are required to deal with various environmental and political agencies, and are expected to meet high standards of 'best practice ratings'.

The following section develops the present theme further by linking ways in which a network of people and companies can profit by a new knowledge-based economics and expand the capacity of the human mind bioethically.

The power of the individual

Our individual contributions towards solving global problems might seem trivial compared with their size, but nonetheless we must not be prevented from making them. It is encouraging to know that from small beginnings, such as buying environmentally friendly products and recycling waste, global change can develop. Single individuals can be standard bearers for change. The founder and chairman of 'Clean Up Australia', Ian Kiernan ('Captain Yukky'), for example, has been honoured with public accolades and awards for his exceptional proactivity and leadership qualities; these include Australian of the Year in 1994, Officer of the Order of Australia (AO) in 1995, and as one of Australia's 100 'living treasures' in 1997. In 1998 he was awarded

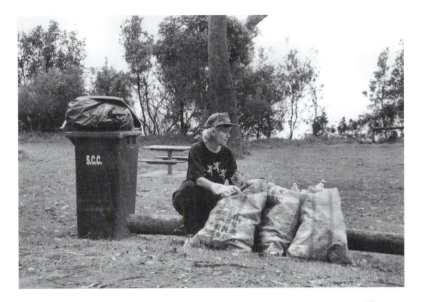

Figure 15.1 Clean Up Australia Sunday. Author with her 'yukky' spoils collected from the side of a typical Australian country road over a distance of 0.7 kilometres.

the prestigious United Nations Sasakawa Environment Prize for leadership in the local and global environmental settings. His status now gives Kiernan power with politicians, corporations and the public. However, this Aussie hero, living treasure, one-time ocean adventurer, was not born to privilege but has worked hard to become an environmental celebrity and a green powerbroker. It all started in 1987 with the one-off idea called 'Clean Up Sydney Harbour Day', which was a tearaway success, drawing 40 000 litter-collecting volunteers.

In 1989 the idea then expanded to what is now 'Clean Up Australia Day', drawing annually 500 000 volunteers (Fig. 15.1). In 1991 the United Nations Environment Program asked Ian Kiernan to replicate the event on a global level. 'Clean Up the World' has grown to encompass some 40 million volunteers in 120 countries during one weekend.

One individual's dream to clean up a harbour progressed to clean up a country, paving the way to clean up the world – it is all possible given goodwill and cooperation. 'I want to be a hard-hitting organization that is in partnership with the people, that business listens to, that governments pay attention to, so that we go and fix the bloody problems', said Kiernan in an interview for *Good Weekend* (28 February 1998). The giant Washington DC based cable network, the Discovery Channel (one of Clean Up's sponsors) is running special programmes promoting 'Clean Up the World'. This campaign, which aims to have every nation involved, is a smart new foray into on-air environmentalism and testimony to one man's infectious belief that humans can triumph over remarkable challenges.

Another example of extraordinary success is 'Earth Hour'. Earth Hour is now an annual global movement originally organized by the World Wide Fund for Nature (WWF) Australia. It all started on 31 March 2007 between 7.30 and 8.30 pm in Sydney, when households and businesses were asked to turn off their lights and non-essential electrical appliances for that hour. As the city darkened, the community delivered a powerful message about the need for action on global warming, particularly significant in the Aussie context with its coal-fired electricity overconsumption. That original event saw over 2.2 million Sydney-siders and over 2100 businesses switching off, leading to a 10.2% energy reduction across the city. As with 'Clean Up Australia Day', first-rate ideas soon take wing and this event too caught the attention of the world. Spectacularly, in March 2008, Earth Hour went global, with 300 000 individuals and over 20 000 businesses participating. Critics maintain that Earth Hour is mere tokenism, but caring for the environment, no matter how small at first, promotes attention which soon becomes an instinctive characteristic of good citizenship. According to EarthHour.org, if the greenhouse reduction achieved in Sydney during Earth Hour was sustained for a year, it would be equivalent to removing 48,616 cars from the road. We need to insure ourselves against unforeseen developments by applying our creative energies from our collective pool of flexible intelligence and sense of responsibility. We would be wise to remind ourselves that just as diversity of species provides biological stability, so diversity of ideas provides cultural security.

Stewardship of Mother Earth – in defence of the global commons

Environmental science, in its broadest terms, is the science of the complex interrelatedness that occurs among the terrestrial, atmospheric, aquatic and living (biospheric) environments, and includes disciplines such as chemistry, biology, ecology, sociology and governance. From the scientific perspective, technological advances should be viewed in terms of how they might adversely affect the environment and how they might also serve environmental rehabilitation. The reactive, gut-level approach, of 'going back to nature' by shunning all technological development is not a viable option because our global environment needs technological assistance to solve its existing health problems.

The biology of ecosystems is strongly expressed through its feedback systems (Chapter 12). Positive feedback is when an action tends to amplify itself, and is essential in maintaining lively reactivity to change. Negative feedback, on the other hand, occurs when a system automatically adjusts to minimize/ normalize a change or disturbance. Thus, in broad terms, healthy systems maintain stability – homeostasis – in dynamic environments by balancing both positive (amplifying) and negative (dampening) feedback mechanisms. By means of homeostatic mechanisms, we reach a state of equilibrium such that physiological processes can proceed at optimum rates through maintaining constant temperature, balancing our internal chemical composition and preserving specialized functions, including emotional stability. When scientists refer to 'vicious' climatic cycles they have in mind uncontrolled positive feedback in which normal deviations of the climate are amplified beyond the point where compensating feedback systems would normally kick in; thus in the climate example, greater heat leads to even greater heat. Another example of detrimental positive feedback is provided by soil erosion. When topsoil is removed by deforestation, water run-off forms gullies, and as topsoil is lost it becomes harder to grow vegetative cover, making the land prone to even more erosion. Left to natural devices, rivers and their floodplains tend to adapt in ways that compensate for increased river flow, thus minimizing environmental harm from flooding. Ruthless, ill-considered exploitation of the environment, such as farming of marginal land without proper conservation practices, and the insensitive exploitation of water, energy and mineral resources, inevitably results in environmental deterioration.

An overarching concern is that the Gaian (next section) system currently has a number of subsystems going into positive feedback where adverse changes are amplified. The time has come for the entire humanity to learn to live in harmony with its local environments, actively utilizing all available avenues, including bio-friendly technologies, to protect what is left of the Earth's biodiversity and the essential habitats upon which it depends. As with multiple-entry bookkeeping practices, resource utilization economics go beyond monetary values and conventional supply/demand relationships by including other economic aspects of resource usage. These additional aspects include pollution, gratuitous war-generated destruction of environments, general deleterious effects on existing life support systems, and other broadly based environmentally interconnected economic concerns. Other aspects of resource utilization consist of intangibles such as culture, knowledge, beauty, ethical insights and general satisfaction with life. These tangibles and intangibles need careful consideration when allocating value to resource development. Gaia is a post-Darwinian evolutionary theory that posits a set of homeostatic mechanisms as devices for self-maintenance of the Earth's environment which is uniquely suitable for the maintenance of life as we know it. Gaia closely illustrates how ignorant resource management may shift Earth's climate and chemical composition to a range unsuitable for all life forms as we know them.

Gaia – Earth's evolving physiology

The Earth system behaves as a single, self-regulating system, comprised of physical, chemical, biological and human components. The interactions and feedbacks between the component parts are complex and exhibit multi-scale temporal and spatial variability.[2]

The English scientist, James Lovelock, embraced the Greek name of the ancient Earth goddess, Gaia, to describe an evolutionary system by which global properties such as atmospheric and oceanic composition and climate set the constraints that bring stability to the living Earth. Lovelock first presented his revolutionary idea at a scientific meeting in 1969 and his theory has since been under intense scrutiny. Gaia challenges the reductionist view of the world by proposing that the world is one living system in which land, sea, sky and life (the biosphere) interact to actively maintain optimal conditions for the maintenance of life. The essence of this theory is that the physical and chemical conditions of the Earth's surface, atmosphere and oceans are kept continuously fit and comfortable for life by the presence of life itself.

Gaia stands in direct contrast to conventional wisdom which holds that life, as it evolved, adapted to the existing planetary conditions, but does not conflict with modern understanding of biogeochemical cycles where the Earth and the biosphere evolved together, forming a self-regulating, dynamically stable whole. Of Gaia's possible mechanisms or organization we have scant knowledge; the theory may, however, be supported to the extent where it can now be demonstrated, with the aid of numerical models and computers, that a diverse web of predators and prey facilitates a more stable and stronger ecosystem than a few more self-contained species, or a shorter food chain of very limited mix. These models also demonstrate that life can automatically be involved in regulating the climate without any kind of conscious, teleological involvement. Lovelock defines Gaia as 'a biological cybernetic system with homeostatic tendencies'. In this it is similar to the homeostatic mechanism underlying the body's adaptive response to stress, which balances the energy

---

[2] Lovelock, J. (2006). *The Revenge of Gaia*. London: Allen Lane, p. xii.

needs of the whole organism by master control of the individual needs of its subsystems. Thus, both Gaia and the living body are seen to be self-regulating, self-sustaining systems, continually adjusting their physical, chemical and biological processes in order to maintain optimal conditions for life and, at the same time, their continued evolution. If the planet functions as a single, indivisible evolutionary process, then its constituent parts, particularly the biosphere, cooperate in achieving a global homeostasis which can dynamically respond to internal and external challenges. Gaia, then, is a single, natural, highly stable system which reflects the totality of spatiotemporal information passed on from generation to generation of living things.

Gaia has to regulate temperature by the amount of carbon dioxide in the atmosphere – too much and the Earth gets hotter, too little and the Earth could freeze over – so biodiversity becomes critically important for maintaining a habitable Earth, and *Homo sapiens* is just one among many creatures. Any single kind of organism in isolation has the potential of disturbing Gaia's homeostasis. For instance, in a world with a preponderance of respirers, carbon dioxide would rise, but in a world of genetic diversity some symbionts would take care of the waste by cycling chemical elements through the components of the biogeochemical cycle (Chapter 12). At its simplest, cellular metabolism is fuelled by two forms of energy transformations. Through the process of photosynthesis, organic carbon and oxygen are produced from CO_2, water and chemical energy from the Sun. Through the process of respiration, biological energy, CO_2 and water are produced from organic carbon and oxygen. Organisms capable of photosynthesis include certain bacteria, cyanobacteria (blue–green algae), algae, non-vascular (primitive) plants and vascular (higher) plants. All organisms respire to fuel the sum of their chemical reactions upon which life depends, but photosynthesis is able to balance the respiratory CO_2 output of all groups of organisms, photosynthetic or non-photosynthetic.

Increased stability provided by biodiversity can be interpreted in mechanistic terms if we accept that there may be mechanisms controlling global homeostasis, where independent homeostatic systems are merged and coordinated in the interests of the greater whole. The world is a cooperative network of all its systems which has properties and powers much greater than the sum of its parts. Gaia is in harmony with and strongly reinforces some previously described ecological principles; namely, that cooperation within and between species, rather than conflict and competition, is the norm. Evolution has much more to do with complex symbiotic systems and mutual cooperation than with competition between individuals and species. In recent times, humankind has placed Gaia under many stresses. By adding greenhouse gases into the air and replacing natural ecosystems with low diversity agriculture, we are hitting

Earth with a 'double whammy' – we are interfering with global temperature regulation by turning up the heat and, simultaneously, removing the natural systems that help to regulate stability.

What is immediately evident is that Gaia is a powerful challenge to our view of the world. If, indeed, living things and the planet interact as one, we have to reassess our environmental responsibilities. In a world where established ecosystems experience continued disturbance, such as heat or drought, those species able to tolerate extreme conditions will adapt and be selected – the rest will become extinct, and the global properties, such as atmospheric and oceanic composition and climate, will stabilize to suit those that have completed their process of adaptation. Scientists have documented how the Earth has homeostatically adjusted to varying levels of carbon dioxide over the past 10 million years to maintain in the atmosphere constant quantities of oxygen, methane and nitrogen at levels that support life as we know it. Present atmospheric pollution with carbon dioxide and methane is similar to the natural release of these greenhouse gases 55 million years ago when comparable quantities of carbon entered the atmosphere. Then, the temperature rose about 8°C in the temperate northern regions and 5°C in the tropics; the consequences of this heating lasted 200 000 years. According to Lovelock, the period we are in now is close to a crisis point for Gaia. More than ever, we have to take care not to violate principles of sustainability which address the needs of the biosphere and the global commons of air, water and soil. *Homo sapiens* has evolved consciousness and gained intelligence; now this dominant species must also acquire wisdom in order to become accountable for the consequences of violating the principles of 'the common good', and to stop risking the survival of life on Earth as we know it. If we accept that human wellbeing and the health of the global commons are interchangeable, then we must also abide by the Gaian principles as described below.

Gaia's three principles

If natural systems are committed to the elimination of excessive randomness by virtue of the fact that they function cybernetically, it may be possible to identify a mechanism(s) by which the basic stability or homeostasis is controlled. Lovelock postulated that Gaia is characterized by three major principles.

The first principle is to keep conditions constant for the maintenance of all life

Our present relationship with Nature is based on the assumption of human superiority over all other living things. This egotistical assumption rests on the fact that we are empowered by our intelligence, and thus technology, to manipulate and exploit our planet and its biota for our own immediate human purposes. The sociobiologist Richard Dawkins has gone so far as to state that both major and minor technological advances can be regarded as analogous to mutations (a change in the genetic constitution of some cells and their progeny). This simple biological analogy can be extended further. The living body can cope with a certain number of mutations, and the older we become the more mutations we carry but, up to a critical point, are still able to function perfectly well. The cumulative effect of mutations is ageing, and ageing (or the 'stress' of life, if you like) weakens our ability to effectively homeostase, predisposing the body to eventual deterioration. Most mutations are deleterious to the organism; other mutations, however, are the raw material driving evolution. Given more knowledge of the functional mechanism of Gaia, there may be room for optimism that, with the aid of beneficial 'technological' mutations, we may facilitate, not harm, the essential global homeostatic process. The ability to respond adaptively to environmental change is essential for survival on this changing planet. With greenhouse-driven global warming, ozone depletion and other serious environmental problems having no ready solutions, climate could change radically in the near future.

The second principle is that Gaia has vital organs

It is suggested that the essential part of Gaia resides in the tropics, on the floors of the continental shelves, and in the soil below the surface. The destruction of reefs, such as the Great Barrier Reef in northern Australia, will have cascading effects, not only on fish species throughout the tropical oceans, but also on the shores and harbours now physically protected from erosion and wave action. If this Gaian principle is true, the reefs are also involved in the crucial task of regulating the salt content of the oceans by acting as evaporation lagoons between the open sea and the tropical shores. The humid tropical forests, likewise, through their capacity to transpire large volumes of water vapour, keep the climate cool. Their replacement by monocultures could precipitate uncontrolled climatic fluctuations. Thus, the fate of the tropical forests will be the major factor that determines the biological health of Earth in the future. These vital, but dwindling, ecosystems are also the greatest single reservoirs of biotic diversity, and thus future evolutionary potential, on the planet.

Scientists have long known that single-celled organisms – bacteria, fungi and protozoa – thrive on all parts of the Earth's surface. Their habitats range from the boiling hot waters of thermal springs to the freezing cold Arctic and Antarctic climes. Longstanding scientific dogma has also held that, deep inside, the Earth is essentially sterile. This belief has been shown to be wrong, because hundreds of thousands of metres below the Earth's crust there are thriving life forms. The study of rock core samples has clearly indicated that subsurface microorganisms are ubiquitous. Scientists have already catalogued and preserved more than 9000 strains of microorganisms from diverse subsurface environments, and reported a unique assortment of bacteria and about 100 types of fungi. These organisms were classified as living only if they were able to be grown in the laboratory. Various bacteria have been recovered from core formations with temperatures as high as 75°C and from depths extending to 2.8 km below the Earth's surface. Other organisms are capable of growing at 110°C in deep-sea volcanic vents, and some may be able to withstand temperatures as high as 140°C, at least for short periods. So, given a tolerance of 110°C, where the temperature rises about 15 degrees per kilometre of depth, allows microbial life to extend, on average, about 7 km below the sea floor. Equally for the exposed continental crust, where the temperature typically increases by about 25 degrees per kilometre, microscopic life could, on average, reach about 4 km down into the Earth's crust.

The richness of deep subsurface life, of course, depends not only on tolerable temperatures but also on the capacity of the local environment to support growth and reproduction. Life's crucial prerequisites include the presence of water, sufficient space in the pores of the rock, and available nutrients such as carbon, nitrogen, phosphorus and trace metals which all organisms need to synthesize their cellular constituents, including DNA and proteins. The environment also has to offer some form of fuel to provide the energy required for ongoing activity. It is of interest to note that, unlike autotrophic (self-sufficient) plants which photosynthesize using solar energy, many autotrophic bacteria capture their energy from inorganic chemical reactions involving iron or sulphur. These deep crust dwellers would very quickly be poisoned by oxygen – the element essential for life on the surface. More study of subsurface communities will tell us how life may have functioned on the early Earth before photosynthesis evolved. It may also provide us with a preview of how life might continue in the event of the irreparable destruction of Gaia's vital organs, which reside on the Earth's surface.

> *The third principle is that Gaian responses to change are governed by the rules of cybernetics*

As discussed above, Earth's climate and chemical composition are uniquely favourable for life as we know it. For example, the oxygen levels in the atmosphere have been constant for thousands of years. Such strongly homeostatic processes, however, give the least warning of undesirable trends;

that is, by the time a malfunction is noticed, inertial drag will bring things to a worse state before an equally slow improvement can set in. Population growth has inbuilt inertia where population numbers will, for a time, continue to increase still further, before the effects of any controlling measures become apparent. A major concern, when dealing with equilibria, is the possibility that systems that are homeostatically controlled may, if disturbed too far, react violently and be destabilized by erratic or sustained oscillations. If such effects occurred, then the extent of global warming or the depletion of the protective ozone shield may deviate greatly from present extrapolations. It may be suicidal for the politicians, whose view extends only to the next election, to decree, based on present measurements, a CO_2 reduction by a specified amount by the year, say, 2020. Such a short-sighted view looks at the situation now, but the situation now is what will have an effect many decades hence. The more we know, the better we shall understand how far we can freely avail ourselves of Gaia's vital organs – the oceans and the Earth's living surfaces and depths.

To summarize Lovelock's theory regarding the relationship of atmosphere to biosphere, we need to accept the contention that living things, once they appeared on our planet, took charge of the global environment in a creative way. In other words, instead of passively riding the planet, they became fully-fledged partners in the shaping of the Earth, its rocks, waters and soil. In time, all species in the planetary biomass act symbiotically to further enhance the total life-giving potentiality of their planet. Natural hierarchies (like our own bodies) arise out of the evolutionary process, but once selected the constituent parts (cells, organs, mind and consciousness) hold together symbiotically. The body, in turn, inhabits a biosphere filled with plants, other animals, microbes and natural forces. The body also inhabits a society and a culture. Once the members of a species have attained a sufficient degree of individuation, they become participating partners within ecosystems where diversity, not unity, is the basis of health (Fig. 15.2).

Scientists estimate that tens of millions of species exist, but they have described only 1.4–1.5 million of them. The importance of such diversity far supersedes our basic human obsession with the exploitation to extinction of the essential resources we use for creating our food, medicine and other processed raw materials. If we degrade the fundamental homeostatic properties of the living Earth herself, we risk permanently changing this previously comfortable Earth to a new biosphere unfavourable for us, but perfectly comfortable for our life form successors.

Environmental destruction is a threat that can only be overcome if the people of all nations work together. Our oceans and our atmosphere will only

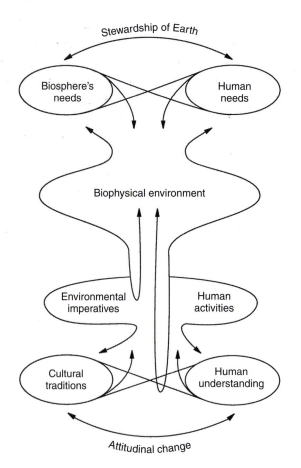

Figure 15.2 Earth's biological, physical, cultural and spiritual components interact as one self-sustaining organism that appears to create the physiological conditions to promote life's succession.

be saved by the aggregate of the world's actions, which must involve cooperation on a previously unparalleled scale. Pooling knowledge and resources internationally will allow faster progress towards scientific understanding of environmental problems and their bioethical solutions. Our role as custodians of our planet is the starting point for the ethical imperative of stewardship, which must underlie all environmental policies. It is humanity's obligation to conserve and protect our planetary life support systems prudently and conscientiously. To all intents and purposes, to be fully human we must consider ourselves as earthlings sharing a common globalized heritage, and respect life on Earth in all its rich diversity. We have a genetic responsibility to look after our planet, which we do not own but hold in trust.

Living within Nature's bounty

The thesis that we, as humankind, are in a holistic relationship with Nature herself should provide us with a meaning of life. The life sciences have provided us with many ecosystems-based insights and adaptive strategies, which increase the chance of survival in the long term. If we prepared ourselves with a greater operational ecological consciousness, we should be able to develop adaptive cultural rules by which we can live. Rules based on Nature's scheme of reciprocity should be simpler to understand and to follow, compared to abiding by a theoretical list of ethical prescriptions. We can learn, for instance, from the rainforests, where, although their soils are poor with few nutrients, they are among the most diverse biomes on Earth. Natural symbiotic relationships between microorganisms, plants and animals have co-evolved in tune so that the whole has become almost perfect in its efficiency and creativity.

The fundamental design principles of Nature are based on cooperation, biological feedback, adaptation to changing conditions and promoting ecological diversity. Human survival themes might ideally echo this pattern and include more cooperation and less conflict, living within our ecological means, and living in harmony with ourselves and the environment. Humans have long had sufficient brain power and, with recently acquired scientific understanding and renewed bioethical awareness, are, if they so wish, facilitated to increase their survival fitness. All that is really required is for us to grow up emotionally, exploit our brain's vast potential, and ethically manage our own fitness as a species. We can no longer accept the killing of our own and other species in local and national coordinated warfare fuelled by ideological competition as being a necessary and inevitable part of life. Our innate and flexible intelligence, however, can still rescue us because within our collective biological nature exist strong survival instincts such as justice, empathy, love and respect for the freedom and lives of others. Refinement of these positive biological instincts can provide us with the necessary assets for the present struggle for adaptive survival.

Our relationship with the biosphere is complex and unique but, after all is said and done, it is also the primal relationship encoded in our genes. There are several basic instinctive human responses to the natural world; responses such as pleasure, love, awe and reverence, for instance, are universally aroused by the beauty and mystery of the non-human. The reactivation of such responses, dormant in times of acute stress, underpin more recent kinds of ecological thinking, which suggest that we should think more in terms of living in harmony with Nature rather than on the basis of its conquest and its exploitation

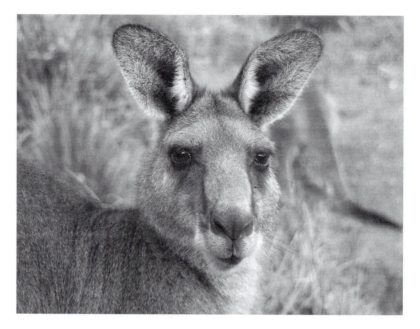

Figure 15.3 We should think more in terms of living in harmony with Nature and its creatures rather than on the basis of their conquest and overexploitation. Eastern grey young male kangaroo, *Macropus giganteus*, at Pebbley Beach, south coast of New South Wales, Australia.

(Fig. 15.3). A cerebral change based on identification with Nature would have powerful effects because such a shift may herald a move from the traditional cold 'ethic of duty' to a warmer, more mature 'ethic of care'. Such a transition would also alleviate human alienation due to living outside Nature, to one of being 'at home'. In other words, the transition back to 'love of life' as recently identified by Macer.

The superb Paleolithic cave paintings at Lascaux and Altamira and the stunning Dreamtime depiction in Aboriginal rock art are testaments to our long knowledge of and sympathy for the biosphere. Our ancestors studied the animals they hunted and knew a tremendous amount about the environment they lived in; they also respected Nature and its creatures (many were also their deities) and their ethical right to exist alongside humankind. Animism probably served as an adaptive ecological mechanism by impressing a bioethical restraint upon overexploitation and abuse. Tribal folk had to honour and respect the attributes of the animals they cohabited with; for example, all living creatures are part of the Dreaming; some are more powerful than others but all are important in the scheme of life for the Australian Aboriginal people.

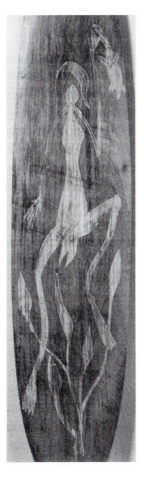

Figure 15.4 Indigenous Australians see their place alongside that of plants, birds, insects and mammals. Traditional Aboriginal 'picture painting' on wood by female elder (artist's name withheld).

Indigenous Australians believe that they have been in Australia since the Dreamtime, or Creation, when their land was shaped by their spiritual ancestors. These ancestors, or first people, journeyed across the country creating the landforms, plants, animals and people diversity. They brought with them laws to live by: ceremony, kinship and ecological knowledge. They taught Aboriginal people how to live in the land and look after the country (Fig. 15.4). Our vanished ancestors practised totemism that allowed them to be related to plants or animals – fish, insects and so forth – through the kinship systems. Kinship means that individuals and clans alike are responsible for the survival of their major totems, with whom they have a specific spiritual relationship.

We have had to revisit the origins of *Homo sapiens* to evaluate both our evolutionary success and future prospects. It was creative intelligence that gave rise to the will to initiate planning, make purposeful use of the imagination, and solve problems by reasoning. Creativity, the basis of freedom, gave rise to technology, art and, as a result of reasoning and moral reflection, ethical rules. Creativity has also resulted in powerful destructive technologies, but the genetic gift of natural justice, or ethics, can, if we choose, secure our further evolution and maintain the biosphere. If we are to sustain ourselves and the biosphere, we require a global ethic. Bioscience ethics, by bridging applied science and applied bioethics, facilitates biological understanding useful in the development of ethically responsible decision-making in tune with present-day reality. *Homo sapiens* has sufficient resourcefulness to apply its collective intelligence and adaptive responsibility to secure the future of all living organisms. Diversity of species provides biological stability; diversity of ideas provides cultural security.

Principles of bioscience ethics for discussion

- The Gaia theory challenges the reductionist view of the world by positing that she is a self-regulating, self-sustaining system continually adjusting physical, chemical and biological processes in order to maintain optimal conditions for life and its continued evolution. It is also evident that our survival in the union of life depends on a more generously directed altruism – one where our considerable power is deployed in justice and decency. Can an appreciation of Gaia's modus operandi play a fundamental role in the evolution of such a new altruism?
- A major responsibility of the modern bioethicist is to integrate current scientific insights of practical and cultural significance with traditional wisdom. The responsibility of the bioscience ethicist is to ensure that such scientific information is not omitted or corrupted in the process. Is a working knowledge of biological systems essential before the philosophy of ethics can adequately be re-addressed?
- Given our increasing understanding of natural phenomena, the future should be positive, with unprecedented opportunities to shape up our extant mores and enjoy a healthy, invigorating existence. What do you consider are the implications of natural ecological limits for human rights and social justice?

Further reading

Chapter 1: Human origins, natural selection and the evolution of ethics

Beauchamp, T. & Childress, J. (1994). *Principles of Biomedical Ethics*, 4th edn. New York: Oxford University Press.

Dawkins, R. (1989). *The Selfish Gene*. Oxford: Oxford University Press.

Farah, M. & Wolpe, P. (2004). Monitoring and brain function: new neuroscience technologies and their ethical implications. *Hastings Center Report* **34**, 35–45.

Fehr, E. & Renninger, S. (2005). The Samaritan paradox. *Scientific American Mind* **14**, 15–21.

Grant, E. (1996). *The Foundations of Modern Science in the Middle Ages: Their Religious, Institutional and Intellectual Contexts*. Cambridge: Cambridge University Press.

Harenski, C. & Hamann, S. (2006). Neural correlates of regulating negative emotions related to moral violations. *NeuroImage* **30**, 313–24.

Hayakawa, T., Altheide, T. & Varki, A. (2005). Genetic basis of human brain evolution: accelerating along the primate speedway. *Developmental Cell* **8**, 2–4.

Illes, J. & Racine, E. (2005). Imaging or imagining? A neuroethics challenge informed by genetics. *American Journal of Bioethics* **5**, 5–18.

Koenig, M., Young, L., Adolphs, R. *et al.* (2007). Damage to the prefrontal cortex increases utilitarian moral judgements. *Nature* **446**, 908–11.

Macer, D. (1998). *Bioethics is Love of Life: An Alternative Textbook*. Tsukuba (Japan): Eubios Ethics Institute.

Maclean, P. (1990). *The Triune Brain in Evolution: Role in Paleocerebral Functions*. New York: Plenum Press.

Mekel-Bobrov, N., Gilbert, S., Evans, P. *et al.* (2005). Ongoing adaptive evolution of ASPM, a brain size determinant in *Homo sapiens*. *Science* **309**, 1720–2.

Mendez, M. (2006). What frontotemporal dementia reveals about the neurobiological basis of mortality. *Medical Hypotheses* **67**, 411–18.

Moser, A. (2000). The wisdom of Nature in integrating science, ethics and the arts. *Science & Engineering Ethics* **6**, 365–82.

Plagnol, V. & Wall, J. (2006). Possible ancestral structure in human populations. *PLoS Genetics* **2**, 972–9.

Pollard, I. (2003). Choose between cooperation and annihilation: A mental mapping project towards a more generously directed altruism. *Eubios Journal of Asian & International Bioethics* **13**, 44–8.

Pollard, I. (2004). Meditation and brain function: A review. *Eubios Journal of Asian & International Bioethics* **14**, 28–33.

Pollard, I. (2007). High tech neuroscience, neuroethics and the precautionary principle. In *Asia-Pacific Perspectives on Ethics of Science and Technology*. Bangkok: UNESCO, pp. 37–43. Ethics2.pdf URL: http://www2.unescobkk.org/elib/publications/137/

Potter, V.-R. (1971). *Bioethics: Bridge to the Future*. Englewood Cliffs, New Jersey: Prentice-Hall.

Rogers, D. & Ehrlich, P. (2008). Natural selection and cultural rates of change. *Proceedings of the National Academy of Sciences* **105**, 3416–20.

Singer, P. (1981). *The Expanding Circle*. New York: Farrar, Straus & Giroux.

Tattersall, I. (1997). Out of Africa again . . . and again? *Scientific American* **276**, 46–53.

Van der Dennen, J., Smillie, D. & Wilson, D. (eds). (1999). *The Darwinian Heritage and Sociobiology*. Westport: Greenwood Press.

Wei-hsun Fu, C. & Wawrytko, S. (1991). *Buddhist Ethics and Modern Society: An International Symposium*. Westport: Greenwood Press.

Wolf, S. (ed.) (1996). *Feminism and Bioethics: Beyond reproduction*. New York: Oxford University Press.

Chapter 2: Sex determination, brain sex and sexual behaviour

Binstock, T. (2001). An immune hypothesis of sexual orientation. *Medical Hypotheses* **57**, 583–90.

Bogaert, A. (2006). Biological versus nonbiological older brothers and men's sexual orientation. *Proceedings of the National Academy of Sciences* **103**, 10 771–4.

Cohen-Bendahan, C., Buitelaar, J., van Goozen, S. & Cohen-Kettenis, P. (2004). Prenatal exposure to testosterone and functional cerebral lateralization: a study in same-sex and opposite-sex twin girls. *Psychoneuroendocrinology* **29**, 911–16.

Cummings, K. (2007). *Katherine's Diary: The Story of a Transsexual*. Trescott: Beaujon Press.

Gooren, L. (2006). The biology of human psychosexual differentiation. *Hormones & Behavior* **50**, 589–601.

Henningsson, S., Westberg, L., Nilsson, S. *et al.* (2005). Sex steroid-related genes and male-to-female transsexualism. *Psychoneuroendocrinology* **30**, 657–64.

Jones, R. & Lopez, K. (2006). Sexual differentiation. In *Human Reproductive Biology*, 3rd edn. San Diego: Academic Press, pp. 127–48.

Kitchin, W. (2003). The fundamental right to be free of arbitrary categorization: The brain sciences and the issue of sex classification. *Washburn Law Journal* **42**, 257–68.

Lummaa, V., Pettay, J. & Russell, A. (2007). Male twins reduce fitness of female co-twins in humans. *Proceedings of the National Academy of Sciences* **104**, 10 915–20.

Muscarella, F., Fink, B., Grammer, K. & Kirk-Smith, M. (2001). Homosexual orientation in males: Evolutionary and ethological aspects. *Neuroendocrinology Letters* **22**, 393–400.

Pol, H., Cohen-Kettenis, P., Van Haren, N. *et al.* (2006). Changing your sex changes your brain: influences of testosterone and estrogen on adult human brain structure. *European Journal of Endocrinology* **155**, S107–14.

Swaab, D. (2007). Sexual differentiation of the brain and behavior. *Best Practice & Research Clinical Endocrinology & Metabolism* **21**, 431–44.

Chapter 3: Inappropriate lifestyle and congenital disability in children: basic principles of growth, toxicology, teratogenesis and mutagenesis

Barker, D. (2004). The developmental origins of chronic adult disease. *Acta Paediatrica* Suppl. **93**, 26–33.

Binetti, P. (2004). The right to be born and the need to be born healthy: Questions in medical ethics. *Clinical Therapeutics* **155**, 89–95.

Fawcett, L. & Brent, R. (2006). Pathogenesis of abnormal development. In R. Hood (ed.). *Developmental and Reproductive Toxicology: A Practical Approach*, 2nd edn. Boca Raton: Taylor & Francis, pp. 61–92.

Gluckman P., Hanson, M., Spencer, H. & Bateson, P. (2005). Environmental influences during development and their later consequences for health and disease: implications for the interpretation of empirical studies. *Proceedings of the Royal Society* **B 272**, 671–7.

Jaenisch, R. & Bird, A. (2003). Epigenetic regulation of gene expression: how the genome integrates intrinsic and environmental signals. *Nature Genetics* **33**, 245–54.

Kapoor, A., Dunn, E., Kostaki, A., Andrews, M. & Matthews, S. (2006). Fetal programming of hypothalamo-pituitary-adrenal function: prenatal stress and glucocorticoids. *Journal of Physiology* **572**, 31–44.

Kunz, L. & King, J. (2007). Impact of maternal nutrition and metabolism on health of the offspring. *Seminars in Fetal & Neonatal Medicine* **12**, 71–7.

Maloney, C. & Rees, W. (2005). Gene-nutrient interactions during fetal development. *Reproduction* **130**, 401–10.

Myatt, L. (2006). Placental adaptive responses and fetal programming. *Journal of Physiology* **572**(Pt1), 25–30.

Pollard, I. (2007). Neuropharmacology of drugs and alcohol in mother and fetus. *Seminars in Fetal & Neonatal Medicine* **12**, 106–13.

Ulijaszek, S., Johnston, F. & Preece, M. (1998). *The Cambridge Encyclopedia of Human Growth and Development*. Cambridge: Cambridge University Press.

Zhang, X., Sliwowska, J. & Weinberg, J. (2005). Prenatal alcohol exposure and fetal programming: effects on neuroendocrine and immune function. *Experimental Biological Medicine* **230**, 376–88.

Chapter 4: Substance abuse and parenthood: biological mechanisms – bioethical responsibilities

Al'Absi, M. (ed.) (2007). *Stress and Addiction: Biological and Psychological Mechanisms*. San Diego: Academic Press.

Barker, D. (2006). Adult consequences of fetal growth restriction. *Clinical Obstetrics and Gynecology* **49**, 270–83.

Bech, B., Nohr, E. & Vaeth, M. (2005). Coffee and fetal death: a cohort study with prospective data. *American Journal of Epidemiology* **162**, 983–90.

Belenko, S. & Peugh, J. (1998). Fighting crime by treating substance abuse. *Issues in Science & Technology* **14**, 53–60.

Castle, D. & Murray, R. (2004). *Marijuana and Madness: Psychiatry and Neurobiology*. Cambridge: Cambridge University Press.

Collins, J., David, R., Handler, A., Wall, S. & Andes, S. (2004). Very low birthweight in African American infants: the role of maternal exposure to interpersonal racial discrimination. *American Journal of Public Health* **94**, 2132–8.

Conners, N., Bradley, R., Mansell, L. *et al.* (2004). Children of mothers with serious substance abuse problems: an accumulation of risks. *American Journal of Drug & Alcohol Abuse* **30**, 85–100.

Donohoe, M. (2003). Causes and health consequences of environmental degradation and social injustice. *Social Science & Medicine* **56**, 573–87.

Gilbert, S. (2005). Ethical, legal and social issues: our children's future. *Neurotoxicology* **26**, 521–30.

Gluckman, P., Hanson, M. & Pinal, C. (2005). The developmental origins of adult disease. *Maternal Child Nutrition* **5**, 130–41.

Gordon, H. (2002). Early environmental stress and biological vulnerability to drug abuse. *Psychoneuroendocrinology* **27**, 115–26.

Grove, N., Brough, M., Canuto, C. & Dobson, A. (2003). Aboriginal and Torres Strait Islander health research and the conduct of longitudinal studies: issues for debate. *Australian & New Zealand Journal of Public Health* **27**, 637–41.

Hales, B., Aguilar-Mahecha, A. & Robaire, B. (2005). The stress response in gametes and embryos after paternal chemical exposures: review. *Toxicology & Applied Pharmacology* **207**, 514–20.

Herz, A. (1997). Endogenous opioid systems and alcohol addiction. *Psychopharmacology* **129**, 99–111.

Higgins, S. & Katz, J. (eds.) (1998). *Cocaine Abuse: Behavior, Pharmacology and Clinical Applications*. San Diego: Academic Press.

Hunter, E. & Harvey, D. (2002). Indigenous suicide in Australia, New Zealand, Canada and the United States. *Emergency Medicine* **14**, 14–23.

Hyman, S. (2007). The neurobiology of addiction: Implications for voluntary control of behaviour. *American Journal of Bioethics* **7**, 8–11.

Kofman, O. (2002). The role of prenatal stress in the etiology of developmental behavioural disorders. *Neuroscience & Biobehavioral Reviews* **26**, 457–70.

Kristenson, M., Eriksen, H., Sluiter, J., Starke, D. & Ursin, H. (2004). Psychobiological mechanisms of socioeconomic differences in health. *Social Science & Medicine* **58**, 1511–22.

Lawrence, D. & Harry, G. (2000). Environmental stressors and neuro-immunological processes. *Brain, Behavior & Immunity* **14**, 231–8.

Lemoine, P., Harousseau, H., Borteryu, J. and Menuet, J. (1968). Les enfants de parents alcooliques: Anomalies observees a propos de 127 cas. (The children of alcoholic parents: Anomalies observed in 127 cases). *Quest Medicale* **21**, 476–82.

Lou, H. (1996). Etiology and pathogenesis of attention deficit hyperactivity disorder (ADHD): Significance of prematurity and perinatal hypoxic–haemodynamic encephalopathy. Review. *Acta Paediatrica* **85**, 1266–71.

Maldonado, R. (2003). The neurobiology of addiction. In: W. Fleischhacker and D. Brooks (eds.) *Addiction: Mechanisms, Phenomenology and Treatment. Journal of Neural Transmission* **66**, Suppl. 1–14.

Marinelli, M. & Piazza, P. (2002). Intersection between glucocorticoid hormones, stress and psychostimulant drugs. A review. *European Journal of Neuroscience* **16**, 387–94.

Moon, R. & Fu, L. (2007). Sudden infant death syndrome. *Pediatrics in Review* **28**, 209–14.

Mustillo, S., Krieger, N., Gunderson, E. *et al.* (2004). Self-reported experiences of racial discrimination and Black-White differences in preterm and low-birthweight deliveries: The CARDIA study. *American Journal of Public Health* **94**, 2125–31.

Muthusami, K. & Chinnaswamy, P. (2005). Effect of chronic alcoholism on male fertility hormones and semen quality. *Fertility & Sterility* **84**, 919–24.

Paradies, Y. (2006). A systematic review of empirical research on self-reported racism and health. *International Journal of Epidemiology* **35**, 888–901.

Pollard, I. (2003). From happiness to depression. *Today's Life Science* **15**, 22–6.

Pollard, I. (2005). Bioscience-bioethics and life factors affecting reproduction with special reference to the Indigenous Australian population: Review. *Reproduction* **129**, 391–420.

Riordan, D., Selvaraj, S., Stark, C. & Gilbert, J. (2006). Perinatal circumstances and risk of offspring suicide. *British Journal of Psychiatry* **289**, 502–7.

Rosenberg, L., Palmer, J., Wise, L., Horton, N. & Corwin, M. (2002). Perceptions of racial discrimination and the risk of preterm birth. *Epidemiology* **13**, 646–52.

Smith, A., Fried, P., Hogan, M. & Cameron, I. (2006). Effects of prenatal marijuana on visuospatial working memory: an fMRI study in young adults. *Neurotoxicology & Teratology* **28**, 286–95.

Solowij, N. & Battisti, R. (2008). The chronic effects of cannabis on memory in humans: a review. *Current Drug Abuse Reviews* **1**, 81–98.

Ursin, H. & Eriksen, H. (2004). The cognitive activation theory of stress: a review. *Psychoneuroendocrinology* **29**, 567–92.

Wakschlag, L., Leventhal, B., Pickett., K., Pine, D. & Carter, A. (2006). Elucidating early mechanisms of developmental psychopathology: the case of prenatal smoking and disruptive behavior. *Child Development* **77**, 893–906.

Zenzes, M. (2000). Smoking and reproduction: gene damage to human gametes and embryos. *Human Reproduction Update* **6**, 122–31.

Chapter 5: Fertility awareness: the ovulatory method of birth control, ageing gametes and congenital malformation in children

Billings, E. & Westmore, A. (2000). *The Billing's Method: Using the Body's Natural Signal of Fertility to Achieve or Avoid Pregnancy.* Melbourne: AOD Pty. Ltd.

Blomberg, S. (1980). Influence of maternal distress during pregnancy on fetal malformations. *Acta Psychiatrica Scandinavia* **62**, 315–30.

Bracken, M. & Vita, K. (1983). Frequency of non-hormonal contraception around conception and association with congenital malformations in offspring. *American Journal of Epidemiology* **117**, 281–91.

Cook, R. (1998). Human rights law and safe motherhood. *European Journal of Health Law* **5**, 357–75.

David, H. (1988). Unwantedness: demographic and psychosocial perspectives. In H. David, Z. Dytrych, Z. Matejcek & V. Schuller (eds). *Born Unwanted – Developmental Effects of Denied Abortion.* New York: Springer, pp. 23–30.

Delhanty, J. & Handyside, A. (1995). The origin of genetic defects in the human and their detection in the pre-implantation embryo. In H. M. Charlton (ed.) *Oxford Reviews of Reproductive Biology*, Vol. 17. Oxford: Oxford University Press, pp. 125–57.

Hansen, D., Lou, H. & Olsen, J. (2000). Serious life events and congenital malformations: a national study with complete follow-up. *Lancet* **356**, 875–80.

Jacobs, P. & Hassold, T. (1995). The origin of numerical chromosome abnormalities. In J. C. Hall & J. C. Dunlap (eds). *Advances in Genetics*, Vol. 33. San Diego: Academic Press, pp. 101–33.

Jongbloet, P. (1985). The aging gamete in relation to birth control failures and Down syndrome. *European Journal of Pediatrics* **144**, 343–7.

Jongbloet, P. (1986). Prepregnancy care: background biological effects. In G. Chamberain & J. Lumlay (eds). *Prepregnancy Care – A Manual of Practice.* Portsmouth: John Wiley.

Jongbloet, P. (1992). Aging gametes in relation to incidence, gender, and twinning in Down syndrome. *American Journal of Medical Genetics* **42**, 855.

Jongbloet, P., Poestkoke, A., Hamers, A. & Van ErkelensZwets, J. (1978). Down syndrome and religious groups. *Lancet* **ii**, 1310.

Khoury, M. & Wagener, D. (1995). Epidemiological evaluation of the use of genetics to improve the predictive value of disease risk factors. *American Journal of Human Genetics* **56**, 835–44.

Kincaid-Smith, P. (1995). The fifth freedom. *Bioethics* **9**, 183–91.

Meites, J. & Lu, J. (1994). Reproductive aging and neuroendocrine function. In H. M. Charlton (ed.) *Oxford Reviews of Reproductive Biology*, Vol. 16. Oxford: Oxford University Press, pp. 215–47.

Milstein-Moscati, I. & Becak, W. (1981). Occurrence of Down syndrome and human sexual behavior. *American Journal of Medical Genetics* **9**, 211–17.

Ryder, B. & Campbell, H. (1995). Natural family planning in 1990s. *The Lancet* **346**, 233–4.

Simpson, J., Gray, R., Queenan, J. *et al.* (1988). Pregnancy outcome associated with natural family planning (NFP): Scientific basis and experimental design for an international cohort study. *Advances in Contraception* **4**, 247–64.

Singh, S., Juarez, F., Cabigon, J. *et al.* (2006). *Unintended Pregnancy and Induced Abortion in the Philippines: Causes and Consequences*. New York: Guttmacher Institute.

The Ad Hoc Committee on Genetic Testing/Insurance Issues Background Statement. (1995). Genetic testing and insurance. *American Journal of Human Genetics* **56**, 327–31.

Vince, G. & Cohen, D. (2003). Ovulation revolution. *New Scientist* **179**, 16.

Chapter 6: Understanding child abuse and its biological consequences

Brennan, D., Hellerstedt, W., Ross, M. & Welles, S. (2007). History of childhood sexual abuse and HIV risk behaviors in homosexuals and bisexual men. *American Journal of Public Health* **97**, 1107–12.

Cook, R., Dickens, B. & Bliss, L. (1999). International developments in abortion law from 1988 to 1998. *American Journal of Public Health* **89**, 579–86.

Downie, R. & Randall, F. (1997). Parenting and the best interests of minors. *The Journal of Medicine & Philosophy* **22**, 219–31.

Gibbs, W. (1995). Seeking the criminal element. *Scientific American* **272**, 77–83.

Glander, S., Moore, M., Michielutte, R. & Parsons, L. (1998). The prevalence of domestic violence among women seeking abortion. *Obstetrics & Gynecology* **91**, 1002–6.

Glaser, D. (2000). Child abuse and neglect and the brain – a review. *The Journal of Child Psychology & Psychiatry & Allied Disciplines* **41**, 97–116.

Hall, D. & Lynch, M. (1998). Violence begins at home. *British Medical Journal* **316**, 1551–60.

Hen, R. (1996). Mean genes: review. *Neuron* **16**, 17–21.

Jong, E. (1995). *Fear of Fifty: A Midlife Memoir*. New York: HarperCollins.

Levitt, S. & Donohue, J. (1999). Abortion: The great crime stopper. Australian Broadcasting Corporation, Radio National. http://www.abc.au/rn/talks/lnl/stories/s46307.htm.

Levitt, S. & Dubner, S. (2005). *Freakonomics: A Rogue Economist Explores the Hidden Side of Everything*. London: Penguin Books.

Parson, E. (2000). Understanding children with war-zone traumatic stress exposed to the world's violent environments. *Journal of Contemporary Psychotherapy* **30**, 325–40.

Rantakallio, P., Laara, E., Isohanni, M. & Moilanen, I. (1992). Maternal smoking during pregnancy and delinquency of the offspring: An association without causation? *International Journal of Epidemiology* **21**, 1106–13.

Reiss, A. Jr. & Roth, J. (ed.) (1993). *Understanding and Preventing Violence*. Washington DC: National Academy Press.

Rizzi, R., Cordoba, R. & Maguna, J. (1998). Maternal mortality due to violence. *International Journal of Gynecology & Obstetrics* **63** (Suppl. 1), S19–24.

Schaefer, C. & Geronimo, T. (2000). *A Parent's Guide to Normal Childhood Development, Ages and Stages*. New York: John Wiley & Son.

Sereny, G. (1998). *Cries Unheard: The Story of Mary Bell*. London: Macmillan.

Singer, G., Stern, Y. & Van der Spy, H. (1979). Emotional disturbance in unplanned, versus planned children. *Social Biology* **23**, 254–8.

Tanner, T. (1980). The Church and social responsibility. In J. Cummings & P. Burns (eds). *The Church Now: An Inquiry into the Present State of the Catholic Church in Britain and Ireland*. Dublin: Gill & Macmillan.

Tolan, P. & Guerra, N. (1994). *What Works in Reducing Adolescent Violence*. The Center for the Study and Prevention of Violence, University of Colorado.

Wadsworth, M. (1979). Family structure. In M. Robertson (ed.) *Roots of Delinquency; Infancy, Adolescence and Crime*. Oxford: Oxford University Press, pp. 34–6.

World Medical Association. (1999). Declaration of Ottawa on the right of the child to healthcare. *Bulletin of Medical Ethics* **145**, 9–11.

Yapko, M. (1994). *Suggestions of Abuse*. New York: Simon & Schuster.

Chapter 7: The state of wellbeing: basic principles, coping strategies and individual mastery

Calhoun, J. (1952). The social aspects of population dynamics. *Journal of Mammalogy* **33**, 139–59.

Christian, J. (1975). Hormonal control of population growth. In B. E. Eleftheriou & R. L. Sprott (eds). *Hormonal Correlates of Behavior*. New York: Plenum Press, pp. 295–374.

Clarke, R., Breeze, E., Sherliker, P. *et al.* (1998). Design, objectives, and lessons from a pilot 25 year follow up re-survey of survivors in the Whitehall study of London civil servants. *Journal of Epidemiology & Community Health* **52**, 364–9.

Dolan, P. & Kahneman, D. (2008). Interpretations of utility and their implications for the valuation of health. *Economic Journal* **118**, 215–34.

Goleman, D. (2003). *Destructive Emotions and How We Can Overcome Them: A Dialogue with the Dalai Lama*. London: Bloomsbury.

Kristenson, M., Eriksen, H., Sluiter, J., Starke, D. & Ursin, H. (2004). Psychobiological mechanisms of socioeconomic differences in health. *Social Science & Medicine* **58**, 1511–22.

Marmot, M. & Wilkinson, R. (1999). *Social Determinants of Health*. Oxford: Oxford University Press.

McEwen, B. (1998). Stress, adaptation, and disease. Allostasis and allostatic load. *Annals of the New York Academy of Sciences* **1**, 33–44.

McEwen, B. (2004). Association of depression with medical illness: does cortisol play a role? *Biological Psychiatry* **55**, 1–9.

McEwen, B. & Lasley, E. (2003). Allostatic load: when protection gives way to damage. *Advances in Mind & Body Medicine* **19**, 28–33.

Newberg, A. & Iversen, J. (2003). The neural basis of the complex mental task of meditation: neurotransmitter and neurochemical considerations. *Medical Hypotheses* **61**, 282–91.

Pollard, I. (2004). Meditation and brain function: a review. *Eubios Journal of Asian & International Bioethics* **14**, 28–33.

Pollard, I. (2005). Bioscience-bioethics and life factors affecting reproduction with special reference to the indigenous Australian population. *Reproduction* **129**, 391–402.

Schwartz, J. & Begley, S. (2002) *The Mind & The GBRain: Neuroplasticity and the power of mental force*. Manhattan, US: Regan Books.

Selye, H. (1976). *The Stress of Life*. New York: McGraw-Hill.

Singh-Manoux, A., Adler, N. & Marmot, M. (2003). Subjective social status: its determinants and its association with measures of ill-health in the Whitehall II study. *Social Science & Medicine* **56**, 1321–33.

Stansfeld, S., Fuhrer, R., Shipley, M. & Marmot M. (1999). Work characteristics predict psychiatric disorder: Prospective results from the Whitehall II study. *Occupational Environmental Medicine* **56**, 302–7.

Wooten, P. (1996). Humor: an antidote for stress. *Holistic Nursing Practice* **10**, 49–55.

Yu, T., Tsai, H. & Hwang, M. (2003). Suppressing tumor progression of *in vitro* prostate cancer cells by emitted psychosomatic power through Zen meditation. *American Journal of Chinese Medicine* **31**, 499–507.

Chapter 8: The state of wellbeing: on the end-of-life care and euthanasia

Berglund, C. (1998). *Ethics for HealthCare*. Oxford: Oxford University Press.

Braun U., Beyth, R., Ford, M. & McCullough, L. (2007). Defining limits in care of terminally ill patients. *British Medical Journal* **334**, 239–41.

Brown, N. (1996). The 'harm', in euthanasia. *Australian Quarterly* **68**, 26–35.

Emanuel, E., Fairclough, D. & Emanuel, L. (2000). Attitudes and desires related to euthanasia and physician-assisted suicide among terminally ill patients and their caregivers. *Journal of the American Medical Association* **284**, 2460–8.

Finch, C. (2007). *The Biology of Human Longevity: Inflammation, Nutrition, and Aging in the Evolution of Life Spans*. San Diego, California: Elsevier Ltd.

Kendall, M., Harris, F., Boyd, K. *et al.* (2007). Key challenges and ways forward in researching the "good death": qualitative in-depth interview and focus group study. *British Medical Journal* **334**, 521–4.

Kübler-Ross, E. (1997). *On Death and Dying*. New York: First Touchstone Edition.

Kuhse, H. (1999). A modern myth: That letting die is not the intentional causation of death. In H. Kuhse & P. Singer (eds). *Bioethics: An Anthology*. Oxford: Blackwell, pp. 255–68.

Scott, A. (1999). Autonomy, power, and control in palliative care. *Cambridge Quarterly of Healthcare Ethics* **8**, 139–47.

Takahashi, T. (ed.) (2005). *Taking Life and Death Seriously – Bioethics from Japan. Advances in Bioethics*, Vol. 8. Oxford: Elsevier Ltd.

Tanida, N. (2000). The view of religions toward euthanasia and extraordinary treatments in Japan. *Journal of Religion & Health* **39**, 339–54.

Verhagen, E. & Sauer, P. (2005). The Groningen protocol – Euthanasia in severely ill newborns. *New England Journal of Medicine* **352**, 959–62.

Chapter 9: Current reproductive technologies: achievements and desired goals

Agarwal, A. & Allamaneni S. (2004). The effect of sperm DNA damage on assisted reproduction outcomes. A review. *Minerva Ginecologica* **56**, 235–45.

Angelopoulou, R., Plastira, K. & Msaouel, P. (2007). Spermatozoal sensitive biomarkers to defective protaminosis and fragmented DNA. *Reproductive Biology & Endocrinology* **5**, 36–51.

Auger, J., Kunstmann, J., Czyglik, F. & Jouannet, P. (1995). Decline in semen quality among fertile men in Paris during the past 20 years. *New England Journal of Medicine* **332**, 281–5.

Bower, C. & Hansen, M. (2005). Assisted reproductive technologies and birth outcomes: overview of recent systematic reviews. *Reproduction, Fertility & Development* **17**, 329–33.

Carlsen, E., Giwercman, A., Keiding, N. & Skakkebaek, N. (1992). Evidence for decreasing quality of semen during past 50 years. *British Medical Journal* **305**, 609–13.

Daniels, K. & Haimes, E. (ed.) (1998). *Donor Insemination: International Social Science Perspectives*. Cambridge: Cambridge University Press.

Davies, M., Wang, J. & Norman, R. (2004). What is the most relevant standard of success in assisted reproduction? Assessing the BESST index for reproduction treatment. *European Society of Human Reproduction & Embryology* **19**, 1049–51.

De Geyter, C., De Geyter, M., Steimann, S., Zhang, H. & Holzgreve, W. (2006). Comparative birth weights of singletons born after assisted reproduction and natural conception in previously infertile women. *Human Reproduction* **21**, 705–12.

Eskenazi, B., Wyrobek, A., Sloter, E. *et al.* (2003). The association of age and semen quality in healthy men. *Human Reproduction* **18**, 447–54.

Glover, T. & Barratt, C. (eds). (1999). *Male Fertility and Infertility*. Cambridge: Cambridge University Press.

Harris, J. & Holm, S. (eds). (1999). *The Future of Human Reproduction, Ethics, Choice and Regulation*. Oxford: Oxford University Press.

Kupta, M., Dorn, C., Richter, O., Felberbaum, R. & van der Ven, H. (2003). Impact of reproductive history on *in vitro* fertilization and intracytoplasmic sperm injection outcome: evidence from the German IVF Registry. *Fertility & Sterility* **80**, 508–16.

Lucifero, D., Chaillet, J. & Trasler, J. (2004). Potential significance of genomic imprinting defects for reproduction and assisted reproductive technology. *Human Reproduction Update* **10**, 3–18.

Moskovtsev, S., Willis, J. & Mullen, B. (2006). Age-related decline in sperm deoxyribonucleic acid integrity in patients evaluated for male infertility. *Fertility & Sterility* **85**, 496–9.

Niemitz, E. & Feinberg, P. (2004). Epigenetics and assisted reproductive technology: A call for investigation. *American Journal of Human Genetics* **74**, 599–609.

Plas, E., Berger, P., Hermann, M. & Pflüger, H. (2000). Effects of aging on male fertility. *Experimental Gerontology* **35**, 543–51.

Pukazhenthi, B. & Wildt, D. (2004). Which reproductive technologies are most relevant to studying, managing and conserving wildlife? *Reproduction, Fertility & Development* **16**, 33–46.

Shalev, C. (2000). Rights to sexual and reproductive health: the ICPD and the convention on the elimination of all forms of discrimination against women. *Health & Human Rights* **4**, 38–66.

Swan, S., Elkin, E. & Fenster, L. (1997). Have sperm densities declined? A reanalysis of global trend data. *Environmental Health Perspectives* **5** 1228–32.

Chapter 10: The recombinant DNA technologies

Barker, J. (2004). The Human Genome Diversity Project: 'Peoples', 'populations' and the cultural politics of identification. *Cultural Studies* **18**, 571–606.

Collins, F., Morgan, M. & Patrinos, A. (2004). The Human Genome Project: Lessons from large-scale biology. *Science* **300**, 286–90.

Crofts, C. & Krimsky, S. (2005). Emergence of a scientific and commercial research and development infrastructure for human gene therapy. *Human Gene Therapy* **16**, 169–77.

Jolles, P. (ed.) (2000). *New Approaches to Drug Development*. Basel: Birkhauser Verlag.

Jorde, L. & Wooding, S. (2004). Genetic variation, classification and 'race'. *Nature Genetics* **36**, S28–S33.

Kaprio, J. (2000). Genetic epidemiology. *British Medical Journal* **320**, 1257–61.

Kim-Cohen, J., Caspi, A., Taylor, A. *et al.* (2006). MAOA, maltreatment, and gene–environment interaction predicting children's mental health: new evidence and a meta-analysis. *Molecular Psychiatry* **11**, 903–13.

Knoppers, B. & Chadwick, R. (2005). Human genetic research: Emerging trends in ethics. *Nature* **6**, 75–9.

Livesey, F. & Hunt, S. (eds). (2000). *Functional Genomics*. Oxford: Oxford University Press.

Mastenbroek, S., Twisk, M., Echten-Arends, J. *et al.* (2007). In vitro fertilization with preimplantation genetic screening. *New England Journal of Medicine* **357**, 9–17.

Neumann-Held, E. & Rehmann-Sutter, C. (2006). *Genes in Development: Re-reading the Molecular Paradigm*. Durham, North Carolina: Duke University Press.

Palladino, M. (2006). *Understanding the Human Genome Project*, 2nd edn. San Francisco: Pearson Benjamin Cummings.

Primary Research Papers. Landmark publications are available free online through the journals *Nature* (www.nature.com/genomics) and *Science* (www.scienceonline.org), respectively.

Ridley, M. (2003). *Nature via Nurture: Genes, Experience, and What Makes us Human*. New York: Harper-Collins.

Tishkoff, S. & Kidd, K. (2004). Implications of biogeography of human populations for 'race' and medicine. *Nature Genetics* **36**, S21–27.

Verlinsky, Y., Cohen, J., Munne, S. *et al.* (2004). Over a decade of experience with preimplantation genetic diagnosis. *Fertility & Sterility* **82**, 302–3.

Weatherall, D. (2000). Single gene disorders or complex traits: Lessons from the thalassaemias and other monogenic diseases. *British Medical Journal* **321**, 1117–20.

Witek, R. (2005). Ethics and patentability in biotechnology. *Science in English Ethics* **11**, 105–11.

Chapter 11: Stem cells, nuclear transfer and cloning technology

Cregan, K. (2005). Ethical and social issues of embryonic stem cell technology. *Internal Medicine Journal* **35**, 126–7.

Edwards, J., Schrick, F., McCracken, M. *et al.* (2003). Cloning adult farm animals: a review of the possibilities and problems associated with somatic cell nuclear transfer. *American Journal of Reproductive Immunology* **50**, 113–23.

Forsberg, E. (2005). Commercial applications of nuclear transfer cloning: three examples. *Reproduction, Fertility & Development* **17**, 59–68.

Keller, G. (2005). Embryonic stem cell differentiation: emergence of a new era in biology and medicine. *Genes & Development* **19**, 1129–55.

Lanza, R., Caplan, A., Silver, L. *et al.* (2000). The ethical validity of using nuclear transfer in human transplantation. *Journal of the American Medical Association* **284**, 3175–9.

Martin, C. & Zhang, Y. (2007). Mechanisms of epigenetic inheritance. *Current Opinion in Cell Biology* **19**, 266–72.

Prentice, D. (2003). Stem cells and cloning. *The Benjamin Cummings Special Topics in Biology Series*; M. Palladino (series ed.) San Francisco: Benjamin Cummings.

Serup, P., Madsen, O. & Mandrup-Poulsen, T. (2001). Islet and stem cell transplantation for treating diabetes. *Journal of the American Medical Association* **322**, 29–34.

Silver, L. (1998). *Remaking Eden: Cloning and Beyond in a Brave New World*. London: Weidenfeld & Nicolson.

Strong, C. (1998). Cloning and infertility. *Cambridge Quarterly of Healthcare Ethics* **7**, 279–93.

Thomson, J. (2000). Legal and ethical problems of human cloning. *Journal of Law and Medicine* **8**, 31–4.

Wilmut, I., Schnieke, A. E., McWhir, J., Kind, A. J. & Campbell, K. H. (1997). Viable offspring derived from fetal and adult mammalian cells. *Nature* **358**, 810–13.

Zhang, S., Kubota, C., Yang, L. *et al.* (2004). Genomic imprinting of H19 in naturally reproduced and cloned cattle. *Biology of Reproduction* **71**, 1540–4.

Chapter 12: Human-dominated ecosystems: re-evaluating environmental priorities

Population growth and economic activity – are we overstraining our limits?

Bertazzi, P., Consonni, D., Bachetti, S. *et al.* (2001). Health effects of dioxin exposure: a 20-year mortality study. *American Journal of Epidemiology* **153**, 1031–44.

Brown, L. (2008). *Plan B 3.0: Mobilizing to Save Civilization*. New York: W. W. Norton & Co.

Chapin III, F., Walker, B., Hobbs, R. *et al.* (1997). Biotic control over the functioning of ecosystems. *Science* **277**, 500–4.

Ehrlich, P. (1968). *The Population Bomb*. New York: Ballantine Books.

Flannery, T. (2005). *The Weather Makers: The History of Future Impact of Climate Change*. Melbourne, Australia: The Text Publishing Company.

Karl, T., Nicholls, N. & Gregory, J. (1997). The coming climate: Meteorological records and computer models permit insights into some of the broad weather patterns of a warmer world. *Scientific American* **276**, 54–9.

Mace, M., Hendriks, C. & Coenrads, R. (2007). Regulatory challenges to the implementation of carbon capture and geological storage within the European Union under EU and international law. *International Journal of Greenhouse Gas Control* **1**, 253–60.

Makandya, A. & Wilkinson, P. (2007). Electricity generation and health. *Energy & Health* **370**, 979–89.

Mathews, J. (2007). Seven steps to curb global warming. *Energy Policy* **35**, 4247–59.

Matson, P., Parton, W., Power, A. & Swift M. (1997). Agricultural intensification and ecosystem properties. *Science* **277**, 504–9.

Pollard, I. (1994). Population dynamics, stress and the general theory of adaptation. In *A Guide to Reproduction, Social Issues and Human Concerns*. Cambridge: Cambridge University Press, pp. 225–48.

Pollard, I. (1994). Extinctions and the conservation of endangered species. In *A Guide to Reproduction, Social Issues and Human Concerns*. Cambridge: Cambridge University Press, pp. 249–73.

Rosenfield, A. & Schwarz, K. (2005). Population and development – Shifting paradigms, setting goals. *New England Journal of Medicine* **352**, 647–9.

Seddon, G. (1997). *Landprints: Reflections on Place and Landscape*. Cambridge: Cambridge University Press.

Stern, N. (2007). *Stern Review on the Economics of Climate Change*. Cambridge: Cambridge University Press.

Sunyer, J. & Grimalt, J. (2006). Global climate change, widening health inequalities, and epidemiology. *International Journal of Epidemiology* **35**, 213–16.

Tsai, W. (2005). Environmental risk assessment of hydrofluoroethers (HFEs). *Journal of Hazard Materials* **17**, 69–78.

Understanding living cycles and anticipating environmental policies rather than relying on remedial measures

Azariah, J. (1995). The Book of Genesis and environmental ethics, biodiversity and the food deficit. *Eubios Journal of Asian & International Bioethics* **5**, 6–10.

Brown, B. (2004). *Memo for a Saner World*. Melbourne (Australia): Penguin Group.

Colborn, T., Dumanoski, D. & Peterson Myers, J. (1996). *Our Stolen Future: Are We Threatening our Fertility, Intelligence, and Survival?* Middlesex: Dutton Penguin.

Congdon, R. & Lamb, D. (1990). Essential nutrient cycles. In L. Webb & J. Kikkawa (eds) *Australian Tropical Rainforests: Science, Values, Meaning*. Melbourne, Australia: CSIRO Publication.

Cowan, P. & Tyndale-Biscoe, H. (1997). Australian and New Zealand mammal species considered to be pests or problems. *Reproduction, Fertility & Development* **9**, 27–36.

Dobson, A., Bradshaw, A. & Baker, A. (1997). Hopes for the future: Restoration ecology and conservation biology. *Science* **277**, 515–22.

Douglas, A. (1995). The ecology of symbiotic microorganisms. In M. Begon & A. Fitter (eds). *Advances in Ecological Research*, Vol. 26. London: Academic Press, pp. 69–103.

Frankham, R., Ballou, J. & Briscoe, D. (2009). *Introduction to Conservation Genetics*. 2nd edn. Cambridge: Cambridge University Press.

Gross, L. (2006). Assessing ecosystem services to identify conservation priorities. *PLoS Biology* **4**, 1877–98.

Guerrier, Y., Alexander, N., Chose, J. & O'Brien, M. (eds). (1995). *Values and the Environment: A Social Science Perspective*. Chichester: Wiley & Sons.

Manahan, S. (1997). *Environmental Science and Technology*. Boca Raton: CRC Lewis.

Millennium Ecosystem Assessment. (2005). *United Nations Environmental Programme*, five volume set. Washington DC: Island Press.

Vandermeer, J. (1996). *Deconstructing Biology: Genetics and Ecology in the New World Order*. Chichester, UK: J. Wiley & Sons.

Wann, D. (1995). *Deep Design: Ecological Design by Sim van der Ryn and Stuart Cowan*. Washington DC: Island Press.

Chapter 13: Human-dominated ecosystems: reclaiming the future for following generations

Alonso-Magdalena, P., Morimoto, S., Ripoll, C., Fuentes, E. & Nadal, A. (2006). The estrogenic effect of bisphenol-A disrupts the pancreatic ß-cell function *in vivo* and induces insulin resistance. *Environmental Health Perspectives* **114**, 106–12.

Bretveld, R., Thomas, C., Scheepers, P., Zielhuis, G. & Roeleveld, N. (2006). Pesticide exposure: the hormonal function of the female reproductive system disrupted? *Reproductive Biology & Endocrinology* **4**, 30–8.

Carson, R. (1962). *Silent Spring*. Back Bay, Boston, Massachusetts: Houghton Mifflin.

Colborn, T., Dumanoski, D. & Peterson Myers, J. (1996). *Our Stolen Future: Are We Threatening our Fertility, Intelligence, and Survival?* Middlesex: Dutton Penguin.

Conover, M. & Hunt, G. (1984). Female–female pairing and sex ratios in gulls: An historical perspective. *Wilson Bulletin* **96**, 619–25.

Dasgupta, P. (1995). Population, poverty and the local environment. *Scientific American* **272**, 26–31.

Hardin, G. (1968). The tragedy of the commons. *Science* **162**, 1243–8.

Hardin, G. (1970). Parenthood: Right or privilege. *Science* **169**, 1.

Heilmann, C., Grandjean, P., Weihe, P., Nielsen, F. & Budtz-Jørgensen, E. (2006). Reduced antibody responses to vaccinations in children exposed to polychlorinated biphenyls. *PLoS Medicine* **3**, 1352–8.

Hutson, J., Baker, M., Terada, M., Zhou, B. & Paxton, G. (1994). Hormonal control of testicular descent and the cause of cryptorchidism. *Reproduction, Fertility & Development* **6**, 151–6.

Jacobson, J., Jacobson, S. & Humphrey, H. (1990). Effects of *in utero* exposure to polychlorinated biphenyls and related contamination on cognitive functioning in young children. *Journal of Pediatrics* **116**, 38–43.

Jacobson, J., Jacobson, S. & Humphrey, H. (1990). Effects of exposure to PCBs and related compounds on growth and activity in children. *Neurotoxicology and Teratology* **12**, 319–26.

Karalliede, L., Feldman, S., Henry, J. & Marrs, T. (eds). (2001). *Organophosphates and Health*. London: Imperial College Press.

Lichtenfels, A., Gomes, J., Pieri, P. *et al.* (2007). Increased levels of air pollution and a decrease in the human and mouse male-to-female ratio in São Paula, Brazil. *Fertility & Sterility* **87**, 230–2.

Meyer, F. (1989). High levels of PCBs in breast milk of Inuit women from Arctic Quebec. *Bulletin of Environmental Contamination & Toxicology* **43**, 641–6.

Milinski, M., Semmann, D. & Krambeck, H. (2002). Reputation helps solve the 'tragedy of the commons'. *Nature* **24**, 424–6.

Pollard, I. (1994). Hormonal contributions to errors of sexual differentiation. In *A Guide to Reproduction, Social Issues and Human Concerns*. Cambridge: Cambridge University Press, pp. 307–19.

Pluim, H., Vijlder, J., Olie, K. *et al.* (1993). Effects of pre- and postnatal exposure to chlorinated dioxins and furans on human neonatal thyroid hormone concentrations. *Environmental Health Perspectives* **101**, 504–8.

Roeleveld, N. & Bretveld, R. (2008). The impact of pesticides on male fertility. *Current Opinion in Obstetrics & Gynecology* **20**, 229–33.

Sharpe, R. & Skakkebaek, N. (1993). Are estrogens involved in falling sperm counts and disorders of the male reproductive tract? *Lancet* **341**, 1392–5.

Sigiura-Ogasawara, M., Ozaki, Y., Sonta, S., Makino, T. & Suzumori, K. (2005). Exposure to bisphenol-A is associated with recurrent miscarriage. *Human Reproduction* **20**, 2325–9.

Somers, C., Yauk, C., White, P., Parfett, C. & Quinn, J. (2002). Air pollution induces heritable DNA mutations. *Proceedings of the National Academy of Sciences* **99**, 15 904–7.

Wigle, D. & Lanphear, B. (2005). Human health risks from low-level environmental exposures: no apparent safety thresholds. *PLoS Medicine* **2**, 1232–4.

Zala, S. & Penn, D. (2004). Abnormal behaviours induced by chemical pollution: a review of the evidence and new challenges. *Animal Behaviour* **68**, 649–64.

Chapter 14: Human-dominated ecosystems: warfare = fitness enhancement or losing strategy?

Bismuth, C., Borron, S., Baud, F. & Barriot, P. (2004). Chemical weapons: documented use and compounds on the horizon. *Toxicology Letters* **149**, 11–18.

Geller, S. & Singer, D. (1998). *Nations at War: A Scientific Study of International Conflict*. Cambridge: Cambridge University Press.

Gilbert, S. (2005). Ethical, legal, and social issues: our children's future. *NeuroToxicology* **26**, 521–30.

Hinde, R. (ed.) (1991). *The Institution of War*. London: Macmillan.

Macer, D. (1998). *Bioethics is Love of Life: An Alternative Textbook*. Tsukuba (Japan): Eubios Ethics Institute.

Parson, E. (2000). Understanding children with war-zone traumatic stress exposed to the world's violent environments. *Journal of Contemporary Psychotherapy* **30**, 325–40.

Patten, J. (2000). Reciprocal altruism and warfare: a case from the Ecuadorian Amazon. In Cronk, L., Chagnon, N. & Irons, W. (eds) *Adaptation of Human Behavior*. New York: Aldine de Gruyter.

Richardson, M. (1995). *The Effects of War On the Environment: Croatia*. London: E & FN Spon.

Robins, N. & Pye-Smith, C. (1997). The ecology of violence. *New Scientist* **153**, 12–13.

Tonge, J. (2005). After Kosovo, Afghanistan and Iraq: what is the future for the UN? *Medicine, Conflict and Survival* **21**, 48–54.

Toole, M. (1995). Mass population displacement: a global public health challenge. *Infectious Disease Clinics North America* **9**, 353–65.

UNHCR: The UN Refugee Agency. (2006). The State of the World's Refugees 2006. Freely available online at http://www.unhcr.org/static/publ/sowr2006/toceng.htm

Wertz, D. (1998). Genetics and 'germ warfare'. *Gene Letter* **2**, 26–8.

Chapter 15: Human-dominated ecosystems: reworking bioethical frontiers

Dugatkin, L. (1997). *Cooperation Among Animals: An Evolutionary Perspective*. New York: Oxford University Press.

Fredrickson, J. & Onstott, T. (1996). Microbes deep inside the Earth. *New Scientist* **275**, 68–73.

French, H. (1992). From discord to accord. *World Watch* **5**, 26–36.

Gross, L. (2006). Assessing ecosystem services to identify conservation priorities. *PLoS Biology* **4**, 1877–98.

Kiuchi, T. & Shireman, W. (2002). *What We Learned in the Rainforest: Business Lessons from Nature: Innovation, Growth, Profit, and Sustainability at 20 of the World's Top Companies*. San Francisco: Berrett-Koehler Publishers.

Lewin, R. (1996). All for one, one for all. *New Scientist* **152**, 28–32.

Lovelock, J. (1986). Gaia: the world as living organism. *New Scientist* **112**, 25–8.

Lovelock, J. (2006). *The Revenge of Gaia*. London: Allen Lane (Imprint of Penguin Books).

Macer, D. (1998). *Bioethics is Love of Life: An Alternative Textbook*. Tsukuba: Eubios Ethics Institute.

Manahan, S. (1997). *Environmental Science and Technology*. Boca Raton: CRC Lewis.

Spinney, L. (1997). The unselfish gene. *New Scientist* **156**, 28–32.

Wakeford, T. & Walters, M. (eds). (1995). *Science for the Earth: Can Science Make the World a Better Place?'* Chichester: John Wiley & Sons.

Weisman, A. (2007). *The World Without Us*. London: Virgin Books.

Wymer, W. & Samu, S. (2003). *Nonprofit and Business Sector Collaboration: Social Enterprises, Cause-related Marketing, Sponsorships, and Other Corporate-nonprofit Dealings*. Binghamton: Best Business Books.

Index